Management of Prader–Willi Syndrome

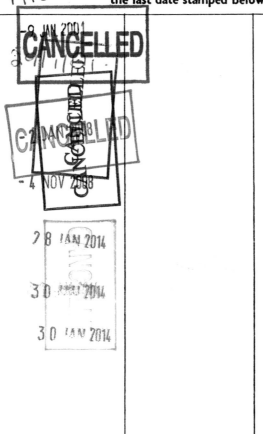

Louise R. Greenswag   Randell C. Alexander

Editors

Management of Prader–Willi Syndrome

Second Edition

With 57 Illustrations

Under the Sponsorship of The Prader–Willi Syndrome Association

Springer-Verlag

New York Berlin Heidelberg London Paris
Tokyo Hong Kong Barcelona Budapest

Louise R. Greenswag, R.N., PH.D.
Adjunct Professor, College of Nursing
Program Consultant for Prader–Willi Syndrome
Iowa Child Health Specialty Clinics
University Hospital School
Division of Developmental Disabilities
The University of Iowa Hospitals and Clinics
Iowa City, Iowa 52242, USA

Randell C. Alexander, M.D., PH.D.
Department of Pediatrics
University Hospital School
The University of Iowa Hospitals and Clinics
Iowa City, Iowa 52242, USA

Library of Congress Cataloging-in-Publication Data.
Management of Prader-Willi syndrome / [edited by] Louise R. Greenswag,
    Randell C. Alexander. – 2nd ed.
        p.   cm.
    Includes bibliographical references and index.
    ISBN 0-387-94373-0. – ISBN 3-540-94373-0
    1. Prader-Willi syndrome.   I. Greenswag, Louise R.
II. Alexander, Randell C.
    [DNLM: 1. Prader-Willi Syndrome.   QS 675 M266 1995]
RJ520.P7M36   1995
618.92′0043 – dc20
DNLM/DLC
for Library of Congress   94-29757

Printed on acid-free paper.

Production coordinated by Chernow Editorial Services, Inc. and managed by Terry Kornak; manufacturing supervised by Jacqui Ashri.
Typeset by Best-set Typesetter Ltd., Hong Kong.
Printed and bound by Edwards Brothers, Inc., Ann Arbor, Michigan.
Printed in the United States of America.

9 8 7 6 5 4 2 1

ISBN 0-387-94373-0 Springer-Verlag New York Berlin Heidelberg
ISBN 3-540-94373-0 Springer-Verlag Berlin Heidelberg New York

To children with Prader–Willi syndrome and their families,
and to
Sidney Greenswag and Carol Alexander
for their encouragement and patience

In Memoriam

HANS ZELLWEGER (1909–1990)

Since the publication of the first edition of this book, our teacher and dear friend, Hans Zellweger, M.D., Professor Emeritus of Pediatrics at The University of Iowa College of Medicine, died. An international pioneer in medical genetics, he is remembered as a role model by a generation of pediatricians around the world for his leadership in the study of human genetics and the care of children with developmental disabilities.

A consummate scholar, Dr. Zellweger took a very special interest and concern in children with Prader–Willi syndrome and their families. We were most fortunate to have had the benefit of his personal friendship, knowledge, encouragement, and support in the development of the first edition of this book.

He was a brilliant, courtly, compassionate, gentle man who had profound respect for the simple dignity of a child, and this text is respectfully dedicated to his memory.

LOUISE R. GREENSWAG, R.N., PH.D.
RANDELL C. ALEXANDER, M.D., PH.D.

Preface

Confronting the complex issues associated with Prader–Willi syndrome puts us in mind of a thousand-piece puzzle where, at first glance, all the parts look much alike but are, in fact, very different. We were pleased that the publication of the initial book in 1988 clarified some of the more confusing aspects of this syndrome and that it became a comprehensive resource for information and enhancement of services. This second volume reflects the considerable advances in research, case finding, and multi-disciplinary management that have evolved.

The Prader–Willi Syndrome Association (USA), with its membership of dedicated parents and professionals and its network of state chapters and allied organizations, is pleased to support this second edition. Our sincere thanks to Louise R. Greenswag and Randell C. Alexander for their significant contribution to transforming more pieces of the puzzle into a more complete picture.

THE OFFICERS AND BOARD OF DIRECTORS
PRADER–WILLI SYNDROME ASSOCIATION (USA)

Acknowledgments

This second edition is the result of recognition by the Prader–Willi Syndrome Association (USA) of significant advances in genetic research, the development of diagnostic criteria, and the expanding horizons of management of this unusual birth defect. We are deeply indebted to this exceptional organization of parents and professionals for its generous financial support in the preparation and publication of the text and for its personal support and encouragement.

We wish to acknowledge the authors of each chapter, who took the time graciously and without remuneration to contribute their expertise despite heavy professional obligations. Their personal commitment in addition to their scholarly and practical insights gave us an extra measure of encouragement.

Very special thanks are due Marci Wooff and Deb Herman for their assistance "par excellence," and for their patience and perseverance during the technical preparation and refinement of all facets of the text. Appreciation is extended to The University of Iowa Hospitals and Clinics —The Department of Pediatrics, Divisions of Medical Genetics and Developmental Disabilities, The Iowa Child Health Specialty Clinics, and to William Day, Executive Medical Editor, Springer-Verlag, New York for his interest and support.

We wish to pay special tribute to the many children born with Prader–Willi syndrome and their extraordinary families. Our lives are enriched by their presence and we owe them a singular debt of gratitude because they have allowed us access to their lives and brought us to a deeper understanding of their struggles.

LOUISE R. GREENSWAG, R.N., PH.D.
RANDELL C. ALEXANDER, M.D., PH.D.

Contents

PART III   The Interdisciplinary Process: Psychosocial Aspects

PART IV   Socialization

PART V   Delivery of Services

PART VI   A Network of Caring

Contributors

RANDELL C. ALEXANDER, M.D., PH.D. Department of Pediatrics, University Hospital School, The University of Iowa, Iowa City, Iowa 52242, USA

HARVEY H. BUSH, 1244 Melrose Way, Vista, California 92083, USA

SUZANNE B. CASSIDY, M.D. Center for Human Genetics, Case Western Reserve University, Cleveland, Ohio 44106, USA

MARY CATALETTO, M.D. Associate Director, Division of Pediatric Pulmonary, Department of Pediatrics, Winthrop University Hospital, Mineola, New York, 11501, USA

IRA COLLERAIN, PH.D. Chief Psychologist, Denton State School, and Adjunct Professor, University of North Texas, Denton, Texas 76202-0368, USA

NANCY CONDON, B.A., M.B.A. Director of Residential Services, Texas Department of Mental Health, Mental Retardation Denton State School, Denton, Texas 76202-0368, USA

MARY ALICE DEUSTERHAUS-MINOR, M.S. Physical Therapist Assistant Program, Stanford-Brown College, Hazelwood, Missouri 63142, USA

DEBORA A. DOWNEY, C.C.C.-S.P. Department of Pediatrics, University Hospital School, The University of Iowa, Iowa City, Iowa 52242, USA

LOUISE R. GREENSWAG, PH.D., R.N. Adjunct Professor, College of Nursing; Program Consultant for Prader–Willi Syndrome, Iowa Child Health Specialty Clinics, University Hospital School, Division of Developmental Disabilities, The University of Iowa Hospitals and Clinics, Iowa City, Iowa 52242, USA

JEANNE M. HANCHETT, M.D. Rehabilitation Institute of Pittsburgh, Pittsburgh, Pennsylvania 15217, USA

JAMES W. HANSON, M.D. National Vaccine Program Office, Washington DC 20201, USA

AL HEINEMANN, 121 Sage Meadow, Maryland Heights, Missouri 63043, USA

GILA HERTZ, PH.D., A.B.S.M. Associate Director, Sleep Disorders Center, Winthrop University Hospital, Mineola, New York 11501, USA

LORI A. HILMER, M.S.W. Division of Developmental Disabilities, University Hospital School, The University of Iowa, Iowa City, Iowa 52242, USA

VANJA A. HOLM, M.D. Child Development and Mental Retardation Center, The University of Washington, Seattle, Washington 98195, USA

SONDRA B. KASKA, J.D. Iowa Protection and Advocacy Services, Inc., Iowa City, Iowa 52244, USA

FRANZ KLUTSCHKOWSKI, ED.D. Psychologist, Denton State School, and Adjunct Professor, Cook County Community College, Denton, Texas 76202-0368, USA

CLAUDIA L. KNUTSON, C.C.C.-SP., M.A. University Hospital School, The University of Iowa, Iowa City, Iowa 52242, USA

KATHY KOBILIS, B.A. Program Manager, Woods Services, Inc., Langhorne, Pennsylvania 19047, USA

PHILLIP D.K. LEE, M.D. Assistant Professor of Pediatrics, Pediatric Endocrinology and Metabolism Section, Endocrinology Consultant, Texas Children's Hospital, Prader–Willi Syndrome Clinic, and Director of Research and Scientific Affairs, Diagnostic Systems Laboratories, Inc., Webster, Texas 77598, USA

JEANNE LEHRER, PH.D. Psychologist, Woods Services, Inc., Langhorne, Pennsylvania 19047, USA

KAREN LEVINE, PH.D. Spalding Rehabilitation Hospital, Boston, Massachusetts 02114, USA

ELIZABETH TRUE LLOYD, O.T.R. 4945 North 26th Street, Arlington, Virginia 22207, USA

BEATE MAIER, PH.D. Rehabilitation Institute of Pittsburgh, Pittsburgh, Pennsylvania 15217, USA

STEWART MAURER. Vice-President, Prader–Willi Syndrome Association (USA), Indianapolis, Indiana 46280, USA

MARY M. MULLIGAN. Humboldt Workshop, Inc., Humboldt, Iowa 50548, USA

ARTHUR J. NOWAK, D.M.D. Department of Pediatric Dentistry, College of Dentistry and Medicine, The University of Iowa, Iowa City, Iowa 52242, USA

SHARON OMROD. Director, Community Based Services, Training School, Vineland, New Jersey 08360, USA

ANNA MARIE SAPORITO, M.ED., C.R.C., C.V.E. Rehabilitational Counsellor and Vocational Evaluator, Community Rehabilitation Service of Pittsburgh, Pittsburgh, Pennsylvania 15227, USA

CURTIS J. SHACKLETT, J.D. 6175 South Quincy, Tulsa, Oklahoma 74136

PATRICIA L. SHAW, B.A. Residential Director, Laura Barker School, 211 Oak Street, Northfield, Minnesota 55057, USA

JACK SHERMAN, M.D. Director, Pediatric Clinic, Nassau County Medical Center, East Meadow, New York 11554, USA

SANDRA L. SINGER. Director, Oakwood Residence, Inc., Minneapolis, Minnesota 55410, USA

SCOTT SPREAT, ED.D. Clinical Services Administrator, Woods Services, Inc., Langhorne, Pennsylvania 19047, USA

DIANE D. STADLER, M.S., R.D./L.D. Division of Developmental Disabilities and Division of Medical Genetics, University Hospital School, The University of Iowa, Iowa City, Iowa 52242, USA

LINDA THORNTON. Coordinator, Prader–Willi Syndrome Association (NZ), Paierau Road, Masterton, New Zealand

JANALEE TOMASESKI-HEINEMANN, M.S.W. 121 Sage Meadow, Maryland Heights, Missouri 63043, USA

DON C. VAN DYKE, M.D. Department of Pediatrics, University Hospital School, The University of Iowa, Iowa City, Iowa 52242, USA

ROBERT H. WHARTON, M.D. Spalding Rehabilitation Hospital, Boston, Massachusetts 02114, USA

BARBARA Y. WHITMAN, PH.D. Cardinal Glennon Children's Hospital/ KCDC, St. Louis, Missouri 63104, USA

Introduction

Having recognized a need to provide a comprehensive resource of information and common sense guidelines, it was with considerable pride that we introduced a definitive text on the management of Prader–Willi syndrome (PWS). The time has now come to examine what has transpired since that first edition was published. Our intent has not changed. Now as then, our objective is to emphasize the need for professionals to develop sensitive, consistent, on-going interventions that optimize the development and adaptation of individuals with PWS and respond to their changing needs. As a consequence of successful management, the life span of this population has dramatically increased and their human potential has been expanded.

Why is this second edition so timely? There are several reasons. First, the boundaries of what we know about PWS have expanded considerably. For instance, an explosion of technological breakthroughs in the field of genetics has resulted in significant refinement in our understanding of genetic mechanisms and advances in diagnosis. New information about endocrinological processes and how they apply to PWS warrants the extra attention in this edition. And, even after the focus and format for this edition was designed, we decided that recent research in sleep disorders should be reported. Second, medical interventions now include administration of growth hormones and the use of psychotropic medications is under investigation. Third, in the past few years there have been important changes in the assessment process. Experience has taught us that the importance of interdisciplinary collaboration cannot be underestimated if effective management strategies are to be forthcoming. And finally, when crises occur, when, where, and how to intervene are major challenges.

This second edition remains fundamentally a "how-to" book. It is our effort to offer an updated resource for professionals, independent practitioners, and care-providers attentive to the best interests of affected children. It was gratifying to learn that the first edition received worldwide distribution. With the exception of chapters incorporating United States legal standards regarding protection and advocacy, education, and criteria for establishment of residential programming, we continue to endeavor to address management issues that cross countries and cultures. Historical, diagnostic, medical, and genetic information is provided to orient the reader. Current research, clinical, social, family, and community issues are explored. The balance of the text suggests pragmatic guidelines for management. Because the syndrome's multifaceted characteristics require support from a variety of professionals, sections of the book, written by specialists, offer information and insight for those less knowledgeable in a given discipline. Designed for clarity and conciseness in communicating ideas, the text also represents a diversity of approaches to management. This diversity itself is reflected in the format and individual writing styles of each author. We are grateful for their contributions and for their personal interest in advancing the concept of multidisciplinary collaboration.

Although PWS must be considered within the context of other developmental disabilities, the nature of this condition requires a unique approach to services. This is by no means an effort to diminish the needs of other children, but rather an attempt to address problems specific to PWS. Clearly, the syndrome is an eating rather than a weight disorder. Service providers must be aware that the overpowering hunger drive that these individuals experience is an organically caused, physiological fact of life. Unlike those with exogenous obesity, the persons with PWS *never* feel full. Left alone, children with the syndrome will literally eat themselves to death. Although the hunger drive may not be evident early in life, the typical affected individual begins to compulsively search for food much as a drug addict seeks out heroin. But, unlike the withdrawal of an addictive drug, total withdrawal of food is fatal. The presence of this lack of satiety is compounded by the fact that most affected individuals lack the cognitive capacity to comply with unsupervised food intake regimens.

Most individuals with PWS are diagnosed and followed at major academic genetic centers that serve as ongoing resources for interdisciplinary services such as the clinic at the University of Iowa Affiliated Program. Early intervention before initial weight gain is critical. Until very recently services focused primarily on weight reduction because parents tended to seek help only *after* their children became grossly obese. Now, as more cases are diagnosed earlier, in the preobesity stage, nutritional management potentially can prevent marked weight gain (although the absence of obesity does not preclude the presence of the syndrome).

While supervision of food intake is a major component of management, the psychosocial dimensions of the syndrome require equal attention because most individuals with PWS tend to become more emotionally labile as they grow older. Usually affable in early childhood, over time they begin to demonstrate bizarre and inappropriate behaviors, regardless of the presence or absence of obesity. However, in between these episodes of acting out, they may be pleasant, friendly, and gentle for long periods of time. Children, who previously died young due to complications of obesity, now face unique problems as developmentally disabled adults; services are required to meet their psychosocial, residential, and vocational needs.

The book is divided into six parts and, to sharpen the perceptions of the reader to the "human dimensions" of PWS, selected personal experiences of parents are integrated throughout.

I. Physiological and Genetics Considerations: Chapter 1 presents an overview of Prader–Willi syndrome, its history, etiology, clinical characteristics, and differential diagnosis. Genetic aspects are introduced in Chapter 2 and Chapter 3 discusses endocrinological management.

II. The Interdisciplinary Process: Health Aspects: Chapter 4 discusses the multidisciplinary team approach to management. Chapters 5–8 describe interventions in the fields of medicine, nursing, dentistry, nutrition, and physical and occupational therapies.

III. The Interdisciplinary Process: Psychosocial Aspects: Chapter 9 addresses psychological management with new information on psychopharmacology. Chapters 10–12 contain current strategies in the disciplines of speech and language, education, and social services.

IV. Socialization: Chapter 13 presents information regarding psychosexuality.

V. Delivery of Services: Chapter 14 offers information about protection and advocacy services. Options for residential and vocational programming are presented in Chapters 15 and 16. A model for crisis intervention is described in Chapter 17.

VI. A Network of Caring: Chapter 18 sensitively portrays the human dimension of PWS with a case description. Chapter 19 sheds light on the emotional aspects of having a child with PWS from two parents' points of view. The National Prader–Willi Syndrome Association (USA) is described in Chapter 20 and its expanding role as a resource for parents and professionals is discussed.

The final sections consist of a glossary of terms, suggested readings, and appendices. Tables, diagrams, and photographs are used throughout the book to illustrate and emphasize the content.

We continue to believe that direct services to individuals with PWS and their families have "come of age." We hope that the descriptions and prescriptions chronicled here will provide a cornerstone for effective care.

LOUISE R. GREENSWAG, R.N., PH.D.
RANDELL C. ALEXANDER, M.D., PH.D.

Part I
Physiological and Genetics Considerations

This baby was several weeks overdue when born. It was a difficult forced labor with intravenous medicines and breaking the water. I was kept medicated for days and never knew what was happening. I was told nothing [in the hospital] and very little when I went home. We left the baby there for a few days. He had difficulty nursing and seldom cried. He was a funny kind of dusky color and cried weakly. We were told at the clinic we took him to when he was about 3 years old that it was "hypothalamus" [sic]. It was a nightmare not knowing the problem or what to do.

We wish we knew for sure if it [PWS] is in our genes. We worry about our normal son. Can we have a PW child?

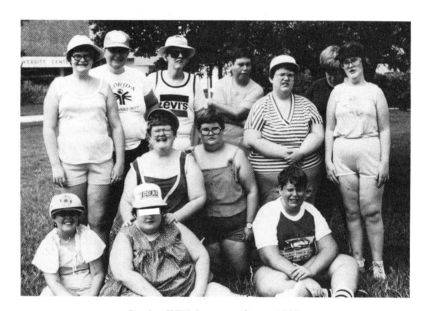

Prader-Willi Summer Camp 1980.

1
Overview

RANDELL C. ALEXANDER, DON C. VAN DYKE, and
JAMES W. HANSON

Prader–Willi syndrome (PWS) is a recognizable pattern of altered growth and development. While the etiology and pathogenesis remain unclear, it is beginning to yield to the application of molecular-genetic technology. Affected persons face life as potentially overweight, short, sexually immature, developmentally delayed individuals with poor gross motor skills. Usually at least mildly retarded, stubborn, egocentric, and emotionally labile, they rarely develop the ability to cope independently with their insatiable hunger and require environmental restrictions to prevent life-threatening obesity. Although individuals with PWS and their family face many of the same problems as others who are developmentally disabled, the unique characteristics of the syndrome—behaviors and gross obesity due to uncontrollable hunger—require special care and services.

Although PWS is not a common disorder, it is no longer considered rare. Estimates of the incidence vary between 1:10,000 and 1:25,000, placing this disorder among the more frequently recognized malformation syndromes. According to the Prader–Willi Syndrome Association, (USA) over 5,000 cases of PWS have been identified throughout the world. Males and females are equally affected, and syndrome has not been shown to be associated with specific racial/ethnic groups, socioeconomic classes, or geographic regions.

However, PWS is an important condition for reasons other than frequency or the complexity of management issues. This unique disorder manifests abnormalities of growth, learning, and physical development that may provide clues to understanding many larger issues such as eating disorders and weight control, the neurophysiology of behavior, patterns of genetic inheritance, and the genetic control of morphogenesis.

History

The first report of PWS was published in 1956 by Prader, Labhart, and Willi (Prader, Labhart, & Willi, 1956a). Although primarily interested in endocrinology, these authors described an unusual pattern of other

3

abnormalities: diminished fetal activity, profound poor muscle tone (hypotonia), feeding problems in infancy, underdeveloped sex organs (hypogonadism and hypogenitalism), short stature and retarded bone age, small hands and feet, delayed developmental milestones, characteristic faces, cognitive impairment, onset of gross obesity in early childhood due to insatiable hunger, and a tendency to develop diabetes in adolescence and adulthood when weight was not controlled. A second report followed that same year (Prader, Labhart, Willi, & Fanconi, 1956b). By 1961, 14 cases had been studied in Switzerland (Prader, Labhart, & Willi, 1961) and six in England (Laurance, 1961). Prader, Labhart, and Willi published a follow-up in 1963 of their original nine cases and elaborated on the role of diabetes mellitus and mental retardation in the clinical picture (Prader, Labhart, & Willi, 1963).

Landmark studies included follow-up accounts of earlier cases by Gabilan and Royer (1968), Zellweger and Schneider (1968), and Dunn (1968). These reports indicated orthopedic, dental, and developmental characteristics that could assist in differential diagnosis and strongly suggest that the PWS syndrome has two clearly identifiable phases. Hall and Smith (1972) gave a detailed account of 32 PWS patients that not only supported earlier diagnostic criteria, but also described behavior and personality problems that appeared to intensify with age. Medical problems associated with PWS have been discussed by Kriz and Clonniger (1981), Holm and Laurnen (1981), Bray, Dahms, Swerdloff, et al. (1983), and Cassidy (1984).

A compendium of current findings that had been presented to the 1979 national conference of the Prader–Willi Syndrome Association was published (Holm, Sulzbacher, & Pipe, 1981) and Cassidy wrote a comprehensive monograph in 1984. A study of 232 individuals with PWS, age 16 and over, indicated that with appropriate nutritional control, the life expectancy of this population has been extended, that emotional liability increases with age and is independent of the presence of adult obesity, that psychosocial adaptation to adulthood requires special management, and that the presence of PWS has a profound impact on family life (Greenswag, 1987).

Etiology and Pathogenesis

The etiology and pathogenesis of PWS was poorly understood until very recent advances in cytogenetics and molecular genetics. These advances are now beginning to provide some insight into the fairly complicated clinical picture of the syndrome, the expression of which may be the final pathway of different etiologies. Approximately 70% of patients with the clinical presentation of PWS have been shown to have a deletion of the proximal part of the long arm of chromosome 15, described as 15q11, q13. The remaining 30% have an apparently normal 15th chromosome.

Molecular studies have shown that for patients with PWS who have deletions these deletions are from the paternally derived chromosome 15. In individuals with PWS with nondeletion, they have been shown to have two maternally derived chromosomes 15. In essence, PWS shows a deletion in the paternal influence described as genomic imprinting of vital segments of chromosome 15. Thus, absence of the paternal 15 chromosomal material suggests that this material is necessary to produce phenotypic and behavioral normalcy. Unique parental disomy may result in pathology because genomic parental imprinting for normalcy has not occurred (see Chapter 2).

Although the vast majority of cases of PWS occur as sporadic events in families, several familial recurrences have been documented. Gabilan and Royer (1968) detailed two cases in the same family (a brother and sister) and another case from related parents. There have been subsequent reports of PWS in siblings (Bolanos, Lopez-Amor, Vasquez, et al., 1974; Cohen, Hall, Smith, et al., 1973; Endo, Tasaska, Matsuura, et al., 1976). Hall and Smith (1972) reported an instance of affected first cousins and Jancar (1971) and Evans (1969) reported two brothers, one of whom had a normal twin sister. Brissenden and Levy (1973) and Ikeda, Asaka, Inouye, et al. (1973) reported instances of monozygotic twins. DeFraites, Thurmon, Farhadian (1975) identified one family with five cases of PWS and suggested that the syndrome arose as an autosomal recessive trait. Lubinsky, Zellweger, Greenswag, et al. (1987) described a family of four siblings (two female, two male) with PWS and no normal children; this diagnosis was made clinically on the basis of history, physical findings, and behavior in three of the children (the other had died at 10 months with a similar history). At that time, no cytogenetic abnormality, detectable molecular deletion, or uniparental disomy (P. Rogan, personal communication) was identified in either the siblings or their parents. Molecular analysis of two siblings from this family has since confirmed the clinical diagnosis of PWS, by showing that both have an imprinting mutation (Nicholls, 1994). Thus, both siblings, but not the parents, have DNA methylation typical of PWS at three imprinted loci spanning 1.5 Mb within 15q11–q13 (*D15S9, D15S63, SNRPN*). In addition, a very small deletion was found in both affected siblings and the father just upstream and overlapping the *SNRPN* promoter (Saitoh, Rogan, & Nicholls, personal communication). The findings in this USA family are similar to those in another family from Scandinavia (Sutcliffe, 1994; Saitoh, Mutirangura, Kuwano, et al., 1994). The father is a phenotypically silent carrier of the deletion, and thus almost certainly inherited the deletion from his mother. However, this deletion leads to prevention of resetting the imprint in the male germline, so all his children inheriting the deletion have PWS. Further studies on the mechanism of imprinting are in process.

If PWS is, in fact, a sequential pattern of altered growth, development, and function stemming from a single localized area of damage in the fetus

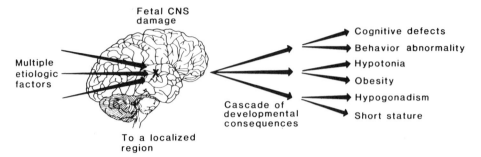

FIGURE 1.1. Pathogenetic model of PWS: sequence.

arising in the central nervous system (Hanson, 1981), it could be predicted that a host of factors, both genetic and environmental, might cause this disorder. A few genetic problems (monogenic or cytogenetic) occurring in a portion of families could explain the low recurrence risk overall, with a few exceptional families presenting with unusual recurrence patterns. Furthermore, this model of causation would predict wide variability in phenotypic outcome based upon the exact location, extent, and timing of the proposed defect in fetal nervous system morphogenesis. It may be expected that within the familial cases, this variability would be difficult to demonstrate since the definition of a case would require modification. The family reported by Clarren and Smith (1977) may illustrate this problem.

On the other hand, PWS may be regarded as a true malformation syndrome. This implies a more restricted (and very probably genetic) group of causal factors that each affects a single (or a few) biochemical or developmental process(es) in a group of tissues leading to the observed range of phenotypic consequences (pleiotrophy) (see Figure 1.1). This pathogenetic model suggests a more restricted case definition, but also allows for some variability both between and within families. Although a few families with monogenic disorders concealed within the larger population of PWS could explain the observed recurrence patterns, cytogenetic rearrangements (at either the microscopic or molecular level) afford a more robust explanation. Deletions and other unbalanced rearrangements of a chromosome could well affect more than a single genetic locus ("contiguous gene disorder"), producing variable consequences. Indeed, "balanced" chromosomal rearrangements in a parent (inversions, translocation, etc.) might account for occasional recurrences in a few families. An alternative explanation for occasional recurrences among children of apparently normal couples is gonadal mosaicism. Answers as to which, if any, of these alternate explanations of PWS may be correct await clarification. It seems likely that such answers may be of substantial interest for such diverse areas of medical science as endocrinology, nutrition, neurophysiology, psychology, and morphogenesis.

Although the cause of PWS may not be clear-cut, the observed abnormalities may result from a localized primary disturbance in the development of the brain above the spinal cord, such as a defect in the hypothalamic–pituitary axis (Gorlin, Pindborg, & Cohen, 1976; Hanson, 1981). Afifi and Zellweger (1969) and Tze, Dunn, and Rothstein (1981) also suggested the presence of a fat metabolism defect. Schwartz, Brunzell, and Bierman (1979) believed that the level of the lipoprotein lipase enzyme may be one of the critical mechanisms by which the brain regulates the number, size, and metabolism of fat cells in the body, and suggested a biochemical explanation for the presence of PWS.

The number of alterations in the body's homeostatic mechanisms (regulatory functions) in PWS implicates the hypothalamus as the probable site of major brain dysfunction. For example, both the satiety and the feeding centers are located in the hypothalamus, and appetite disturbance may be a function of overactivity or underactivity of one of these centers or a problem in the balance between the two. The hypothalamus also helps to regulate production of growth and sex hormones.

Sleep, breathing, and body temperature may also be affected, either in this area or in adjacent brain structures. Sleep disorders in PWS occur both day and night and may represent different mechanisms (Appendix A). The hypothalamus and adjoining areas are also responsible for activity levels and the propensity for vomiting. To date, neither computed tomography scans of the brain, magnetic resonance imaging, nor autopsy results have yielded any specific defect or abnormality. It is possible that flaws exist in specific types or balances of neurotransmitters regulating brain cell-to-cell communication. Positive emission tomography (PET) scans have yet to be used to investigate whether a functional defect could be detected. Other abnormalities seem to reflect problems with areas of the brain that are either more diffuse or less clearly understood.

Intelligence, behavior problems, and speech and language skills (cognitive functions) may represent somewhat more global differences in brain functioning. Future research may establish an underlying biochemical defect or microstructural abnormality in the brain that would account for the characteristic symptoms.

Natural History and Clinical Manifestations

Natural History

The diagnostic picture of an individual with PWS appears to change as the child matures (Hoefnagel, Costello, & Hatoum, 1967), and only recently have diagnostic criteria been well established (Holm, Cassidy, Butler, et al., 1993). Zellweger (1969) divided the syndrome into two

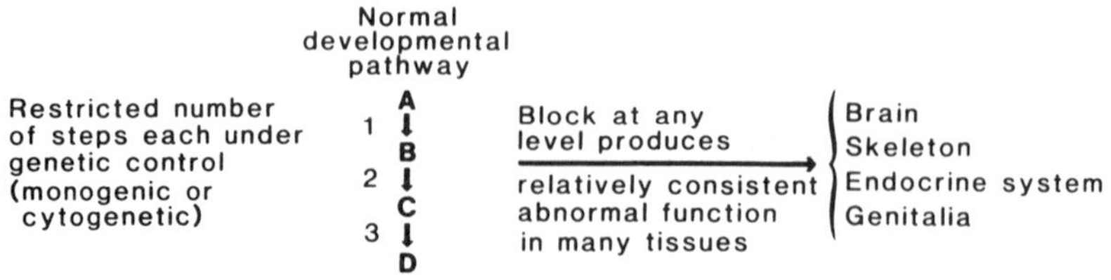

```
                          Normal
                      developmental
                        pathway
Restricted number          A
of steps each under    1   |      Block at any        ⎧ Brain
genetic control            B      level produces      ⎪ Skeleton
(monogenic or          2   |      ─────────────────→  ⎨ Endocrine system
cytogenetic)               C      relatively consistent⎪ Genitalia
                       3   |      abnormal function    ⎩
                           D      in many tissues
```

FIGURE 1.2. Pathogenetic model of PWS: syndrome.

phases, the first of which occurs in the prenatal and neonatal period and early infancy. (Figure 1.2).

Phase I

Compared with a normal fetus, the PWS child is less active *in utero*, is more likely to be delivered in a breech or shoulder position, and may have an excessive amount of amniotic fluid (Hall & Smith, 1972). The diminished fetal activity and high breech presentation suggest that profound hypotonia may be present early in fetal life. The neonatal phase is marked by below-average weight, poor suck, reflexes that are difficult to elicit, extreme hypotonia, lethargy, small genitalia (more noticeable in males), and skeletal anomalies of the head (Zellweger, 1984). Sometimes the severe lack of muscle tone (amyotonia) will "mimic flaccid paralysis" (Zellweger, 1981). Because of poor muscle tone, these babies have little facial expression, a weak cry, and tend to present with feeding problems for weeks or months, necessitating special feeding techniques. These limp, floppy, difficult-to-feed infants may be labeled as having "failure to thrive" and may be mistakenly diagnosed as having some form of congenital hypotonia or muscular dystrophy. The hypotonia eventually resolves itself to the point where the infant can feed, although suck remains weak and feeding times are prolonged. Another consequence of the hypotonia is that motor development is often delayed even beyond that expected due to limited cognition. However, some time after the first year of life, the degree of hypotonia diminishes and motor function begins to improve.

Phase II

In the second phase an uncontrollable hunger drive insidiously emerges, usually between the ages of 2 and 3 years. At this time, the children begin to gorge themselves and, unless restricted, become grossly obese (Zellweger, 1981). Although the insatiable hunger drive may be present earlier (in the first phase), it is masked by the hypotonia. It is important to note that children with PWS do not merely overeat but are compulsively obsessed with food, demonstrate bizarre food-seeking behaviors, and during early years may eat nonfood items. Unable to satisfy their ravenous hunger, their life is "one endless meal" (See, 1976). Zellweger (personal conversation, 1989) hypothesized two food-seeking behaviors: those individuals who constantly forage and those who only gorge when food is available. Also, early in the second phase, relieved parents, who initially struggled with earlier feeding problems, are delighted when their children appear eager to eat. Unfortunately, all too quickly these toddlers may bloom into poorly coordinated, grossly overweight, impulsive, temperamental children with whom families must learn to cope. Although PWS children are initially friendly and affectionate, their behaviors appear to deteriorate as they mature (Cassidy, 1984). Their emotional ability is characterized by placid affability and sudden, severe, unpredictable, uncontrollable outbursts of anger, hindering psychosocial adaptation (Greenswag, 1987).

The body fat of individuals with PWS characteristically is distributed in the adipose tissue of the trunk and thighs while the lower arms and legs remain lean; the hands and feet are unusually small (Holm, 1981; Nugent & Holm, 1981). On growth curve records (see Appendix B), the child is short and bone age is significantly delayed; when the epiphyses fuse, final stature is small (Dunn, 1968); Nugent & Holm, 1981). When the physiological hunger drive is left unmanaged, gross obesity and death result (Zellweger, 1981).

Diagnostic Criteria

The differential diagnosis of Phase I of Prader–Willi is an effort to separate Prader–Willi syndrome from other infantile hypotonias. These include congenital myotonic dystrophy, Zellweger's syndrome, atonic diplegia, Werdnig–Hoffman (spinal muscle atrophy), congenital myopathies, benign congenital hypotonias, and in some cases CNS anoxia. Clinical findings helpful in the differential diagnosis are muscle tone, strength and mass, reflexes, oral motor mechanism, and general CNS status. Laboratory studies helpful in some cases are electromyelogram and muscle biopsy. The differential diagnosis of Prader–Willi syndrome is listed in Table 1.1.

Consensus diagnostic criteria have recently been developed by a group of national and international experts based on 113 patients (Holm et al., 1993). Three categories of diagnostic criteria for Prader–Willi syndrome were developed: major, minor, and supportive. Major criteria and minor criteria were valued on a point system with one point assigned to major and one half to minor. Supportive criteria were not included on the point system. Because changes in clinical presentation occur over time, the scoring system varies depending on age. For children 3 years old and younger, five points are required for diagnosis, four coming from the

TABLE 1.1. Differential diagnosis of Phase I Prader-Willi syndrome versus other infantile hypotonias. (Zellweger, 1988).

	Prader-Willi	Cogenital myotonic dystrophy	Zellweger syndrome	Atonic diplegia	Werdnig-Hoffmann spinal muscular atrophy	Congenital myopathies	Benign congenital hypotonia
Muscle tone	Atonia improving	Atonia improving, myotonia appears later on	Persistent atonia	Atonia improving, spasticity appears later on in some cases	Progressively decreasing	Decreased but no progression	Decreased but improving
Muscle strength	Slightly decreased	Decreased	Decreased	Very decreased	Progressively decreasing	Decreased	Good
Muscle mass	Slightly decreased	Decreased	Decreased	Decreased	Progressive decrease to severe muscular atrophy	Decreased, often severe atrophy	Usually good, sometimes decreased
Tendon reflexes	Initially absent, later on present	Initially absent, later on present	Absent or weak	Hyperactive, Babinski positive	Weak, later absent	Absent or (rarely) weak	Normal but difficult to alicit
Sucking/swallowing	Difficult for weaks or months	Difficult for months	Difficult throughout life in most cases	—	Good; difficulties may occur in advanced stages	Usually good, rarely difficult	Normal
Mental status	Lethargic for weeks or months	Lethargic for months	Lethargic nonresponsive throughout life	Slow motor development	Alert	Alert	Alert
Electromyogram	Normal	Normal	Normal	Normal	Abnormal	Abnormal	Abnormal
Muscle biopsy	Normal	Normal or nonspecific myopathy	Normal; mitochondrial myopathy in exceptional cases	Normal	Abnormal	Abnormal	Abnormal
Other manifestations	Dysmorphic features, hypothermia, hypogonadism, microgenitale in boys, chromosome abnormality in over 50%	Clubfeet, abnormal diaphragm present	Clubfeet, hepatomegaly, abnormal ocular findings, convulsions, dysmorphic features	Convulsions present, slow development	Normal intelligence with severe muscle weakness	—	Normal development, easy fatigability
Infant mortality	Low	High	Very high, rarely survive to age of 2 years	Low	High	Higher than usual	Not increased

major group. For individuals, 3 years of age to adulthood, a total score of eight is necessary with five or more points coming from the major criteria group. Diagnostic criteria of Prader–Willi are listed in Table 1.2.

Management

Case management begins with the recognition of the presence of PWS by the parents, family, and all care providers who must understand that the syndrome will not disappear, and cannot be corrected, and that intervention means the management of clinical symptoms.

Individuals with PWS undergo significant developmental changes over time and, although professionals working with families naturally focus on their own disciplines, they must be aware of how the syndrome impacts on other spheres of both the child's and family's existence. As is true for all low-incidence handicapping conditions, when there is extensive lack of professional experience, the knowledge of parents should be drawn on when creating management strategies. Even in cases when diagnosis is made early and excessive weight gain is avoided, extensive on-going interdisciplinary intervention is essential. Specific strategies should emphasize genetic counseling, prevention of obesity, behavior management, environmental controls, planned activities, special educational and vocational services, and psychotherapeutic support and guidance for future planning.

It is very difficult to discourage food foraging habits since the insatiable hunger drive does not appear to diminish. Effective nutritional intervention requires considerable time, planning, and commitment. Acquiring accurate baseline data, education of care providers, environmental control, and frequent monitoring of growth curves and calorie intake are essential. When individuals are diagnosed early, greater opportunities exist to avoid initial weight gain (see Chapter 7). Although, early diagnosis was noted to have a positive effect on subsequent weight and behavior management during early schooling, it is not certain if these effects continue later in life (Greenswag & Alexander, 1990).

Individuals with PWS have special educational needs, the planning for which should take into account their cognitive limitations. In this respect, their parents share concerns similar to those of parents of children with other handicapping conditions (see Chapter 11).

Prader, Labhart, and Willi (1963) described their patients as good-natured children with silly, contented facial expressions. Others described younger children as placid, affectionate, and outgoing (Cassidy, 1984; Hanson, 1981). However, as indicated earlier, behavioral problems appear to intensify with age. Zellweger and Schneider (1968) suggested that definitive behavioral changes take place between the ages of 3 and 5 as the universal symptom of insatiable hunger emerges. Greenswag and

TABLE 1.2. Consensus diagnostic criteria for Prader–Willi syndrome.[a,b]

Major criteria
1. Neonatal and infantile central hypotonia with poor suck, gradually improving with age
2. Feeding problems in infancy with need for special feeding techniques and poor weight gain/failure to thrive
3. Excessive or rapid weight gain on weight-for-length chart (excessive is defined as crossing two centile channels) after 12 months but before 6 years of age; central obesity in the absence of intervention
4. Characteristic facial features with dolichocephaly in infancy, narrow face or bifrontal diameter, almond-shaped eyes, small-appearing mouth with thin upper lip, down-turned corners of mouth (3 or more required)
5. Hypogonadism—with any of the following, depending on age:
   a. Genital hypoplasia (male: scrotal hypoplasia, cryptorchidism, small penis and/or testes for age (<5th percentile); female: absence or severe hypoplasia of labia minora and/or clitoris
   b. Delayed or incomplete gonadal maturation with delayed pubertal signs in the absence of intervention after 16 years of age (male: small gonads, decreased facial and body hair, lack of voice change; female: amenorrhea/oligomenorrhea after age 16)
6. Global developmental delay in a child younger than 6 years of age; mild to moderate mental retardation or learning problems in older children
7. Hyperphagia/food foraging/obsession with food
8. Deletion 5q11–13 on high resolution (>650 bands) or other cytogenetic/molecular abnormality of the Prader–Willi chromosome region, including maternal disomy

Minor criteria
1. Decreased fetal movement or infantile lethargy or weak cry in infancy, improving with age
2. Characteristic behavior problems—temper tantrums, violent outbursts and obsessive/compulsive behavior; tendency to be argumentative, oppositional, rigid, manipulative, possessive, and stubborn; perseverating, stealing, and lying (5 or more of these symptoms required)
3. Sleep disturbance or sleep apnea
4. Short stature for genetic background by age 15 (in the absence of growth hormone intervention)
5. Hypopigmentation—fair skin and hair compared to family
6. Small hands (<25th percentile) and/or feet (<10th percentile) for height age
7. Narrow hands with straight ulnar border
8. Eye abnormalities (esotropia, myopia)
9. Thick viscous saliva with crusting at corners of the mouth
10. Speech articulation defects
11. Skin picking

Alexander (1990) showed the onset of obesity to be at approximately 2 to 3 years while behavioral problems usually emerge at age 4. Stubbornness and hyperactivity replace affability; repetitive and incessant chattering, verbal aggressiveness, and self-assaultive acts are observed; erratic, unpredictable rages increase; signs of depression and, in rare instances, psychotic episodes may occur (Hall & Smith, 1972; Zellweger, 1984).

TABLE 1.2. *Continued*

Supportive findings (increase the certainty of diagnosis but are not scored)
  1. High pain threshold
  2. Decreased vomiting
  3. Temperature instability in infancy or altered temperature sensitivity in older children and adults
  4. Scoliosis and/or kyposis
  5. Early adrenarche
  6. Osteoporosis
  7. Unusual skill with jigsaw puzzles
  8. Normal neuromuscular studies

[a] Reproduced from Holm et al., by permission of *Pediatrics 91*, 398, 1993.
[b] Scoring: Major criteria are weighted at one point each. Minor criteria are weighed at one half point. Children 3 years of age or younger: five points are required for diagnosis, four of which should come from the major group. Children 3 years of age to adulthood: total score of eight is necessary for the diagnosis. Major criteria must comprise five or more points of the total score.

Constant efforts to satisfy hunger seem to result in aggressive and bizarre food-seeking activities such as foraging, hoarding, and gorging (Byrt, 1969a,b; Dunn, Tze, Alisharin, et al., 1981; Marshall, Wallace, Elder, et al., 1981). Older children and adolescents frequently appear to develop serious personality problems ranging from being secretive and manipulative to being dull, lethargic, and indifferent (Hall & Smith, 1972; Kollrack & Wolff, 1966). When normal secondary sex characteristics fail to develop in adolescence, feelings of loneliness and isolation increase.

Day and night sleep problems are frequently present and may require medical intervention. Daytime sleepiness and sleep difficulties have been reported by some authors in over 90% of individuals with Prader–Willi syndrome. In some cases, children tend to fall asleep during certain daytime activities. A study by Hertz and Cataletto (Appendix A) implicates the possible presence of nocturnal sleep abnormalities in Prader–Willi syndrome that may cause a decrease in oxygen saturation, which may play a role in daytime sleepiness. Obviously, obesity and a small upper airway could lead to sleep apnea, which also may be another cause for a decrease in oxygen saturation (Appendix A).

Greenswag (1984) indicated that emotional instability is a predictable problem that limits psychosocial adaptation in adolescence and adulthood, appears to function independently of weight, and complicates case management. For older persons with PWS, lack of social experience and limited interpersonal skills and relationships seem to intensify as a result of poor physical skills and increased antisocial behaviors (see Chapter 9). Although the danger of pregnancy does not exist, concerns about sexuality, sexually transmitted diseases, and a desire for independent living increase during the teen years. Once schooling is completed, responsibility for social and vocational experiences falls to the family.

Parents/care providers face a future of restricted life (locked food) and erratic behavior. Future planning including residential options becomes an important concern (see Chapter 15).

Future Trends

Recent advances in genetic theory have spawned considerable research activity about PWS. With more precise delineation of a specific chromosomal defect, molecular probes may aid in more accurate diagnoses, and a better understanding of the pathophysiology leading to PWS characteristics may be achieved. The unique physiological aspects of sleep (e.g., sleep-disordered breathing and excessive daytime sleepiness) are currently an area of heightened interest in the scientific community (see Appendix A). In addition to major medical and weight management concerns, the psychosocial aspects of the syndrome need considerable study since little is known about the nonmedical aspects of this birth defect and their significance for PWS person and their family. After diagnosis, what does the future hold for these individuals? Certainly, the functional, emotional, and social patterns of a large group of individuals with PWS need to be investigated in order to enhance their capacity to contribute as productive members of society.

References

Afifi, A.K., & Zellweger, H. (1969). Pathology of muscular hypotonia in Prader-Willi syndrome: Light and electron microscope study. *Journal of the Neurological Sciences, 9,* 49–61.

Bolanos, F., Lopez-Amor, E., Vasquez, G., Losker, R., & Morato, T. (1974). Hypothalmic-pituitary-gonadal function in two siblings with Prader-Willi syndrome. *Revista de Investigacion Clinica, 26,* 53–62.

Bray, G., Dahms, W., Swerdloff, R., Fiser, R., Atkinson, R., & Carrell, R. (1983). The Prader-Willi syndrome: A study of 40 parents and a review of the literature. *Medicine, 62,* 59–80.

Brissenden, J.E., & Levy, E.P. (1973). Prader-Willi syndrome in infant monozygotic twins. *American Journal of Diseases of Children, 126,* 110–112.

Byrt, R. (1969a). A patient with suspected Prader-Willi syndrome at a mental subnormality hospital. 1. *Nursing Times, 65*(39), 1234–1235.

Byrt, R. (1969b). A patient with suspected Prader-Willi syndrome at a mental subnormality hospital. 2. *Nursing Times, 65*(40), 1260–1263.

Cassidy, S.B. (1984). Prader-Willi syndrome. *Current Problems in Pediatrics, 14,* 1–55.

Clarren, S.K., & Smith, D.W. (1977). Prader-Willi syndrome: Variable severity and recurrence risk. *American Journal of Diseases of Children, 131,* 798–800.

Cohen, M.M., Hall, B.D., Smith, D.W., Graham, C.D., & Lampert, K.J. (1973). A new syndrome with hypotonia, obesity, mental deficiency, and facial, oral, ocular and limb abnormalities. *The Journal of Pediatrics, 83,* 280–285.

DeFraites, E.B., Thurmon, T.F., & Farhadian, H. (1975). Familial Prader-Willi syndrome. *Birth Defects: Original Article Series*, *11*(4), 123–126.

Dunn, H.G. (1968). The Prader-Willi syndrome: Review of the literature and report of nine cases. *Acta Paediatrica Scandinavica Supplement*, *186*, 1–38.

Dunn, H.G., Tze, W.J., Alisharin, R.M., & Schulzer, M. (1981). Clinical experience with 23 cases of Prader-Willi syndrome. In V.A. Holm, S.J. Sulzbacher, & P.L. Pipes (Eds.), *The Prader-Willi syndrome* (pp. 69–88). Baltimore: University Park Press.

Endo, M., Tasaka, N., Matsuura, N., & Matsuda, I. (1976). Laurence-Moon-Biedl syndrome and Prader-Willi syndrome in a single family. *European Journal of Pediatrics*, *123*(4), 269–276.

Evans, P.R. (1969). The Prader-Labhart-Willi syndrome. *Developmental Medicine and Child Neurology*, *11*, 380–382.

Gabilan, J.C., & Royer, P. (1968). Le syndrome de Prader, Labhart, et Willi (etude de onze observations). *Archives Francasises de Pediatrie*, *25*, 121–149.

Gorlin, R.J., Pindborg, J.J., & Cohen, M.M., Jr. (1976). Prader-Willi syndrome. In *Syndromes of the head and neck* (2nd ed., pp. 618–621). New York: McGraw-Hill.

Greenberg, F., & Ledbetter, D. (1988). Deletions of proximal 15q without Prader-Willi syndrome (abstract). *Proceedings of the Greenwood Genetics Center*, *7*, 238–239.

Greenswag, L.R. (1984). *The adult with Prader-willi syndrome: A descriptive investigation*. Doctoral thesis, The University of Iowa. (DA 056952, University Microfilms Internation, Ann Arbor, MI).

Greenswag, L.R. (1987). Adults with Prader-Willi syndrome: A survey of 232 cases. *Developmental Medicine and Child Neurology*, *29*, 145–152.

Greenswag, L.R., & Alexander, R.C. (1990). Early diagnosis in Prader-Willi syndrome: Implications for managing weight and behavior. *Dysmorphology and Clinical Genetics*, *4*(1), 8–12.

Hall, B.D., & Smith, D.W. (1972). Prader-Willi syndrome. A resume of 32 cases including an instance of affected first cousins, one of whom is of normal stature and intelligence. *The Journal of Pediatrics*, *81*, 286–293.

Hanson, J. (1981). A view of etiology and pathogenesis of Prader-Willi syndrome. In V.A. Holm, S.J. Sulzbacher, & P.L. Pipes (Eds.), *The Prader-Willi syndrome* (pp. 45–53). Baltimore: University Park Press.

Hoefnagel, D., Costello, P.J., & Hatoum, K. (1967). Prader-Willi syndrome. *Journal of Mental Deficiency Research*, *11*, 1–11.

Holm, V.A. (1981). The diagnosis of Prader-Willi syndrome. In V.A. Holm, S.J. Sulzbacher, & P.L. Pipes (Eds.), *The Prader-Willi syndrome* (pp. 27–44). Baltimore: University Park Press.

Holm, V.A., & Laurnen, E.L. (1981). Prader-Willi syndrome and scoliosis. *Developmental Medicine and Child Neurology*, *23*, 192–201.

Holm, V.A., Sulzbacher, S.J., & Pipes, P.L. (Eds.). (1981). *The Prader-Willi syndrome*. Baltimore: University Park Press.

Holm, V.A., Cassidy, S.B., Butler, M.G., Hanchett, J.M., Greenswag, L.R., Whitman, B.Y., & Greenberg, F. (1993). Prader-Willi syndrome; Consensus diagnostic criteria. *Pediatrics*, *91*, 398–402.

Ikeda, K., Asaka, A., Inouye, E., Kaihara, H., & Kinoshita, K. (1973). Monozygotic twins concordant for Prader-Willi syndrome. *Japanese Journal of Human Genetics*, *18*, 220–225.

Jancar, J. (1971). Prader-Willi syndrome (hypotonia, obesity, hypogonadism, growth and mental retardation). *Journal of Mental Deficiency Research, 15*, 20–29.

Kollrack, H.W., & Wolff, D. (1966). Paranoid-halluzinatorische Psychose bei Prader-Labhart-Willi-Franconi-Syndrome. *Acta Paedopsychiatrica Scandinavica, 33*, 309–314.

Kriz, J.S., & Clonninger, B.J. (1981). Management of a patient with Prader-Willi syndrome by a dental-dietary team. *Special Care Dentist, 1*(4), 179–182.

Laurence, B.M. (1961). Hypotonia, hypogonadism and mental retardation in childhood. *Archives of Disease in Childhood, 36*, 690.

Lubinsky, M., Zellweger, H., Greenswag, L., Larson, G., Hansmann, I., & Ledbetter, D. (1987). Familial Prader-Willi syndrome with normal chromosomes. *American Journal of Medical Genetics, 28*, 37–43.

Marshall, B.D., Jr., Wallace, C.J., Elder, J., Burke, K., Oliver, T., & Blackman, R. (1981). A behavioral approach to the treatment of Prader-Willi syndrome. In V.A. Holm, S.J. Sulzbacher, & P.L. Pipes (Eds.), *The Prader-Willi syndrome* (pp. 185–199). Baltimore: University Park Press.

Nicholls, R.D. (1994). New insights reveal complex mechanisms involved ingenomic imprinting. *Am J Hum Genet, 54*(5), 733–740.

Nugent, J.K., & Holm, V. (1981). Physical growth in Prader-Willi syndrome. In V.A. Holm, S.J. Sulzbacher, & P.L. Pipes (Eds.), *The Prader-Willi syndrome* (pp. 269–280). Baltimore: University Park Press.

Prader, A., Labhart, A., & Willi, H. (1956a). Ein Syndrom von Adipositas, Kleinwuchs, Kryptorchismus and Oligophrenie nach myotonieartigem Zustand in Neugeborenenalter. *Schweizerische Medizinische Wochenschrift, 86*, 1260.

Prader, A., Labhart, A., Willi, H., & Fanconi, G. (1956b). Ein Syndrome von Adipositas, Kleinwuchs, Kryptorchismus und Idiotie bei Kindern und Erwachsenen, die als Neugeborene ein myatonie-artiges Bild geboten haben. *Proceedings of the VIII International Congress on Pediatrics, Copenhagen*, pp. 1260–1261

Prader, A., Labhart, A., & Willi, H. (1961). Das syndrom von Imbezilllitat, Adipostas, Muskelhypotonie, Hypogenitalismus, Hypogonadismus und Diabetes Mellitus mit "Myatonic"-Anamnese. In *Proceedings of the Second International Congress on Mental Retardation, Vienna, Austria, 1961*. Basel: S. Karger.

Prader, A., Labhart, A., & Willi, H. (1963). Das syndrom von Imbezilllitat, Adipostas, Muskelhypotonie, Hypogenitalismus, Hypogonadismus und Diabetes Mellitus mit "Myatonic"-Anamnese. *Second International Congress on Mental Retardation, Vienna, 1961*. Basel: S. Karger.

Saitoh, S., Mutirangura, A., Kuwano, A., Ledbetter, D.H., & Niikawa, N. (1994). Isochromosome 15q of maternal origin in two Prader-Willi syndrome patients previously diagnosed erroneously as cytogenetic deletions. *Am J Med Genet, 50*(1), 64–67.

Schwarz, R., Brunzell, J., & Bierman, E. (1979). Elevated adipose tissue lipoprotein-lipase in the pathogenesis of obesity in Prader-Willi syndrome. *Clinical Research, 27*(2), 137–143.

See, C. (1976). For some children life is one endless meal. *Today's Health*, vol. 1, 15–17, 50–51.

Sutcliffe, J.S. (1994). Deletions of a differentially methylated CpG island at the SNRPN gene define a putative imprinting control region. *Nature Genet, 8*, 52–58.

Tze, W.J., Dunn, H.G., & Rothstein, R.L. (1981). Endocrine profiles and metabolic aspects of Prader-Willi syndrome. In V.A. Holm, S.J. Sulzbacher, & P.L. Pipes (Eds.), *The Prader-Willi syndrome* (pp. 281–291). Baltimore: University Park Press.

Zellweger, H. (1969). The HHHO or Prader-Willi syndrome. *Birth defects: Original Article Series, 5*(2), 15–17.

Zellweger, H. (1981). Diagnosis and therapy in the first phase of Prader-Willi syndrome. In V.A. Holm, S.J. Sulzbacher, & P.L. Pipes (Eds.), *The Prader-Willi syndrome* (pp. 55–68). Baltimore: University Park Press.

Zellweger, H. (1984). The Prader-Willi syndrome. *Journal of the American Medical Association, 25*(4), 18–35.

Zellweger, H. (1988). Differential diagnosis in Prader-Willi syndrome. In L. Greenswag & R. Alexander (Eds.), *Management of Prader-Willi syndrome* (pp. 20–21). New York: Springer-Verlag.

Zellweger, H., & Schneider, H.J. (1968). Syndrome of hypotonia-hypomentia-hypogonadism-obesity (HHHO) or Prader-Willi syndrome. *American Journal of Diseases of Children, 115*, 558–598.

2
Genetics of Prader–Willi Syndrome

SUZANNE B. CASSIDY

Historical Aspects

Since Prader–Willi syndrome (PWS) was first described in 1956, many of its features have been recognized as arising from insufficient function of the hypothalamus (Prader, Labhart, & Willi, 1956). This part of the brain plays a major role in the control of so-called homeostatic, or baseline, functions, among them hunger, thirst, sleep–wake cycles, and temperature regulation. The hypothalamus also releases hormones that travel to the pituitary gland (the "master gland" at the base of the brain), controlling the release of other hormones such as those that stimulate growth (growth hormone), sex hormones (gonadotropins), and thyroid hormones to control basal metabolic rate. Thus, an animal such as a cat that has had its hypothalamus destroyed will have many of the functional abnormalities seen in PWS, as will a previously normal person with acquired damage to the hypothalamus due to an injury, stroke, or tumor. Even the personality characteristics seen in PWS, including the temper tantrums, may result. Because the hypothalamus was a logical place to look for a structural defect in PWS, the few reported autopsy studies focused on that part of the brain. Unfortunately, no gross or microscopic abnormalities of it could be visualized to explain the clinical features of the disorder.

Ignorance of the cause of PWS remained for many years. It had been observed that the likelihood of typical PWS recurring in a family was very small: reportedly less than 3–5%, according to the few reports in the medical literature. Nonetheless, this complex multisystem disorder, which usually includes mental retardation, suggested a genetic condition, most likely due to a single gene mutation or a chromosomal disorder. In fact, in a small percentage of cases, an apparently balanced rearrangement of the chromosomes, called a Robertsonian translocation, was found (Figure 2.1). Such translocations usually occurr between chromosomes in which the major constriction (centromere) is very near the tip (telomere) of the chromosome, rather than near the middle of the chromosome, including numbers 13, 14, 15, 21, and 22. Hawkey and Smithies (1976) noted that

18

most such Robertsonian translocations found in individuals with PWS involved chromosome 15. However, in this type of translocation, it is believed that no transcribed (genetically active) chromosome material is lost or altered, merely that two chromosomes have become "stuck" together, losing only a small amount of information that codes for the organization of subcellular organelles called nucleoli. This information is present on multiple chromosomes, so its absence on one or two is believed to have no effect. While it did not explain the cause of PWS, the frequent involvement of chromosome 15, in such transactions, was a hint.

Chromosomal Deletion in PWS

At the end of the 1970s, a new technique called prometaphase or high-resolution chromosome banding was developed for analyzing chromosomes in more detail. This allowed much greater visibility of fine chromosome structure. Taking the aforementioned "hint" about chromosome 15, Ledbetter, Riccardi, Airhart, et al. (1981), using this new technique, reported the presence of a small deletion within the long arm of chromosome 15 [del 15(q11–q13)] in approximately half the people with PWS whom they studied (Figure 2.2). Since all 46 chromosomes come in pairs, with one member of each pair inherited from each parent, the blood chromosomes of some parents of people with PWS were studied for the presence of this deletion. In the families studied, neither parent was found to have the deletion, indicating that it is a new change in the affected individual (a *de novo* deletion) which occurred at or before the time of conception. Subsequently, researchers studied series of patients to further delineate the exact location and frequency of the deletions, which, depending on the criteria used for diagnosis of the syndrome, were found in 50–100% of tested patients. Recent summaries of these studies suggested that approximately 60–70% of clinically typical patients have the deletion (reviewed in Butler, 1990; Ledbetter & Cassidy, 1988). The remainder (except for a few with Robertsonian translocations) appeared to be chromosomally normal. Several of these studies also sought to identify clinical differences between patients with and without the deletion. Those studies using careful criteria for diagnosis showed that the only difference was in the proportion of patients with hypopigmentation (fair coloring for the family), which was more frequent in the patients with deletions than in those without (Butler, 1990). The significance of this finding was not understood until several years later.

Although parental chromosomes look normal when a deletion is found in a child with PWS, Butler and Palmer (1983) used minor normal variations in chromosome structure (chromosomal polymorphisms) to identify the fact that the deletion occurs in the chromosome 15 inherited from the father. This finding has subsequently been confirmed in other

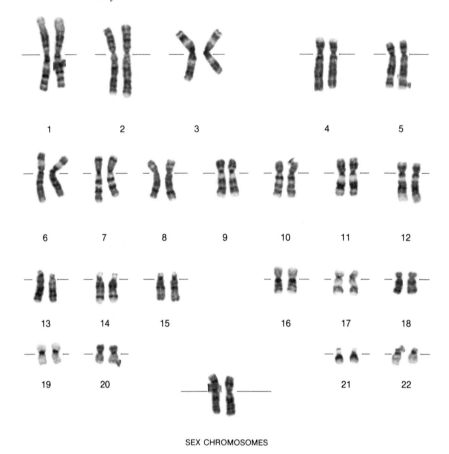

FIGURE 2.1. (A) Normal routine karyotype. (B) Robertsonian translocation involving chromosome 15 in a patient with PWS. (Photo courtesy of Stuart Schwartz, Ph.D., Case Western Reserve University.)

reports (reviewed in Butler, 1990) and most recently through use of molecular genetic technology (Nicholls, 1993). This became particularly intriguing when it was recognized that a proportion of patients with a clinically very distinct disorder, Angelman syndrome, had the same or a very similar chromosomal deletion, and that with Angelman syndrome the deletion occurs in the chromosome 15 inherited from the mother (Donlon, 1988; Knoll, Nicholls, Magenis, et al., 1989). In both disorders, the parent from whom the deleted chromosome 15 was inherited has normal chromosome 15s in their blood, and it is presumed that the deletion occurred as a new mutation in the one sperm (in PWS) or the one egg (in Angelman syndrome) that resulted in the affected child.

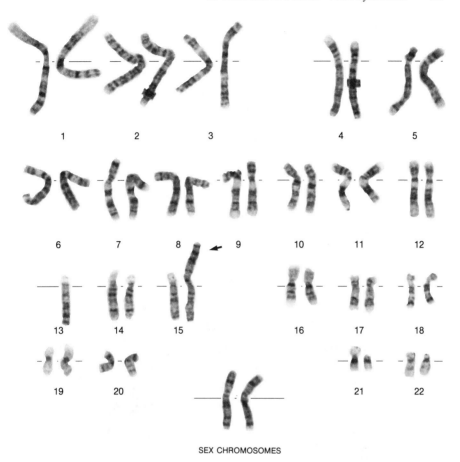

SEX CHROMOSOMES

FIGURE 2.1. (B)

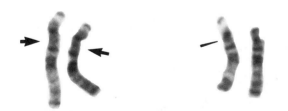

FIGURE 2.2. Pairs of 15s illustrating deletion. The arrows show band 15q11–q13, which is not present in the right-hand member of the right-hand pair. The left-hand pair is normal. (Photo courtesy of Stuart Schwartz, Ph.D., Case Western Reserve University.)

Angelman Syndrome

Angelman syndrome is a relatively newly recognized condition (Angelman, 1965). It is marked by severe mental retardation with absence of speech, unsteady jerky gait, hyperactivity, seizure disorder with characteristic EEG changes (high amplitude spike and slow waves), and frequent paroxysms of laughter. There are also characteristic dysmorphic features (Figure 2.3), including a small head with flattened back, flat cheekbones, large mouth with widely spaced teeth and frequent tongue protrusion, and prominent chin; hypopigmentation is common. This condition is easily distinguished clinically from PWS, even though the children are somewhat hypotonic as infants (Clayton-Smith & Pembrey, 1992). Approximately 50–60% of patients with Angelman syndrome have a deletion of chromosome 15 long arm in the same place as most people with PWS have their deletion (Knoll et al., 1989) based on high-resolution analysis.

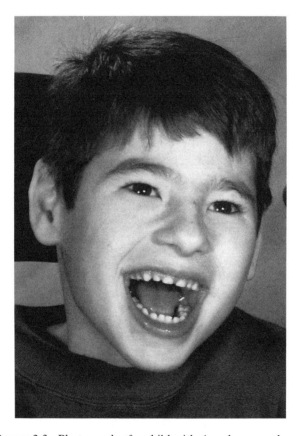

FIGURE 2.3. Photograph of a child with Angelman syndrome.

Uniparental Disomy

Recognition of the reason why some people with PWS have normal chromosomes while others have a deletion came in 1989, when Nicholls and colleagues used molecular genetic markers to study the 15q11–13 region. This technology allows detection of small differences in DNA structure not visible with chromosomal analysis. Whereas chromosomal techniques rely upon subjective interpretation of the structure of chromosomes, molecular techniques are objective chemical reactions. As expected, it was determined that some people who do not have a deletion visible with chromosomal techniques do have a deletion using molecular techniques. However, this represented only a small proportion of cases without a visible deletion. More interestingly, it was also determined that the remaining patients without a deletion had two maternally derived chromosome 15q regions and no paternally derived chromosome 15q (Nicholls, Knoll, Butler, et al., 1989). This situation is called uniparental disomy, and although unprecedented before it was found in PWS, it was theorized by Engel in 1980 to explain some unexplained genetic phenomena. Thus, instead of inheriting one paternal and one maternal chromosome 15, people with PWS who do not have a deletion lack the same paternal genetic material because they did not inherit a paternal chromosome 15 at all. Instead they received two maternal ones. The chromosomes themselves are normal in number and structure, but the inheritance pattern is wrong. Sometimes, due to maternal disomy, the child with PWS has two of the same member of the maternal chromosome 15 pair (isodisomy), sometimes both members of the maternal chromosome 15 pair (heterodisomy), and sometimes a combination of both. But this does not affect the end result since all the chromosome 15s are normal. *In effect, whether there is a paternal deletion or maternal uniparental disomy, the paternal contribution to a specific important region of chromosome 15 long arm associated with PWS is missing.*

Although the cause of uniparental disomy is not yet known, it has been shown that this type of chromosome maldistribution is similar in origin to that causing Down syndrome, which results from the presence of three copies of chromosome 21 (called trisomy 21), instead of the normal two. This process is called nondisjunction, because the two members of one parent's chromosome pair fail to separate, or disjoin, when the egg or sperm (which normally each contain only one member of each pair) is formed. This process was documented in a few cases of PWS (Cassidy, Lai, Erickson, et al., 1992) in which very early fetal trisomy 15 (the presence of three 15s) was detected by a prenatal diagnosis technique called chorionic villus sampling, which consists of taking a sample of the early developing fetal placenta at around 10 weeks of pregnancy. In these cases, when the fetal chromosomes were again checked at 16–18 weeks of pregnancy by amniocentesis, the number of chromosomes was normal and there were only two copies of chromosome 15. Thus, one member of the trisomy 15 was lost. At birth, the baby was hypotonic and had feeding problems, and maternal uniparental disomy for chromosome 15 was found, confirming PWS. Other information suggests that this is the most common cause of maternal disomy in PWS. As in Down syndrome, parents who have a child with PWS on the basis of maternal disomy tend to be older, on average, than mothers in the general population, or than mothers of children with PWS due to paternal 15 deletion (Clayton-Smith & Pembrey, 1992). There may also be other as yet undocumented mechanisms by which uniparental disomy can occur.

An occasional case of nondeletion Angelman syndrome also has uniparental disomy, but in these cases it is paternal disomy. Thus, Angelman syndrome results from absence of the *maternal* contribution to the long arm of chromosome 15, whether by deletion or disomy, the opposite situation from that seen in PWS. However, in about 30–40% of people with Angelman syndrome, neither deletion nor disomy can be documented, and such patients have one chromosome 15 from each parent. These cases are probably due to a change in a single gene. Such a situation has not been found in PWS as yet. For further discussion of the genetics of Angelman syndrome, see Nicholls (1993).

A diagrammatic summary of the genetic aspects of PWS and Angelman syndrome is shown in Figure 2.4. It illustrates the genetic composition of individuals with these two disorders, as described above.

Testing for Genetic Composition in PWS and Angelman Syndrome

Since there is more than one genetic alteration causing both PWS and Angelman syndrome, testing to confirm a diagnosis is not simple. Few laboratories today are able to perform all the tests needed to identify both deletion and uniparental disomy for either disorder.

Deletion testing by high-resolution cytogenetic analysis can be done in many chromosome analysis labs, but is not always accurate. Since it depends on visual inspection, sometimes a deletion is missed, and, even more upsetting, sometimes an apparent deletion is found when neither PWS nor Angelman syndrome is present clinically. These deletions are usually not found when more sophisticated testing based on DNA analysis is done.

A new technique has been developed in the last few years that detects the chromosome 15 deletion in a simple and accurate way. The technique is called fluorescence *in situ* hybridization, abbreviated FISH. A DNA probe, or segment of DNA that can combine with the genetic material normally present in 15, is tagged with fluorescence and allowed to mix with a blood chromosome preparation. If the normal genetic constitution in 15 is present, there will be a fluorescent spot on both chromosome 15s.

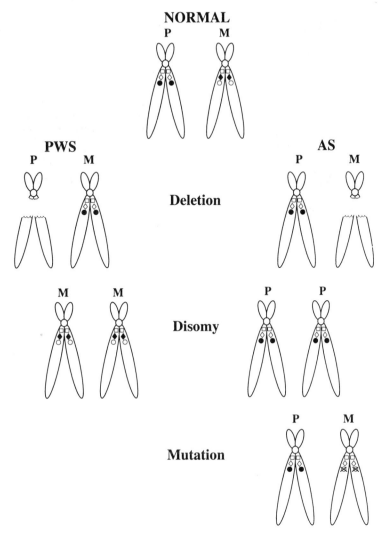

FIGURE 2.4. The genetics of PWS and Angelman syndrome. Square, albinism gene; diamond, Prader–Willi syndrome genes; circle, Angelman syndrome genes. Blackened symbols indicate inactivation of genes (see page 27).

If one chromosome has a deletion, only one of the chromosome 15s will have such a spot, because the DNA in the relevant segment of the other chromosome is missing (Figure 2.5). This is an easy and accurate test for the deletion associated with either syndrome.

Disomy testing currently requires more sophisticated and complex molecular genetic analysis. A deletion is first ruled out by the usual tests, then samples from both parents and the patient are obtained in order to

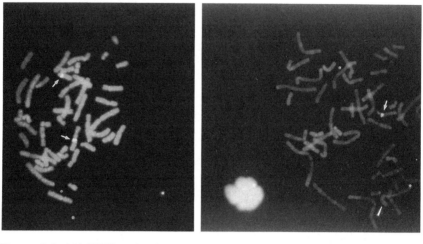

FIGURE 2.5. (A) FISH probes in a normal cell with two fluorescent spots showing the presence of band 15q11–q13. (B) FISH probes in a cell of a patient with PWS due to deletion 15q; one chromosome 15 lacks a fluorescent spot and is deleted. (Photo courtesy of Stuart Schwartz, Ph.D., Case Western Reserve University.)

compare a number of DNA markers all along chromosome 15. If the child has inherited chromosome 15 DNA markers from both parents, then uniparental disomy is not present. If the child has only chromosome 15 DNA markers found in the mother, then maternal uniparental disomy is present, and confirms the presence of PWS. Conversely, if only the father's DNA markers for chromosome 15 are present, then the child has paternal uniparental disomy, confirming Angelman syndrome. This type of testing is available in only a few places around the country, and sometimes FISH studies are not available in the same location. It is anticipated that advances in technology will allow both types of testing to be available in several laboratories in the near future.

Genetic Imprinting

The genetic findings in PWS and Angelman syndrome can best be explained by a phenomenon called genetic (or genomic) imprinting. This is a process whereby genes or groups of neighboring genes are modified differently, and therefore expressed differently, depending upon the sex of the parent from whom they were inherited. This imprinting does not alter the gene itself and it is a reversible process. Rather, some genes are normally inactivated and prevented from being expressed even though the DNA structure itself is not changed.

Genetic imprinting had been recognized for several years in other animals and in plants, but PWS and Angelman syndromes were the first of several human disorders in which it has been identified. Normally the maternally derived copies of chromosome 15 in the region critical for PWS are inactivated, and only the paternally derived 15 region is expressed in cells (Figure 2.4). When the paternal copy of this region is missing by deletion or by complete absence of chromosome 15 as in maternal disomy, there is no active copy and, therefore, abnormality in development results in PWS. The converse is true in 60–70% of cases of Angelman syndrome, which result from the absence or imprinting of the needed maternal active genes. It is believed that imprinted genes may be "shut off" by a reversible chemical reaction, such as attachment of a methyl group. Studies are ongoing to help delineate mechanisms of imprinting and explain how the same genetic information, when modified differently, has as different an outcome as it does in PWS and Angelman syndromes.

Genetic Structure of Chromosome Region 15q11–13

Since the advent of molecular genetic techniques in the mid-1980s, considerable progress has been made in dissecting out the structure of the genetic information in the region of chromosome 15 critical for producing (or preventing) PWS and Angelman syndromes. But there is still a long way to go before the exact genes whose effect is missing or abnormal in these conditions are identified. It has been known since the first description of the deletion that the important area of chromosome 15 is between bands labeled q11 and q13. Recent molecular studies demonstrate that about 95% of deletions seen in PWS or Angelman syndrome have the same breakpoints. It has been determined that the loci (genetic locations) of the gene or genes for PWS and Angelman syndrome are different, but are very close together, and that the usual deletion for either disorder encompasses a larger genetic segment than both loci (Figure 2.6). It has also been learned that a gene for a form of albinism, or genetic hypopigmentation, is present between the usual deletion breakpoints on 15 but is not part of either the PWS or Angelman syndrome critical regions and is not imprinted. This explains why some people with PWS and some with Angelman syndrome with deletion have hypopigmentation. Thus, even though Angelman syndrome and PWS are caused by the same chromosomal deletion, it may be merely a matter of proximity and perhaps not a genetic relationship.

Molecular studies also suggest that three or four different genes are usually deleted or inactive in order to cause PWS, while it may be that only one or two genes need be missing or inactive to cause Angelman syndrome. However, the normal functions of these genes are still not

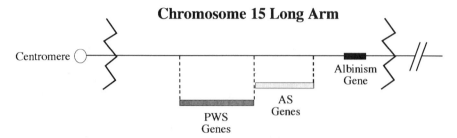

FIGURE 2.6. Simplified diagram of the genetic region of chromosome 15 relevant to PWS and Angelman syndromes. Jagged lines indicate breakpoints.

known. Candidate genes within these two critical regions are being identified and tested for the possibility of having a major impact in causing one disorder or the other. Some candidate genes have been eliminated as having important functions in PWS even though they are within the deleted segment.

Over the next several years, it is anticipated that much will be learned about precisely what causes the alterations that result in PWS. Certainly, dramatic progress has occurred in the past and considerable, active, ongoing research is likely to produce additional advances. Such knowledge would allow for the possibility of specific treatment(s), further understanding of the causes of individual problems seen within the complex pattern called PWS, and, in the more distant future, perhaps lead to prevention of the condition.

Recurrence Risks

Although there is a theoretical possibility of recurrence of PWS within a family, no reports of recurrence among siblings has been reported in which the affected individual had either a chromosomal deletion or maternal uniparental disomy of 15. The report of an occasional family in which more than one child was affected with PWS suggests that there may be a recurrence risk that is more than negligible. However, there have been only a few such families reported and none of those tested has had either a deletion or uniparental disomy. In these families there is a possibility that an abnormality in the process of genetic imprinting may be caused by a single gene defect. Hopefully, further study of these few families will identify ways that people might be tested to see if they may be at risk for recurrence. Within those families who have PWS without deletion or disomy, while there is the potential for a higher incidence of recurrence, there is still too little information available to speculate on the degree of risk at the present time.

At this point it is safe to say that parents who have a child with PWS on the basis of a chromosome 15 deletion or maternal disomy have a less than 1% chance of having another affected child. When a chromosomal translocation is present, the theoretical risk may be a bit higher, but only if the translocation is also present in one of the parents. Even in this situation, the risk is theoretical, since no such recurrence has been documented. Prenatal testing for chromosome 15 deletion by FISH or uniparental disomy of chromosome 15 is possible by amniocentesis or chorionic villus sampling for the purpose of reassurance.

If individuals with PWS on the basis of 15q deletion were fertile, it would be possible for them to pass on the deletion. If the affected individual were a male, there would be the theoretical 50% risk that his offspring would have PWS. If the affected individual were a female, there would be a similar risk that the child would have Angelman syndrome. However, to date there have been no reported cases of children born to individuals with PWS, and infertility is the rule.

Genetic Counseling

Medical geneticists are physicians trained to provide expert diagnosis of genetic disorders such as PWS. Such professionals can be found at virtually all medical schools and major medical centers. In addition, clinical services for families of individuals with PWS should involve genetic associates or genetic counselors who have a masters degree in genetics and can be certified by the American Board of Medical Genetics. Through a counseling process, these professionals can provide families with supportive information about the diagnosis, natural history, and potential outcomes associated with this defect. This process includes describing the characteristics of the syndrome, the associated findings, the genetic basis (with careful explanation), the recurrence risk, and current methods for prenatal detection (including the risks and benefits of all testing procedures). The goal of genetic counseling is to assist families to understand, anticipate, and cope with this complex disorder.

Managing PWS is challenging and assistance is needed to determine the best approaches. Grasping the unusual genetic features of PWS often requires basic instruction in human genetics and should include those aspects that distinguish PWS but that are not often taught in schools. It is part of the genetic counseling process with families of children with PWS to stress that chromosome alterations are common and that there is nothing that either parent did or did not do prior to or during the pregnancy that caused the chromosomal alteration seen in PWS. In other words, it is no one's fault and no one could have predicted it. It is an accident of the complex process of getting genetic information from the parents to the child. Even though the likelihood of recurrence within the family is small, decisions about having other children and about the possibility of prenatal diagnosis for reassurance should be addressed. Frequently, the anxiety associated with news of the diagnosis precludes family members from hearing and/or absorbing the facts provided by the geneticist. The genetic counselor often will be requested to reiterate information initially provided by the medical geneticist, clarify that there is no way to predict the occurrence of this genetic error, discourage inaccurate interpretation, and allay fears.

Genetic counseling is nondirective; family members are not told what to do, since all families have different moral, ethical, religious, and experiential backgrounds. The families, not the counselors, must live with their decisions and need support whatever their choices. Information is provided about family support organizations and appropriate management. If difficulty is encountered in finding the appropriate genetics assistance in a specific area, the central offices of the genetics organizations can be reached at (301) 571-1825.

Summary

The genetics of PWS are unique, and in recent years knowledge about causes and testing has greatly increased. Approximately 70% of people who are clinically typical have a deletion within the proximal long arm of the paternally-derived member of the chromosome 15 pair [del 15(q11–q13)]. The remainder have maternal uniparental disomy for chromosome 15 also resulting in the absence of the paternal contribution to this region. Genetic imprinting explains the fact that a clinically distinct disorder, Angelman syndrome, results from a maternal deletion or paternal uniparental disomy in the same region. PWS is probably due to the absence or lack of expression of three or four genes within this critical region. Progress is rapidly being made toward identifying the specific effects of these genes, with a view to compensating for their effects.

References

Angelman, H. (1965). "Puppet" children: A report on three cases. *Developmental Medicine and Child Neurology*, 7, 681–683.

Butler, M.G. (1990). Prader-Willi syndrome: Current understanding of cause and diagnosis. *American Journal of Genetics*, 35, 319–332.

Butler, M.G., & Palmar, C.G. (1983). Parental origin of chromosome 15 deletion in Prader-Willi syndrome. *Lancet*, 1, 285–286.

Cassidy, S.B., Lai, L.W., Erickson, R.P., Magnuson, I., Thomas, E., Gendron, R., & Herrmann, J. (1992). Trisomy 15 with loss of the paternal 15 as a cause of Prader-Willi syndrome due to maternal disomy. *American Journal of Human Genetics*, 51, 701–708.

Clayton-Smith, J., & Pembrey, M.E. (1992). Angelman syndrome. *Journal of Medical Genetics*, *29*, 412–415.

Donlon, T.A. (1988). Similar molecular deletions on chromosome 15q11.2 are encountered in both the Prader-Willi and Angelman syndromes. *Human Genetics*, *80*, 322–338.

Engel, E. (1980). A new genetic concept: Uniparental disomy and its potential effect, isodisomy. *American Journal of Medical Genetics*, *6*, 137–143.

Hawkey, C.J., & Smithies, A. (1976). The Prader-Willi syndrome with a 15/15 translocation: Case report and review of the literature. *Journal of Medical Genetics*, *13*, 152–157.

Knoll, J.H., Nicholls, R.D., Magenis, E., & Graham, J., Jr. (1989). Angelman and Prader-Willi syndrome share a common chromosome 15 deletion but differ in parental origin of the deletion. *American Journal of Medical Genetics*, *32*, 285–290.

Ledbetter, D.H., & Cassidy, S.B. (1988). Etiology of Prader-Willi syndrome. In M.L. Caldwell & R.L. Taylor (Eds.), *Prader-Willi syndrome: Selected research and management issues* (pp. 13–28). New York: Springer-Verlag.

Ledbetter, D.H., Riccardi, V.M., Airhart, S.D., Strobel, R.J., Keenen, S.B., & Crawford, J.D. (1981). Deletion of chromosome 15 as a cause of the Prader-Willi syndrome. *New England Journal of Medicine*, *304*, 325–329.

Nicholls, R.D. (1993). Genomic imprinting and uniparental disomy in Angelman and Prader-Willi syndrome: A review. *American Journal of Medical Genetics*, *46*, 16–25.

Nicholls, R.D., Knoll, J.H.M., Butler, M.G., Karam, S., & Lalande M. (1989). Genetic imprinting suggested by maternal heterodisomy in nondeletion Prader-Willi syndrome. *Nature* (*London*), *342*, 281–285.

Prader, A., Labhart, A., Willi, H. (1956). Ein Syndrom von Adipositas, Kleinwuchs, Kryptorchismus und Oligophrenie nach Myotonicartigem Zustand in Neugeborenalter. *Schweizerische Medizinische Wochenschrift*, *86*, 1260–1261.

3
Endocrine and Metabolic Aspects of Prader–Willi Syndrome

Phillip D.K. Lee

Several of the typical features of Prader–Willi syndrome (PWS) are consistent with an underlying endocrine or metabolic abnormality. Among these are short stature, central obesity, decreased lean mass, cryptorchidism, and hypogonadism. Although hypogonadotropic hypogonadism is a well-characterized and nearly universal feature of PWS, it is unlikely to account for all of these phenotypic features. Recent data indicate that abnormalities of the growth hormone (GH) and insulin-like growth factor (IGF) systems may also occur in PWS and could account for some of the phenotypic characteristics. The detailed study of endocrine, metabolic, and body composition pathophysiology in PWS is a rapidly developing field, aided by improvements in both diagnostic criteria for PWS and technical methodology. Such studies hold promise for new therapeutic modalities in PWS.

Cryptorchidism, Hypogonadotropic Hypogonadism, and Sexual Development

Pathophysiology

Cryptorchidism is a common finding in male infants with PWS, and has been reported in >90% of phenotypically diagnosed cases (Aughton & Cassidy, 1990; Bray, Dahms, Swerdloff, et al., 1983; Dunn, 1968). Such data may be somewhat biased since cryptorchidism is considered by some authors to be a phenotypic criterion for diagnosis of PWS in males. However, recent data confirm the high frequency of cryptorchidism in chromosomally diagnosed cases of PWS (Hamabe, Fukushima, Harada, et al., 1991; Robinson, Bottani, Xie, et al., 1991).

In PWS-associated cryptorchidism, both testicles are typically present (although one or both may be rudimentary or degenerated) and may be located at the inguinal ring or in the abdominal cavity. In such cases, the scrotum is often bifid or otherwise hypoplastic (Cassidy, 1983; Laurence, 1967). The penis is usually normally formed and may be normal or small in size (Aughton & Cassidy, 1990; Bray et al., 1983; Cassidy, Rubin, & Mukaida, 1987; Greenberg, Elder, & Ledbetter, 1987; Stephenson, 1980). Male accessory ducts and Wolffian structures, including the prostate, are present.

Fetal testicular descent and penile enlargement normally occur after 30 weeks gestation (Hutson & Donahoe, 1986). Therefore, the spectrum of male genital abnormalities found in PWS suggests a late-gestation deficiency in fetal testosterone secretion; a defect in earlier gestation would result in more extensive urogenital malformation. During late gestation, the fetal testicles are stimulated primarily by fetal pituitary, rather than placental, gonadotropins. Therefore, cryptorchidism in PWS is probably reflective of *in utero* deficiencies in the secretion of fetal pituitary gonadotropins: luteinizing hormone (LH) and follicle-stimulating hormone (FSH). The presence of male accessory structures and, more particularly, the absence of female internal structures, indicate that secretion of Müllerian-inhibitory factor (MIF) is probably intact.

No specific abnormalities of female fetal sexual development have been reported in PWS, although detailed studies of late gestational events, such as clitoral and uterine enlargement and labial maturation, have not been reported (Cassidy, 1983). However, no major abnormalities are expected since the development of female genital structures is considered to be less hormone dependent than male genital structures in the human fetus.

In normal human infants, a postnatal gonadotropin surge at 30–60 days leads to a transient increase in gonadal steroid production. Although data are limited, this apparently does not occur in infants with PWS. Furthermore, testicular response to exogenously administered gonadotropin is usually minimal. It should be kept in mind that these data are somewhat biased, since most infants receiving either physiologic or pharmacologic gonadal response testing will have a concomitant cryptorchidism or other external genital defect; usual response patterns in female and noncryptorchid male infants with PWS have not been studied.

After the neonatal period and before puberty, the human pituitary–gonadal axis is normally in a state of hypogonadotropic hypogonadism. However, low levels of both ovarian and testicular hormone secretion in response to intermittent gonadotropin pulses may occur in normal prepubertal children, and could have effects on skeletal growth and body composition. Studies of this phenomenon have been limited primarily by inadequate hormonal assay sensitivity. In children with PWS and hypogonadotropic hypogonadism, neither the gonadotropic nor gonadal steroid pulses would be expected, although low constitutive gonadal hormone secretion could occur.

In both boys and girls with PWS, pubertal changes associated with adrenal androgen secretion, or adrenarche, usually progress normally. These changes include the development of secondary sexual hair (e.g., axillary, pubic, and adult body hair), acne, and a variable degree of phallic (penile or clitoral) enlargement. Although the normal physiologic regulation of adrenarche has not been completely defined, adrenal androgen secretion is stimulated by adrenocorticotropic hormone (ACTH) as well as other factors, such as insulin, insulin-like growth factor I (IGF-I), and, possibly, a pituitary factor termed adrenal-stimulating hormone (ASH) (Miller, 1988).

In children with PWS-associated obesity and in children with non-PWS exogenous obesity, adrenarche may occur early, i.e., onset before age 8 years, in the absence of an identifiable intrinsic abnormality in adrenal androgen secretion (Garty, Shuper, Mimouni, et al., 1982). This condition, termed premature or precocious adrenarche, could be due to increased adrenal exposure to insulin or IGF-I. Children with benign premature adrenarche are typically taller than expected for their age and genetic potential, and have accelerated skeletal maturation. In children with premature adrenarche associated with non-PWS exogenous obesity, adult final height is usually not compromised. Similar data for children with PWS have not been published, although our experience suggests that final height is low for midparental height, as is typical for all children with PWS.

In boys with PWS, regardless or whether cryptorchidism is present or absent, normal puberty shows minimal, if any, natural progression past adrenarche, although isolated cases of normal male puberty have been reported (Vanelli, 1984). Both serum gonadotropin and serum testosterone levels may increase into the normal early-pubertal range; however, further gonadal axis maturation usually does not occur. Boys with PWS rarely progress past Tanner genital stage 2–3 and, in our experience, palpable testes are virtually always <5 mL in volume.

A similar condition of hypogonadotropic hypogonadism in girls with PWS most commonly leads to primary amenorrhea. Although delayed, normal and even precocious menses have been reported in girls with PWS (Bray et al., 1983; Cassidy, 1983; Kauli, Prager-Lewin, & Laron, 1978; Walterspiel, Wolff, & Heinze, 1981), some of these cases may be either factitious (Bray et al., 1983) or associated with an apparent variant syndrome (MacMillan, Kim, & Weisskopf, 1972). In the author's experience, vaginal spotting or bleeding has been observed only in cases of self-inflicted vaginal canal abrasions: It is conceivable that uterine endometrial estrogenization by estrogens formed by peripheral conversion of adrenal androgens could occur and cause bleeding; however, neither normal cyclic pituitary gonadotropin nor normal ovarian estrogen secretion has been convincingly demonstrated in girls with PWS.

Significant breast development, even to full maturation, can occur in girls with PWS. This is presumably due to estrogens derived from adrenal androgen conversion in peripheral tissues and, possibly, low levels of ovarian estrogen secretion. Gynecomastia may occur in boys with PWS-associated obesity, as it does in boys with exogenous obesity. However, this rarely causes significant true mammary gland maturation.

Neither male nor female fertility has been definitively reported in PWS. Most adults with PWS are not married and, presumably, have limited sexual contacts. In addition, spermatogenesis and ovulation are unlikely to be normal in PWS. Testicular biopsy usually shows Sertoli cell-only histology (Bray et al., 1983; Katcher, Bargman, Gilbert, et al., 1977; Wannarachue, Ruvalcaba, & Kelley, 1975) and a single female autopsy case revealed a lack of normal ovarian follicles (Bray et al., 1983).

The etiology for the hypogonadotropic hypogonadism in PWS is not known. Several lines of evidence suggest that, unlike in Kallman syndrome, the defect is not at the pituitary level: (1) the occasional case of normal or precocious puberty (see above), (2) the observation that gonadotropin secretion can be stimulated by clomiphene treatment (Bray et al., 1983; Hamilton, Scully, & Kliman, 1972; Jeffcoate, Laurence, Edwards, et al., 1980; Linde, McNeil, & Rabin, 1982; McGuffin & Rogol, 1975), (3) reports of increased gonadotropin secretion in PWS patients with primary hypogonadism (Seyler, Arunlanantham, & O'Connor, 1979; Wu, Hasen, & Warburton, 1981), and (4) a report of dexamethasone-suppressible hypergonadotropinemia (Shimizu, Negishi, Takahashi, et al., 1990). Furthermore, although a few patients may develop primary hypogonadism (e.g., secondary to cryptorchidism), stimulation of gonadal function by clomiphene or intranasal gonadotropin administration has been reported (Bray et al., 1983; Hamilton, Scully, & Kliman, 1972; Haschke & Hohenauer, 1978; Linde, McNeil, & Rabin, 1982), indicating that a primary gonadal defect may not be intrinsic to the syndrome. It appears, therefore, that the hypogonadotropic hypogonadism in PWS is due to hypothalamic, higher central nervous system, or, possibly, peripheral factors. The defect does not involve a universal disturbance in biological rhythms, since cyclic melatonin secretion is normal (Tamarkin, Abastillas, Chen, et al., 1982; Willig, Braun, Commentz, et al., 1986). A report of a urinary gonadotropin-inhibitory substance in a patient with PWS may be relevant (Harris & Knigge, 1982); however, more detailed information has not been presented.

Diagnostic Procedures

Any male infant with hypotonia and cryptorchidism should be suspected of having PWS. The diagnosis should then be confirmed by specific chromosomal analysis (see Chapter 2). If the chromosomal diagnosis is confirmed, additional testing to confirm hypogonadotropic hypogonadism is probably unnecessary in most cases. However, testing of the gonadal axis may be essential in identifying functional testicular tissue prior to medical or surgical intervention.

Single measurements of serum testosterone in the neonatal period or during the expected secondary gonadotropin surge at 30–60 days of age may, if positive, confirm the presence of functional testicular tissue. In most laboratories, a level of >20–50 ng/dL is indicative of probable testicular testosterone production. Because gonadotropin priming may be necessary for normal testicular hormone secretion and PWS is associated with deficient gonadotropin secretion, normal infantile levels of testosterone are not expected in PWS. Indeed, the measurement of negligible testosterone levels does not preclude the existence of functional testicular tissue.

More extensive testicular evaluation may be indicated prior to surgical intervention. Since orchiopexy is usually not performed in the immediate neonatal period, such testing should be delayed until appropriate. A standard "short" testosterone stimulation test involves daily intramuscular injections of chorionic gonadotropin ($1500 \, U/m^2$/dose) for 3–5 days, with serum testosterone levels measured at baseline and 24 hr after the last injection. However, since gonadotropin priming may be necessary to achieve testicular secretion, a "long" test may be preferable. A typical regimen is chorionic gonadotropin 500–1000 U by intramuscular injection twice a week (e.g., Monday/Thursday) for 5 weeks (10 doses total) with baseline and 24 hr postfinal dose serum testosterone measurements. The baseline level is theoretically not necessary, although it may provide an indication of testicular responsiveness. A post-test testosterone level of >100–200 ng/dL is clearly indicative of testicular activity; levels between 20 and 100 ng/dL are considered equivocal, although there is presumably some amount of functional tissue present. "Long" testing also has the theoretical advantage of causing more prolonged testosterone production, a small "cosmetic" amount of genital growth, testicular enlargement, and possible spontaneous testicular descent. However, these latter effects are rarely, if ever, observed in PWS. Intranasal and subcutaneous gonadotropin administration have also been used for diagnosis and treatment of cryptorchidism; however, reports specific to PWS are limited (Haschke & Hohenauer, 1978; Jaskulsky & Stone, 1987).

Testicular ultrasound or magnetic resonance imaging may also be useful in locating testicular tissue, particularly when the testis are truly nonpalpable. A visualization procedure coupled with chorionic gonadotropin testing is often performed prior to orchidectomy. Brain imaging studies are not particularly useful, since no structural abnormalities of the central nervous system have been identified in PWS (Cacciari, Zucchini, Carla, et al., 1990; Swaab, Hofman, Lucassen, et al., 1993).

Children with PWS-associated obesity often have signs of premature adrenarche, e.g., pubic or axillary hair before 8 years of age (Garty et al., 1982). The overwhelming likelihood is that the adrenarche is related to obesity. The most common organic etiology of premature adrenarche, congenital adrenal hyperplasia, has a population prevalence that is several-fold higher than PWS. However, the joint occurrence of these 2 conditions has an expected prevalence on the order of $<10^{-6}$, and no actual cases have been reported. Likewise, there appears to be no increased occurrence of virilizing adrenal tumors or other rare hyper-androgenic conditions in PWS. If screening for these conditions is desired, e.g., if the child is not obese or has an unusual clinical presentation, a single serum measurement of 17α-hydroxyprogesterone (for adrenal hyperplasia) and testosterone (for other lesions) should be sufficient. Dehydroepiandrosterone (DHEA) and DHEA-sulfate levels are usually within the adrenarchal range and have limited diagnostic use. Adrenal imaging is not indicated unless these tests are abnormal.

Adolescents with PWS will invariably have hypogonadotropic hypo-gonadism, and additional testing is usually not required to confirm the diagnosis. For research purposes or in equivocal cases, serum FSH and LH levels can be measured at timed intervals (e.g., every 15 min for 60–90 min) following intravenous administration of gonadotropin-releasing hormone (Zappulla, Salardi, Tassinari, et al., 1981; Zárate, Soria, Canales, et al., 1973/74). As discussed above, clomiphene priming may help to normalize the gonadotropin response. Measurements of basal serum testosterone or estrogen may occasionally be useful in guiding hormone replacement therapy; e.g., stabilization of testosterone levels at a very subphysiologic level may be used as an indication for replacement therapy.

Fertility testing is rarely, if ever, clinically warranted in PWS. Despite the obesity, there does not appear to be an increased occurrence of polycystic ovarian disease in PWS.

Treatment

In the neonatal and prepubertal period, a short course of low-dose testo-sterone may be used to improve the appearance and function of the penis (Guthrie, Smith, & Graham, 1973). This is particularly indicated if the stretched penile length is $<1.5–2.0$ cm, a situation that could lead to difficulty with toilet training and upright urination, as well as complicate peer relationships (Cassidy, 1983). A suggested regimen is depot testo-sterone (cypionate or enanthate) 25.0 mg by intramuscular injection every 3 to 4 weeks for 3–6 months. A longer course or higher dose is not recommended since either of these could lead to inappropriate virilization and acceleration of skeletal maturation. The child should be examined prior to each dose to gauge clinical response and the necessity for additional doses. Particularly in the obese child, the suprapubic fat pad should be compressed when obtaining a penile length measurement. On occasion, a few strands of pubic hair may be observed during the treatment course, but this invariably disappears after treatment.

Uncorrected cryptorchidism carries a potential risk for testicular degeneration and malignancy, and this risk may be increased if the testis is functional and located in the abdomen. On the other hand, orchiopexy (surgical relocation of the testis in the scrotum) has not been definitively proven to decrease the risk for malignant transformation. Furthermore, despite the high frequency of cryptorchidism, testicular malignancy appears to be rare in PWS, with only a single reported case of seminoma (Robinson & Jones, 1988). Nevertheless, correction of cryptorchidism may have medical and psychological benefits in individual cases.

Spontaneous testicular descent may occur in prepubertal or pubertal boys with PWS (Hamilton, Scully, & Kliman, 1972), perhaps due to the effects of adrenal androgens. In other cases, medical intervention with gonadotropin administration (see preceding section) may be successful in achieving testicular descent (Uehling, 1980), and may facilitate localization of the testis during surgery. Orchiopexy may be particularly difficult in PWS due to the hypoplastic accessory structures and scrotum. Surgery often is delayed until 4 years of age. Either before or after surgery, the testicles may become atretic and essentially nonfunctional. In some cases, removal of the testicular tissue with placement of a prosthesis may be considered.

The need for androgen replacement therapy in boys with PWS is somewhat controversial, although male hypogonadism can lead to decreased muscle mass and osteoporosis. The oral synthetic androgen, oxandrolone, has been used in prepubertal and early adolescents to stimulate linear growth (vide infra), however, at usual doses the androgenic effects of oxandrolone are relatively weak and do not lead to complete masculinization. More potent oral analogues or parenteral administration of testosterone itself may be used to achieve virilization, however, adverse behavioral effects, particularly inappropriate sexual and physically aggressive behavior, may occur. Furthermore, any functioning testicular tissue will be suppressed with this treatment. A more physiologic approach might be used in boys with functional testicular tissue, e.g., intermittent or pulsatile gonadotropin administration (Jaskulsky & Stone, 1987; Jeffcoate et al., 1980; Weninger, Frisch, Widhalm, et al., 1983); however, this modality is somewhat cumbersome and few cases would be expected to show a complete response to this treatment.

An individualized approach to testosterone replacement would seem to be most advisable. Boys with PWS who are only moderately retarded, have reasonable social interactions, and have the ability for emotional control may be ideal candidates for treatment, since the physical changes that occur could enhance their chances for semi-independent social adjustment. In such cases, after the age of 14–15 years (the upper limit for onset of normal pubertal maturation), low dose intramuscular depot testosterone (100 mg each month) can be started, with gradual increases as tolerated to a dose of 200 mg once or twice a month. Such treatment should be coupled with ongoing psychological counseling and behavior monitoring.

Although estrogen replacement is probably beneficial in hypoestrogenemic non-PWS women, benefits have not yet been proven in PWS. However, osteoporosis clearly occurs in untreated women with PWS and, theoretically, could be related to estrogen defiency. Various treatment options are available, the most convenient of which include estrogen patches and low-dose estrogen contraceptives. If estrogen replacement therapy is started, this should be balanced with a progestin to minimize cancer risk and, for practical reasons, an effort should be made to choose a modality that will minimize the amount of menstrual bleeding and spotting. Contraception per se is probably not necessary for most women with PWS; however, the risk for sexually transmitted disease is present and all adolescent and adult women (and men) with PWS should receive appropriate counseling.

There is no specific treatment for premature adrenarche; this condition rarely causes significant clinical or psychological problems. Although obesity is thought to be pathogenetic for this condition, there is no evidence that intensive weight control slows the progress of adrenarche once it has started.

Growth, Growth Hormone, and the Insulin-like Growth Factors

Pathophysiology

Several studies have clearly demonstrated that PWS is associated with decreased childhood linear growth velocity and compromised final adult height (Bray et al., 1983; Butler & Meaney, 1991a,b; Dunn, 1968; Fesseler & Bierich, 1983; Holm & Nugent, 1982; Hooft, Delire, & Casneuf, 1966; Laurence, 1967; Nozaki & Katoh, 1981; Zellweger & Schneider, 1968). Although children with PWS may develop premature adrenarche and increased linear growth for age (Harty, Hollowell, & Sieg, 1993; vide supra), even in these cases, final adult height appears to be compromised, especially if a correction is made for midparental height (Prader, 1981). Thus, PWS is one of only a very few conditions in which obesity is associated with short stature, and is clearly distinguished from exogenous obesity, in which childhood linear growth rate is accelerated and final height is normal or increased (Epstein, Wing, & Valoski, 1985; Epstein, McCurley, Valoski, et al., 1990).

No intrinsic bone or cartilage abnormality has been identified in PWS, and there is no evidence for any specific defect in calcium, phosphorous, or vitamin D metabolism that accounts for the abnormal linear skeletal growth. Although hypogonadism has been postulated to contribute to the abnormal growth pattern, other conditions associated with hypogonadism, such as congenital bilateral anorchia, idiopathic hypogonadotropic hypogonadism, and Klinefelter's syndrome, are not associated with short stature. In some respects, the linear growth abnormality in PWS most closely resembles that in Turner syndrome (gonadal dysgenesis), in which anabolic steroid treatment has also been shown to have limited efficacy (Nilsson, 1989).

The growth pattern in PWS suggests an abnormality in growth hormone (GH) secretion or action. Furthermore, the body composition changes in PWS, including increased adipose and decreased non-bone lean (i.e., muscle) mass, are similar to GH deficiency (Lee, Hwu, Henson, et al., 1993), and are unlike exogenous obesity, in which non-bone lean mass is increased.

Studies of GH secretion using standard provocative stimulation testing have shown a delayed and abnormally low response in PWS (Angulo, Castro-Magana, & Uy, 1991; Bray et al., 1983; Costeff, Holm, Ruvalcaba, et al., 1990; Fesseler & Bierich, 1983; Hwu, Klish, Henson, et al., 1992; Nozaki & Katoh, 1981; Parra, Cervantes, & Schultz, 1973; Theodoridis, Brown, Chance, et al., 1971b). However, this result was postulated to be due to obesity since in exogenous obesity GH response to provocative testing is also blunted (Cacciari, Cicognani, Pirazzoli, et al., 1975; Hasen & Wu, 1982; Lu, Cowell, Jimenez, et al., 1991; Van Vliet, Bosson, Rummens, et al., 1986) and GH secretion has been shown to have an independent negative correlation with estimates of adipose tissue (Iranmesh, Lizarralde, & Veldhuis, 1991). In exogenous obesity, the blunted GH response may be due to feedback suppression of GH release, perhaps mediated by insulin through increased secretion of somatostatin (Iranmesh, Lizarralde, & Veldhuis, et al., 1991; Van Vliet et al., 1986).

The growth stimulating and other metabolic effects of GH are mediated by the insulin-like growth factors, IGF-I and IGF-II, growth factors that are secreted by the liver and other tissues and stimulate the growth of cells (Lee & Rosenfeld, 1988). GH is thought to have minimal, if any, direct growth-stimulating effects; its primary effect is to stimulate IGF production. In true GH deficiency, GH secretion is negligible and IGF levels are very low, leading to decreased linear growth. On the other hand, in exogenous obesity, GH levels are low but IGF levels are normal or high, probably due to stimulation of IGF production by insulin or other factors. IGF-I and II are carried in the bloodstream by several specific binding proteins, especially IGFBP-3. Therefore, measurement of either serum IGF levels or serum IGFBP-3 levels provides an indirect measure of GH secretion and a direct measure of the GH–IGF axis.

It has been reported that IGF-I (somatomedin-C) levels were low in 2 children with PWS, both of whom showed a positive growth response and increased IGF-I levels with GH treatment (Lee, Wilson, Rountree, et al., 1987a; Lee, Wilson, Hintz, et al., 1987a). Low IGF-I levels were also reported by Costeff et al. (1990) in 5 of 6 children with PWS. Recent studies in 12 children with chromosomally confirmed PWS also demonstrated low GH, IGF-I, and IGFBP-3 levels (Hwu et al., 1992; Lee, Hwu, Brown, et al., 1992b). In this cross-sectional study, IGF-I and IGFBP-3 were observed to decline relative to age- and sex-related norms (both IGF-I and IGFBP-3 normally increase during childhood and puberty), such that the levels were invariably below the normal range after 5 years of age. Thus, unlike non-PWS exogenous obesity, levels of IGF, the active component in the GH-IGF system, are abnormally low in PWS.

The suggestion that GH/IGF deficiency is a feature of PWS is further suggested by body composition studies. In exogenous obesity, both fat and non-bone lean (e.g., muscle) mass are increased. Conversely, in true GH deficiency, there is a relative or absolute increase in fat mass and decreased absolute non-bone lean mass. Studies in 12 children with PWS using dual-photon absorptiometry have shown an absolute and relative increase in fat mass and a marked decrease in non-bone lean mass, similar to the pattern seen in GH deficiency, and unlike exogenous obesity (Hwu et al., 1992; Lee et al., 1993).

Therefore, it appears that children with PWS have both GH and IGF deficiencies. These abnormalities, in particular the IGF deficiency, could contribute to both the linear growth abnormality and abnormal body composition in PWS. The etiology of the GH/IGF deficiency is not known. It is unlikely to represent true congenital pituitary GH deficiency, since IGF and IGFBP-3 levels appear to be normal before age 5 years. One possibility is that the GH and IGF deficiencies are separate, e.g., GH secretion is suppressed by incompletely defined obesity-related factors (Weninger, 1983; vide supra), while the low IGF levels may be caused by an as yet undefined peripheral defect in IGF generation. This combination would lead to an overall GH/IGF deficiency with no endogenous compensatory mechanism. Furthermore, since the GH/IGF system is thought to mediate lipolysis and protein synthesis, a deficiency of this system may explain the propensity for the evident substrate shuttling to fat rather than muscle.

Treatment of childhood PWS with GH has been shown to significantly increase linear growth, increase IGF and IGFBP-3 levels, and lead to an absolute and relative increase in non-bone lean mass; bone mineral density may also increase significantly in some cases (Angulo, Castro-Magana, & Uy, 1991; Lee et al., 1987a,b, 1993; Trygstad, 1993; Wu, St Louis, Rubin, et al., 1988). These body composition changes are similar to those observed in non-PWS patients treated with GH (Gregory, Greene, Jung, et al., 1991; Rosenbaum, Gertner, & Leibel, 1989; Zachmann, Fernandez,

Tassinarin, et al., 1980). Levels of the GH-dependent bone matrix protein, osteocalcin, are low prior to therapy and increase during GH treatment (Lee et al., 1993). Anecdotal reports from the parents of treated patients include improved energy levels, appetite control, and improved mental concentration ability; however, these parameters have not yet been objectively measured in relation to treatment. Furthermore, blinded or dose-ranging studies of GH treatment in PWS have not been reported.

Diagnostic Procedures

GH secretion is episodic, and current testing of GH secretion relies on pharmacologic stimulation of GH secretion by several GH secretagogues, including insulin (hypoglycemia), L-DOPA, clonidine, arginine, and glucagon. By convention, a low response to at least 2 known stimuli is required for diagnosis of GH deficiency. Procedures for GH testing are standard in most pediatric centers.

As described above, GH testing is likely to be abnormal in PWS, and this may be related to obesity rather than to PWS itself. To confirm a defect in the GH/IGF system, single serum measurements of IGF-I (Lee & Rosenfeld, 1988; Lee, Wilson, Rountree, et al., 1990) or, preferably, IGFBP-3 (Hasegawa, Hasegawa, Aso, et al., 1993; Lee et al., 1992b), should be obtained. Both IGF-I and IGFBP-3 are relatively stable through the day, and sequential or stimulated testing is not necessary. IGF-I levels should be measured only in an assay that removes interfering IGF-binding proteins; IGFBP-3 levels can be measured without special sample preparation. Both levels should be compared to age- and sex-related normal ranges collected in the same laboratory. A low IGF-I or IGFBP-3 level in a well-nourished individual is indicative of GH/IGF deficiency, especially if stimulated GH levels are also low.

Treatment

Since GH/IGF deficiency in PWS fulfills usual diagnostic criteria, replacement therapy may be medically indicated. However, the relative costs and benefits of treatment must be carefully weighed and discussed with the patient (if possible) and parents/guardians in each individual case. At this time, GH therapy is approved only for use in GH-deficient children with open epiphyses, although studies in adults with GH deficiency and other conditions suggest possible therapeutic benefits (Nilsson, 1989; O'Halloran, Tsatsoulis, Whitehouse, et al., 1993).

Several preparations of recombinant DNA-derived human growth hormone are commercially available. In studies done to date, PWS patients have shown a good response to standard GH doses (Lee et al., 1993), e.g., 0.3 mg/kg/week or 0.05 mg/kg/day by subcutaneous injection.

Lower doses may also be efficacious (Fesseler & Bierich, 1983; Lee et al., unpublished data). However, dose-response studies have not been performed. Although anabolic steroids, such as oxandrolone (Holm, Nugent, Ruvalcaba, et al., 1989; Nugent & Holm, 1981) may have limited linear growth effects as compared to GH, additive effects of low-dose oxandrolone with GH treatment in PWS have been observed (Lee et al., 1987b; Raiti, Trias, Levitsy, et al., 1973); similar to observations in Turner syndrome (Rosenfeld et al., 1992).

Possible side-effects of standard or lower dose GH treatment are few. Reports of increased leukemia risk have not been completely supported by international ongoing follow-up studies. GH is an insulin counter-regulatory hormone, and may cause glucose intolerance in susceptible individuals. This may be especially true in obese individuals with insulin resistance. The author has observed 2 children with PWS who developed clinically significant glucose intolerance (fasting hyperglycemia, glucosuria, elevated glycated hemoglobin levels) while on standard GH doses; this resolved immediately in both cases with cessation of GH treatment. Both patients were >200% ideal body weight. One patient elected to discontinue treatment and the other restarted treatment at 0.025 mg/kg/day (half-dose) without recurrence of the glucose intolerance. Based on this observation, routine monitoring of fasting blood glucose, urine glucose, and/or glycated hemoglobin levels during GH treatment is advised.

Since increased linear growth is not the only expected benefit of GH treatment in PWS, other parameters should also be monitored, including bone density (vide infra), fat, and non-bone lean mass (Lee et al., 1993). Energy expenditure measures may also be useful (Schoeller, Levitsky, Bardini, et al., 1988). Compliance with GH administration can be monitored using serum IGF-I or IGFBP-3 levels.

Osteoporosis

Pathophysiology

Decreased bone mineral density is a frequent finding in PWS, and may contribute to an increased incidence of minor fractures (Cassidy, Rubin, & Mukaida, 1985; Rubin & Cassidy, 1988). Scoliosis is also frequently observed in PWS, and is often attributed to the combination of hypotonia and obesity (Gurd & Thompson, 1981; Holm & Laurnen, 1981). However, scoliosis may occur in infants and nonobese children with PWS, suggesting that obesity may not be a causative factor in all cases (Holm & Laurnen, 1981). Although a contributory role of osteoporosis in the pathogenesis of scoliosis has not been studied, orthopedic reports indicate that the vertebral bones in PWS may be osteoporotic and heal poorly with metal bracing (Rees, Jones, Owen, et al., 1989; Soriano, Weisz, & Houghton, 1988).

An intrinsic abnormality in calcium, phosphorous, vitamin D, or parathyroid hormone metabolism has not been identified in PWS. Dietary calcium deficiency may occur with severe calorie restriction; however, this is unlikely to be major etiologic factor for most individuals with PWS. As discussed in the preceding sections, both hypogonadism and GH/IGF deficiency are probable major factors in the pathophysiology of osteoporosis. Although there are few studies specific to PWS, both male and female hypogonadism has been associated with osteoporosis in adults. Furthermore, GH-deficient adults and children without PWS also have decreased bone mineral density (O'Halloran et al., 1993; Shore, Chesney, Mazess, et al., 1980).

Diagnosis

Dual-photon X-ray absorptiometry (DPA) is currently the preferred method for assessment of bone mineral density, and also provides measurements of bone mineral content and regional body composition (Jensen, Kanaley, Roust, et al., 1993; Lee et al., 1993). DPA involves regional or whole body scanning using a collimated beam of gamma radiation. Recent improvements allow a whole body scan in <10 min, with minimal radiation exposure.

Given the high incidence of osteoporosis in PWS, we recommend regular DPA measurements in postpubertal patients. Younger patients should also be studied if there is clinical evidence of osteoporosis. Lumbar vertebral measurements alone may be obtained to monitor axial skeleton calcification. However, whole body scanning has the additional advantage of providing objective measurements of fat and lean mass.

Ideally, DPA measurements would be interpreted in relation to fracture risk; however, such standards are not yet readily available for PWS. Pending collection of these data, DPA measurements should be compared to age- and sex-matched norms collected on the same instrument. Since heavier individuals would normally be expected to have increased axial bone mineral density, a weight correction would also be ideal; however, these standards are also not yet generally available.

Treatment

Most of the available treatment modalities for osteoporosis have been most extensively tested in normal postmenopausal women. These include dietary calcium and vitamin D supplementation, estrogen replacement therapy, and physical exercise. The efficacy of such treatment has not been completely investigated. This therapeutic uncertainty, coupled with the lack of adequate treatment studies specific to PWS, suggests a need for careful design and monitoring of any treatment modality. Consideration should be given to the following:

1. The prescribed diet should contain adequate calcium intake. If this is not possible within the caloric restraints of the diet, calcium supplements should be prescribed.

2. Vitamin D supplementation is usually not required for individuals with adequate sun exposure. However, fair-skinned individuals may have an increased incidence of osteoporosis, and hypopigmentation is a known feature of a large subset of individuals with PWS (Butler, 1989). In addition, many PWS individuals have lifestyles that do not include adequate sun exposure. Therefore, adequate dietary vitamin D should be ensured.

3. Sex steroid replacement therapy may decrease the risk for osteoporosis. Testosterone replacement in hypogonadal men and estrogen replacement in hypogonadal and postmenopausal women have been shown to improve bone mineral density in non-PWS populations.

4. Finally, GH treatment has been shown to improve bone mineral density in GH deficient adults (O'Halloran et al., 1993).

Treatment of osteoporosis should be individualized with regular monitoring of bone mineral density.

Thyroid Hormone, Cortisol, Prolactin, and Gastrointestinal Hormones

Unlike in Down (Pueschel & Pezzullo, 1985) and Turner (Germain & Plotnick, 1986) syndromes in which there are increased frequencies of autoimmune thyroiditis, no specific abnormality of the thyroid axis has been identified in PWS. In published studies, and in our own investigations, thyroid hormone levels, thyroid-stimulating hormone (TSH) levels, and TSH secretion in response to parenteral thyrotropin-releasing hormone (TRH) are normal (Bray et al., 1983; Calisti, Giannessi, Cesaretti, et al., 1991; Costeff et al., 1990; Lee et al., 1993; Ohashi, Takeda, Morioka, et al., 1980; Tolis, Lewis, Verdy, et al., 1974; Tze, Dunn, & Rothstein, 1981; Weninger et al., 1983). A single case of a patient previously diagnosed with hypothyroidism and later found to have PWS with a mosaic genotype has been reported (Bhate, Robertson, Davison, et al., 1989); however, the diagnosis of hypothyroidism was not specifically investigated and may be in doubt.

Early studies using urinary steroid metabolite measurements indicated a possible defect in ACTH responsiveness and glucocorticoid secretion (Rudd, Chance, & Theodoridis, 1969; Sarren, Ruvalcaba, & Kelley, 1975). However, this has not been confirmed in other studies. Cortisol and adrenocorticotropic hormone (ACTH) levels and cortisol secretion in response to parenteral ACTH are normal in PWS (Bray et al., 1983; Cacciari et al., 1990; Lee et al., 1993; Smith, Neeman, Wulff, et al., 1970).

Basal and TRH-stimulated prolactin levels are normal in PWS (Calisti et al., 1991; Lee et al., 1993; Ohashi et al., 1980; Smith et al., 1970; Tolis et al., 1974).

Pancreatic polypeptide secretion in response to protein has been reported to be deficient in PWS (Tomita, Greeley, Watt, et al., 1989; Zipf, O'Dorisio, Cataland, et al., 1983). This is a potentially important observation, since pancreatic polypeptide may be involved in satiety regulation. However, short-term infusion with pancreatic polypeptide had no measurable clinical effects in children with PWS (Zipf, O'Dorisio, & Berntson, 1990).

Obesity, Glucose Intolerance, and Diabetes Mellitus

Pathophysiology

Glucose intolerance and diabetes mellitus can occur in patients with PWS (Illig, Tschurni, & Vischer, 1975; Laurence, 1967; Laurence, Brito, & Wilkinson, 1981), although the precise incidence is not known. Clinically and biochemically, the usual case of diabetes mellitus in PWS is indistinguishable from obesity-related Type II, non-insulin-dependent diabetes mellitus, which occurs with a prevalence of 0.5% in the general population. This agrees with studies that indicate that the metabolic characteristics of PWS obesity do not differ from usual exogenous obesity (Bray, 1992; Gotlin, Dubois, Mace, et al., 1972).

Unlike Down and Turner syndrome, both of which are associated with an increased occurrence of Type I (insulin-dependent) diabetes mellitus, there does not appear to be any unique risk for diabetes mellitus in PWS, other than that associated with obesity. In the author's experience, diabetes mellitus has not been observed in normal weight or moderately obese patients with PWS. Moreover only a minority of very obese PWS patients develop clinically significant glucose intolerance or diabetes mellitus.

The pathogenesis of obesity-related glucose intolerance and Type II diabetes mellitus is not known, and probably involves more than one mechanism. Postulated abnormalities include defects in insulin secretion and action and possible abnormalities in glucose transport. A reduced amount of insulin receptors has been similarly observed in PWS and non-PWS obese patients (Kousholt, Beck-Nielsen, & Lund, 1983; Nozaki & Katoh, 1981) and is probably secondary to hyperinsulinemia. Increased visceral fat may account for the insulin resistance and predisposition to diabetes mellitus (Björntorp, 1991; Bray, 1992; Caro, 1991).

Nondiabetic children and adults with PWS-associated obesity may have elevated fasting insulin levels and elevated insulin and glucose responses on glucose-tolerance testing similar to patterns in exogenous obesity

(Deschamps, Giron, & Lestradet, 1977; Lautala, Knip, Auckerbloom, et al., 1986; Parra, Cervantes, & Schultz, 1973). We have recently observed increased fasting insulin and decreased postprandial insulin responses in some cases (Lee et al., 1992b), a pattern that resembles that reported for some cases of Type II diabetes mellitus. Much more work is needed to define the pathogenesis of obesity-related glucose intolerance and diabetes mellitus.

Type I, insulin-dependent diabetes mellitus occurs infrequently in PWS, with an incidence that is probably not greater than expected by chance. Anti-islet cell antibodies and other markers of autoimmune islet cell destruction are invariably negative in PWS-associated diabetes mellitus, which is consistent with the diagnosis of Type II diabetes mellitus.

Diagnosis

Diagnosis of diabetes mellitus should follow the guidelines of the American Diabetes Association (1993). Briefly, for Type II diabetes mellitus, a fasting blood glucose of ≥ 140 mg/dL and an abnormal oral glucose tolerance test are considered to be diagnostic. Impaired glucose tolerance (IGT) is characterized by a normal fasting glucose level and an elevated glucose level on oral glucose tolerance testing.

Obese patients with PWS should be screened regularly for clinical and biochemical evidence of glucose intolerance. Clinical signs include increased thirst and urination; however, most cases of Type II diabetes mellitus are relatively asymptomatic. Although fasting blood glucose levels and oral glucose tolerance tests are ideal, these are often impractical for routine screening in this population. A positive urine dipstick for glucose may indicate a need for further testing if positive; however, both false positive and false negative results may occur.

In our experience and as reported by others, total glycated hemoglobin levels measured by boronate affinity chromatography may provide a sensitive marker for glucose intolerance (Lee, Sherman, O'Day, et al., 1992a). This method is not the same as hemoglobin A_1 or A_{1c} measurements, which are relatively insensitive at the lower end of glycemia and are subject to interference by hemoglobin variants. In our clinic, regular measurements of total glycated hemoglobin are routine. An elevated level coupled with an elevated fasting blood glucose level is considered diagnostic of clinically significant glucose intolerance; oral glucose tolerance testing is rarely necessary. Fasting insulin and C-peptide of insulin levels are usually elevated in PWS-associated obesity and diabetes mellitus; these measurements provide little additional diagnostic information.

Ketonuria may be observed in some cases of Type II diabetes mellitus, however, frank ketoacidosis rarely occurs. The occurrence of ketoacidosis should suggest the possibility of Type I, insulin-dependent diabetes mellitus.

Treatment

Treatment guidelines for diabetes mellitus have been established by the American Diabetes Association (1993). The first line of treatment for Type II diabetes mellitus is diet and weight control. In PWS, these treatment elements are usually already in place at the time of diagnosis of diabetes mellitus, and any additional attempts at diet control may be extremely difficult. In addition, lack of appetite control may be especially difficult to treat, and can even override weight loss after gastroplasty (Miyata, Dousei, Narada, et al., 1990). However, since weight reduction is by far the most effective treatment modality for obesity-related Type II diabetes mellitus, every effort should be made to achieve weight control through a combination of calorie restriction and exercise. Appetite suppressants have not been proven to be effective in PWS (Bray et al., 1983; Cassidy, 1983). A ketogenic, protein-sparing fast may be therapeutically beneficial (Bistrian, Blackburn, & Stanbury, 1977); however, long-term treatment studies have not been reported.

Oral hypoglycemic agents have limited efficacy in the absence of adequate weight control. Treatment with long acting sulfonylureas, such as glipizide, may be used in combination with a diet regimen. Insulin treatment is also of questionable benefit, and could compound the tendency toward weight gain. However, in selected cases subcutaneous short-acting (regular) and intermediate-acting (NPH) insulin can provide temporary control of glucose levels. Recently, combination therapy with intermediate or long-acting (e.g., ultralente) insulin and an oral hypoglycemic has been reported to be useful in non-PWS Type II diabetes mellitus. As with single-agent therapy, this treatment is unlikely to be beneficial without adequate weight control.

Treatment of diabetes mellitus is important in reducing the risk for renal, retinal, and macrovascular (e.g., atherosclerotic) disease. Patients with PWS-associated diabetes mellitus should receive regular screening for these complications according to the guidelines of the American Diabetes Association. The relatively low incidence of diabetic retinopathy and nephropathy in PWS may be secondary to the increased mortality and shortened life span due to cardiovascular disease. However, one case of diabetic retinopathy has been reported in a patient with PWS (Savir, Dickerman, Karp, et al., 1974).

Cholesterol and Lipids

No specific intrinsic abnormalities of cholesterol or lipid metabolism have been identified in PWS (Bier, Kaplan, & Havel, 1977; Theodoridis, Albutt, & Chance, 1971). Although increased adipose tissue lipoprotein lipase activity has been reported in patients with PWS (Schwartz, Brunzell,

& Bierman, 1979), the control group for this study was not strictly matched for adiposity. In our experience, cholesterol and fasting lipid levels range from normal to slightly elevated and LDL to HDL ratios are similar to other obese patients, e.g., often in the moderate risk category. These findings are consistent with a dietary etiology and treatment with dietary fat restriction may be indicated. Patients with diabetes mellitus may have cholesterol and lipid abnormalities typical for this disorder. Successful treatment of the diabetes mellitus is usually beneficial.

Patients who are found to have extremely elevated cholesterol or triglyceride levels should be evaluated for the possibility of familial hypercholesterolemia or hypertriglyceridemia, both of which have relatively high prevalence in the general population. Pharmacologic treatment may be indicated in these cases.

Summary

In summary, two endocrine abnormalities may be specific to PWS:

1. Hypogonadotropic hypogonadism, which apparently begins *in utero* and involves the hypothalmic control of gonadotropin secretion rather than pituitary secretory ability itself, accounts for the cryptorchidism as well as abnormalities in sexual maturation. Hypogonadism is probably also a major factor in the development of osteoporosis, and may contribute to other somatic characteristics of the syndrome.

2. A deficiency in GH-related growth factors, particularly IGF-I, may account for the linear growth abnormalities, and may contribute to the osteoporosis and somatic characteristics of the syndrome. The etiology of this deficiency is not certain, and could be related to GH deficiency or to a peripheral defect in IGF generation.

Other endocrine abnormalities in PWS are probably secondary to obesity, including:

1. an increased risk of premature adrenarche,
2. decreased GH secretion, and
3. hyperinsulinism, glucose intolerance, and Type II non-insulin-dependent diabetes mellitus.

Finally, the following endocrine systems are apparently normal in PWS: thyroid, adrenal, and prolactin.

Based on this knowledge, the following elements should be considered in the evaluation and treatment of patients with PWS:

1. Gonadotropin stimulation testing may be useful in evaluating testicular function prior to treatment of cryptorchidism.
2. Weight control is essential in minimizing the risks for premature adrenarche, hyperinsulinism, and glucose intolerance. Obese patients

should be monitored regularly for evidence of clinically significant glucose intolerance.

3. Evaluation of GH/IGF status should be considered after the age of 5 years. Low IGF levels may indicate possible therapeutic efficacy for exogenous GH. Such treatment should include careful monitoring of body composition.

4. Gonadal steroid replacement therapy should be considered for adolescents and adults, and may help to prevent osteoporosis.

5. Routine measurements of bone density should be included for the detection and treatment of osteoporosis.

Although there are many deficits in our knowledge of the pathogenesis of PWS, new information gleaned from the studies reviewed here and ongoing investigations can help to improve the therapeutic outlook for affected individuals.

References

American Diabetes Association (1993). Clinical Practice Recommendations. *Diabetes Care, 16* (suppl 2), 1–118.

Angulo, M., Castro-Magana, M., & Uy, J. (1991). Pituitary evaluation and growth hormone reatment in Prader-Willi syndrome. *Journal of Pediatric Endocrinology, 4,* 167–173.

Aughton, D.J., & Cassidy, S.B. (1990). Physical features of Prader-Willi syndrome in neonates. *AJDC, 144,* 1251–1254.

Bhate, M.D., Robertson, P.E., Davison, E.V., & Brummitt, J.A. (1989). Prader-Willi syndrome with hypothyroidism. *Journal of Mental Deficiency Research, 33,* 235–244.

Bier, D.M., Kaplan, S.L., & Havel, R.J. (1977). The Prader-Willi syndrome: Regulation of fat transport. *Diabetes, 26,* 874–881.

Bistrian, B.R., Blackburn, G.L., & Stanbury, J.B. (1977). Metabolic aspects of a protein-sparing modified fast in the dietary management of Prader-Willi obesity. *New England Journal of Medicine, 296,* 774–779.

Björntorp, P. (1991). Metabolic implications of body fat distribution. *Diabetes Care, 14,* 1132–1143.

Bray, G.A. (1992). Genetic, hypothalamic and endocrine features of clinical experimental obesity. *Progress in Brain Research, 93,* 333–340.

Bray, G.A., Dahms, W.T., Swerdloff, R.S., Fiser, R.H., Atkinson, R.L., & Carrel, R.E. (1983). The Prader-Willi syndrome: A study of 40 patients and a review of the literature. *Medicine, 60,* 59–80.

Butler, M.G. (1989). Hypopigmentation: A common feature of Prader-Labhart-Willi syndrome. *American Journal of Human Genetics, 45,* 140–146.

Butler, M.G., & Meaney, F.J. (1991a). Standards for selected anthropometric measurements in Prader-Willi syndrome. *Pediatrics, 88,* 853–860.

Butler, M.G., & Meaney, F.J. (1991b). Anthropometric study of 38 individuals with Prader-Labhart-Willi syndrome. *American Journal of Medical Genetics, 26,* 445–455.

Cacciari, E., Cicognani, A., Pirazzoli, P., Zappulla, F., Salaerdi, S., & Bernardi, F. (1975). Relationships among the secretion of ACTH, GH, and cortisol during the insulin induced hypoglycemia test in normal and obese child. *Journal of Clinical Endocrinology and Metabolism, 40*, 802–806.

Cacciari, E., Zucchini, S., Carla, G., Pirazzoli, P., Cicognani, A., Mandini, M., Busacca, M., & Trevisan, C. (1990). Endocrine function and morphological findings in patients with disorders of the hypothalamo-pituitary area: A study with magnetic resonance. *Archives of Disease in Childhood, 65*, 1199–1202.

Calisti, L., Giannessi, N., Cesaretti, G., & Saggese, G. (1991). Studio endocrino nella sindrome di Prader-Willi. A propositi di 5 casi. *Minerva Pediatrica, 43*, 587–593.

Caro, J.F. (1991). Insulin resistance in obese and nonobese man. *Endocrine Reviews, 73*, 691–695.

Cassidy, S.B. (1983). Prader-Willi syndrome. *Current Problems in Pediatrics, 14*, 1–55.

Cassidy, S.B., Rubin, K.G., & Mukaida, C.S. (1985). Osteoporosis in Prader-Willi syndrome. *American Journal of Human Genetics, 37*, A49.

Cassidy, S.B., Rubin, K.G., & Mukaida, C.S. (1987). Genital abnormalities and hypogonadism in 105 patients with Prader-Willi syndrome. *American Journal of Medical Genetics, 28*, 922–923.

Costeff, H., Holm, V.A., Ruvalcaba, R., & Shaver, J. (1990). Growth hormone secretion in Prader Willi syndrome. *Acta paediatrica Scandinavica, 79*, 1059–1062.

Deschamps, I., Giron, B.J., & Lestradet, H.J. (1977). Blood glucose, insulin, and free fatty acid levels during oral glucose tolerance tests in 158 obese children. *Diabetes, 26*, 89–93.

Dunn, H.G. (1968). The Prader-Labhart-Willi syndrome: Review of the literature and report of nine cases. *Acta Paediatrica Scandinavica, 186* (suppl), 1–38.

Epstein, L.H., Wing, R.R., & Valoski, A. (1985). Childhood obesity. *Pediatric Clinics of North America, 32*, 363–379.

Epstein, L.H., McCurley, J., Valoski, A., & Wing, R.R. (1990). Growth in obese children treated for obesity. *AJDC, 144*, 1360–1364.

Fesseler, W.H., & Bierich. J.R. (1983). Untersuchungen beim Prader-Labhart-Willi Syndrom. *Monatsschrift für Kinderheilkunde, 131*, 844–847.

Garty, B., Shuper, A., Mimouni, M., Varsano, I., & Kauli R. (1982). Primary gonadal failure and precocious adrenarche in a boy with Prader-Labhart-Willi symptoms. *European Journal of Pediatrics, 139*, 201–203.

Germain, E.L., & Plotnick, L.P. (1986). Age-related antithyroid antibodies and thyroid abnormalities in Turner syndrome. *Acta Paediatrica Scandinavica, 75*, 750–755.

Gotlin, R., Dubois, R., Mace, J., & Myer, W. (1972). Carbohydrate metabolism in the Prader-Willi syndrome. *Clinical Research, 20*, 274 (abstract).

Greenberg, F., Elder, F.F.B., & Ledbetter, D.H. (1987). Neonatal diagnosis of Prader-Willi syndrome and its implications. *American Journal of Medical Genetics, 28*, 845–856.

Gregory, J.W., Greene, S.A., Jung, R.T., Scrimgeour, C.M., & Rennie, M.J. (1991). Changes in body composition and energy expenditure after six weeks' growth hormone treatment. *Archives of Disease in Childhood, 66*, 598–602.

Gurd, A.R., & Thompson, T.R. (1981). Scoliosis in Prader-Willi syndrome. *Journal of Pediatric Orthopedics, 1*, 317–320.

Guthrie, R.D. Smith, D.W., & Graham, C.B. (1973). Testosterone treatment for micropenis during early childhood. *Journal of Pediatrics, 83*, 247–252.

Hamabe, J., Fukushima, Y., Harada, N., Abe, K., Matsuo, N., Nagai, T., Yoshioka, A., Tomoki, H., Tsukino, R., & Niikawa, N. (1991). Molecular study of the Prader-Willi syndrome. Deletion, RFLP, and phenotype analysis of 50 patients. *American Journal of Medical Genetics, 41*, 54–63.

Hamilton, C.R., Jr., Scully, R.E., & Kliman, B. (1972). Hypogonadotropinism in Prader-Willi syndrome: Induction of puberty and spermatogenesis by clomiphene citrate. *American Journal of Medicine, 52*, 322–329.

Harris, J.C., & Knigge, K.M. (1982). Disappearance of a urinary antigonadotropin following HCG administration in Prader-Willi syndrome. *Progress in Clinical and Biological Research, 92*, 273–282.

Harty, J.R., Hollowell, J.G., & Sieg, K.G. (1993). Tall stature, An atypical phenotype in Prader-Willi syndrome. *Clinical Pediatrics, 32*, 179–180.

Haschke, F., & Hohenauer, L. (1978). Endocrine studies in four patients with Prader-Labhart-Willi syndrome during early infancy and childhood. *Pediatric Research, 12*, 1100 (abstract).

Hasegawa, Y., Hasegawa, T., Aso, T., Kotoh, S., Tsuchiya, Y., Nose, O., Ohyama, Y., Araki, K., Tanaka, T., Saisyo, S., Yokoya, S., Nishi, Y., Miyamoto, S., Sasaki, N., Kurimoto, F., Toyama, M., Harada, A., Horie, H., & Stene, M. (1993). Comparison between insulin-like growth factor-I (IGF-I) and IGF binding protein-3 (IGFBP-3) measurement in the diagnosis of growth hormone deficiency. *Endocrine Journal (Japan), 40*, 185–190.

Hasen, J., & Wu, R.H. (1982). Growth hormone secretion in the Prader-Labhart-Willi syndrome. *Fertility and Sterility, 387*, 499 (letter).

Holm, V.A., & Laurnen, E.L. (1981). Prader-Willi syndrome and scoliosis. *Developmental Medicine and Child Neurology, 92*, 201.

Holm, V.A., & Nugent, J.K. (1982). Growth in the Prader-Willi syndrome. *Birth Defects: Original Article Series, 18*, 93–100.

Holm, V.A., Nugent, J.K., Ruvalcaba, R.H., & Costeff, H. (1989). Oxandrolone therapy in six boys with the Prader-Willi syndrome. *Journal of Pediatrics, 114*, 325–327.

Hooft, C., Delire, C., & Casneuf, J. (1966). Le syndrome de Prader-Labhart-Willi-Fanconi: Etude clinique, endocrinologique et cytogenetique. *Acta Pœdiatrica Belgica, 20*, 27–50.

Hutson, J.M., & Donahoe, P.K. (1986). The hormonal control of testicular descent. *Endocrine Reviews, 7*, 270–283.

Hwu, K., Klish, W.J., Henson, H., Brown, B.T., Bricker, J.T., LeBlanc, A.D., Fiorotto, M.L., Greenberg, F., & Lee, P.D.K. (1992). *Endocrine status, growth hormone (GH) therapy and body composition in Prader-Willi syndrome (PWS)*. Presented at the 74th annual meeting of the Endocrine Society, San Antonio, abstract #710.

Illig, R., Tschurni, A., & Vischer, D. (1975). Glucose intolerance and diabetes mellitus in patients with the Prader-Labhart-Willi syndrome. *Modern Problems in Pediatrics, 12*, 203–210.

Iranmesh, A., Lizarralde, G., & Veldhuis, J.D. (1991). Age and relative adiposity are specific negative determinants of the frequency and amplitude of growth hormone (GH) secretory bursts and the half-life of endogenous GH in healthy men. *Journal of Clinical Endocrinology and Metabolism, 73*, 1081–1088.

Jaskulsky, S.R., & Stone, N.N. (1987). Hypogonadism in Prader-Willi syndrome. *Urology, 29*, 207–208.

Jeffcoate, W.J., Laurence, B.M., Edwards, C.R.W., & Besser, G.M. (1980). Endocrine function in the Prader-Willi syndrome. *Clinical Endocrinology, 12*, 81–89.

Jensen, M.D., Kanaley, J.A., Roust, L.R., O'Brien, P.C., Braun, J.S., Dunn, W.L., & Wahner, H.W. (1993). Assessment of body composition with use of dual-energy X-ray absorptiometry: Evaluation and comparison with other methods. *Mayo Clinic Proceedings, 68*, 867–873.

Katcher, M.L., Bargman, G.J., Gilbert, E.F., & Opitz, J.M. (1977). Absence of spermatogonia in the Prader-Willi syndrome. *European Journal of Pediatrics, 124*, 257–260.

Kauli, R., Prager-Lewin, R., & Laron, Z. (1978). Pubertal development in the Prader-Labhart-Willi syndrome. *Acta Pædiatrica Scandinavica, 67*, 763–767.

Kousholt, A.M., Beck-Nielsen, H., & Lund, H.T. (1983). A reduced number of insulin receptors in patients with Prader-Willi syndrome. *Acta Endocrinologica, 104*, 345–351.

Laurence, B.M. (1967). Hypotonia, mental retardation, obesity, and cryptorchidism associated with dwarfism and diabetes in child. *Archives of Diseases in Childhood, 42*, 126–149.

Laurence, B.M., Brito, A., & Wilkinson, J. (1981). Prader-Willi syndrome after age 15 years. *Archives of Disease in Childhood, 56*, 181–186.

Lautala, T., Knip, M., Auckerbloom, H.K., Koubalainen, K., & Martin, J.M. (1986). Serum insulin-releasing activity and the Prader-Willi syndrome. *Acta Endocrinologica, 279* (suppl), 416–421.

Lee, P.D.K., & Rosenfeld, R.G. (1988). Clinical utility of insulin-like growth factor assays. *Pediatrician, 14*, 154–161.

Lee, P.D.K., Wilson, D.M., Rountree, L., Hintz, R.L., & Rosenfeld, R.G. (1987a). Linear growth response to exogenous growth hormone in Prader-Willi syndrome. *American Journal of Medical Genetics, 28*, 865–871.

Lee, P.D.K., Wilson, D.M., Hintz, R.L., & Rosenfeld, R.G. (1987b). Growth hormone treatment of short stature in Prader-Willi syndrome. *Journal of Pediatric Endocrinology, 2*, 31–34.

Lee, P.D.K., Wilson, D.M., Rountree, L., Hintz, R.L., & Rosenfeld, R.G. (1990). Efficacy of insulin-like growth factor I levels in predicting the response to provocative growth hormone testing. *Pediatric Research, 27*, 45–51.

Lee, P.D.K., Sherman, L.D., O'Day, M.R., Rognerud, R.L., & Ou, C.N. (1992a). Comparisons of home blood glucose testing and glycated protein measurements. *Diabetes Research and Clinical Practice, 16*, 53–62.

Lee, P.D.K., Hwu, K., Brown, B., Greenberg, F., & Klish, W. (1992b). Endocrine investigations in children with Prader-Willi syndrome. *Dysmorphology and Clinical Genetics, 6*, 27–28.

Lee, P.D.K., Hwu, K., Henson, H., Brown, B.T., Bricker, J.T., LeBlanc, A.D., Fiorotto, M.D., Greenberg, F., & Klish, W.J. (1993). Body composition studies in Prader-Willi syndrome (PWS): Effects of growth hormone (GH) therapy. In K.J. Ellis & J.D. Eastman (Eds.), *Human body composition. In vitro methods, models and applications* (pp. 201–206). Newark: Plenum Press.

Linde, R., McNeil, L., & Rabin, D. (1982). Induction of menarche by clomiphene citrate in a fifteen year old girl with the Prader-Labhart-Willi syndrome. *Fertility and Sterility, 37*, 118–120.

Lu, P.W., Cowell, C.T., Jimenez, M., Simpson, J.M., & Silink, M. (1991). Effect of obesity on endogenous secretion of growth hormone in Turner's syndrome. *Archives of Disease in Childhood, 66*, 1184–1190.

MacMillan, D.R., Kim, C.B., & Weisskopf, B. (1972). Syndrome of growth resistance, obesity, and intellectual impairment with precocious puberty. *Archives of Disease in Childhood, 47*, 119–121.

McGuffin, W.L., Jr., & Rogol, A.D. (1975). Response to LH-RH and clomiphene citrate in two women with the Prader-Labhart-Willi syndrome. *Journal of Clinical Endocrinology and Metabolism, 41*, 325–331.

Miller, W.L. (1988). Molecular biology of steroid hormones synthesis, *Endocrine Reviews, 9*, 295–318.

Miyata, M.D., Dousei, T., Harada, T., Aono, T., Kitagawa, T., Nose, O., & Kawashima, Y. (1990). Metabolic changes following gastroplasty in Prader-Willi syndrome: A case report. *Japanese Journal of Surgery, 20*, 359–364.

Nilsson, K.O. (1989). What is the value of growth hormone treatment in short children with specified syndromes? Turners syndrome, osteochondrodysplasias, Prader-Willi syndrome, Noonan syndrome. *Acta Pædiatrica Scandinavica, 362* (suppl), 61–68.

Nozaki, Y., & Katoh, K. (1981). Endocrinological abnormalities in Prader-Willi syndrome. *Acta Pædiatrica Japonica, 23*, 301–306.

Nugent, J.K., & Holm, V.A. (1981). Physical growth in Prader-Willi syndrome. In V.A. Holm, S. Sulzbacher, & P.L. Pipes (Eds.), *The Prader-Willi syndrome* (pp. 269–279). Baltimore: University Park Press.

O'Halloran, D.J., Tsatsoulis, A., Whitehouse, R.W., Holmes, S.J., Adams, J.E., & Shalet, S.M. (1993). Increased bone density after recombinant human growth hormone (GH) therapy in adults with isolated GH deficiency. *Journal of Clinical Endocrinology and Metabolism, 76*, 1344–1348.

Ohashi, T., Takeda, K., Morioka, M., Akaeda, T., Kumon, H., Mitsuhata, N., & Ohmori, H. (1980). Endocrinological study on Prader-Willi syndrome: Report of four cases and review of the literature. *Nippon Hinyokika Gakkai Zasshi, 71*, 999–1009.

Parra, A., Cervantes, C., & Schultz, R.B. (1973). Immunoreactive insulin and growth hormone responses in patients with Prader- Willi syndrome. *Journal of Pediatrics, 83*, 587–593.

Prader, A. (1981). The Prader-Willi syndrome: An overview. *Acta Pædiatrica Japonica, 23*, 307–311.

Pueschel, S.M., & Pezzullo, J.C. (1985). Thyroid dysfunction in Down syndrome. *AJDC, 139*, 636–639.

Raiti, S., Trias, E., Levitsy, L., & Grossman, M.S. (1973). Oxandrolone and human growth hormone. Comparison of growth-stimulating effects in short children. *AJDC, 126*, 597–600.

Rees, D., Jones, M.W., Owen, R., & Dorgan, J.C. (1989). Scoliosis surgery in the Prader-Willi syndrome. *Journal of Bone and Joint Surgery, 71*, 685–688.

Robinson, A., & Jones, W.G. (1988). Prader-Willi syndrome. *Alabama Jourunal of Medical Sciences, 25*, 495–496.

Robinson, W.P., Bottani, A., Xie, Y.G., Balakrishman, J., Binkert, F., Machler, M., Prader, A., & Schinzel, A (1991). Molecular, cytogenetic, and clinical investigations of Prader-Willi syndrome patients. *American Journal of Human Genetics, 49*, 1219–1234.

Rosenbaum, M., Gertner, J.M., & Leibel, R.L. (1989). Effects of systemic growth hormone (GH) administration on regional adipose tissue distribution and metabolism in GH-deficient children. *Journal of Clinical Endocrinology and Metabolism, 69*, 1274–1281.

Rosenfeld, R.G., Frane, J., Attie, K.M., Brasel, J.A., Burstein, S., Cara, J.F., Chernausek, S., Gotlin, R.W., Kuntze, J., Lippe, B.M., Mahoney, P.C., Moore, W.V., Saenger, P., & Johanson, A.J. (1992). Six-year results of a randomized prospective trial of human growth hormone and oxandrolone in Turner syndrome. *Journal of Pediatrics, 121*, 49–55.

Rubin, K., & Cassidy, S.B. (1988). Hypogonadism and osteoporosis. In L.R. Greenswag & R.C. Alexander (Eds.), *Management of Prader-Willi syndrome* (pp. 23–33). New York: Springer-Verlag.

Rudd, B.T., Chance, G.W., & Theodoridis, C.G. (1969). Adrenal response to ACTH in patients with Prader-Willi syndrome, simple obesity, and constitutional dwarfism. *Archives of Diseases in Childhood, 44*, 244–247.

Sarren, C., Ruvalcaba, R.H.A., & Kelley, V.C. (1975). Some aspects of carbohydrate metabolism in Prader-Willi syndrome. *Journal of Mental Deficiency Research, 19*, 113–119.

Savir, A., Dickerman, Z., Karp, M., & Laron, Z. (1974). Diabetic retinopathy in an adolescent with Prader-Labhart-Willi syndrome. *Archives of Diseases in Childhood, 49*, 963–964.

Schoeller, D.A., Levitsky, L.L., Bandini, L.G., Dietz, W.W., & Walczak, A. (1988). Energy expenditure and body composition in Prader-Willi syndrome. *Metabolism, 37*, 115–120.

Schwartz, R.S., Brunzell, J.P., & Bierman, E.L. (1979). Elevated adipose tissue lipoprotein lipase in the pathogenesis of obesity in Prader-Willi syndrome. *Transactions of the Association of American Physicians, 92*, 89–95.

Seyler, L.E., Arunlanantham, K., & O'Connor, C.F. (1979). Hypergonadotropic-hypogonadism in the Prader-Labhart-Willi syndrome. *Journal of Pediatrics, 94*, 435–437.

Shimizu, H., Negishi, M., Takahashi, M., Shimomura, Y., Uehara, Y., Kobayashi, I., & Kobayashi, S. (1990). Dexamethasone suppressible hypergonadotropism in an adolescent patient with Prader-Willi syndrome. *Endocrinologica Japonica, 37*, 165–169.

Shore, R.M., Chesney, R.W., Mazess, R.B., Rose, P.G., & Bargman, G.J. (1980). Bone mineral status in growth hormone deficiency. *Journal of Pediatrics, 96*, 393–396.

Smith, J.D., Neeman, J., Wulff, J., & Seely, J.R. (1970). Clinical metabolic study of the Prader-Willi syndrome. *Journal of the Oklahoma State Medical Association, 63*, 234–238.

Soriano, R.M.G., Weisz, I., & Houghton, G.R. (1988). Scoliosis in the Prader-Willi syndrome. *Spine, 13*, 209–211.

Stephenson, J.B.P. (1980). Prader-Willi syndrome: neonatal presentation and later development. *Developmental Medicine and Child Neurology, 22*, 792–799.

Swaab, D.F., Hofman, M.A., Lucassen, P.J., Purba, J.S., Raadsheer, F.C., & Van-de-Nes, J.A. (1993). Functional neuroanatomy and neuropathology of the human hypothalamus. *Anatomy and Embryology*, *187*, 317–330.

Tamarkin, L., Abastillas, P., Chen, H.C., McNemar, A., & Sidbury, J.B. (1982). The daily profile of plasma melatonin in obese and Prader-Willi syndrome children. *Journal of Clinical Endocrinology and Metabolism*, *55*, 491–495.

Theodoridis, C.G., Albutt, E.C., & Chance, G.W. (1971a). Blood lipids in children with the Prader-Willi syndrome: A comparison with simple obesity. *Australian Pædiatric Journal*, *7*, 20–23.

Theodoridis, C.G., Brown, G.A., Chance, G.W., & Rudd, B.T. (1971b). Plasma growth hormone levels in children with the Prader-Willi syndrome. *Australian Pædiatric Journal*, *7*, 24–27.

Tolis, G., Lewis, W., Verdy, M., Friesen, H.G., Solomon, S., Pagalis, G., Pavlatos, E., Fessas, P., & Rochefort, J.G. (1974). Anterior pituitary function in the Prader-Labhart-Willi (PLW) syndrome. *Journal of Clinical Endocrinology and Metabolism*, *39*, 1061–1066.

Tomita, T., Greeley, G., Jr., Watt, L., Doull, V., & Chance, T. (1989). Protein meal-stimulated pancreatic polypeptide secretion in Prader-Willi syndrome of adults. *Pancreas*, *4*, 395–400.

Trygstad, O. (1993). Growth hormone treatment in Prader-Labhart-Willi syndrome. *Pediatric Research*, *33* (suppl), S40 (abstract).

Tze, W.J., Dunn, H.G., & Rothstein, R.L. (1981). Endocrine profiles and metabolic aspects of Prader-Willi syndrome. In V.A. Holm, S. Sulzbacher, & P.L. Pipes (Eds.), *The Prader-Willi syndrome* (pp. 281–291). Baltimore: University Park Press.

Uehling, D. (1980). Cryptorchidism in the Prader-Willi syndrome. *Journal of Urology*, *124*, 103–104.

Vanelli, M.D., Bernasconi, S., Caronna, N., Virdis, R., Terzi, C., & Giovanelli, G. (1984). Precocious puberty in a male with Prader-Labhart-Willi syndrome. *Helvetica Pædiatrica Acta*, *39*, 373–377.

Van Vliet, G., Bosson, D., Rummens, E., Robyn, C., & Wolter, R. (1986). Evidence against growth hormone-releasing factor deficiency in children with idiopathic obesity. *Acta Endocrinologica*, *279* (suppl), 403–410.

Walterspiel, J.N., Wolff, J., & Heinze, E. (1981). Pubertas präcox bei Prader-Labhart-Willi-Syndrom. *Klinische Pädiatrie*, *193*, 120–121.

Wannarachue, N., Ruvalcaba, R.H.A., & Kelley, V.C. (1975). Hypogonadism in Prader-Willi syndrome. *American Journal of Mental Deficiency*, *79*, 592–603.

Weninger, M., Frisch, H., Widhalm, K., & Schernthaner, G. (1983). Endokrine Untersuchungen bei Prader-Labhart-Willi-Syndrom: Pubertätseintritt bei einem 19 Jahre alten Knaben nach Langseitverabreichung eines LHRH-Analogens. *Experimental and Clinical Endocrinology*, *82*, 8–14.

Willig, R.P., Braun, W., Commentz, J.C., & Stahnke, N. (1986). Circadian fluctuation of plasma melatonin in Prader-Willi's syndrome and obesity. *Acta Endocrinologica*, *279* (suppl), 411–415.

Wu, R.H., Hasen, J., & Warburton, D. (1981). Primary hypogonadism and 13/15 chromosome translocation in Prader-Labhart-Willi syndrome. *Hormone Research*, *15*, 148–158.

Wu, R.H., St. Louis, Y., Rubin, K., Cassidy, S.B., Thorpy, M.J., & Saenger, P. (1988). Growth hormone therapy in Prader-Willi syndrome (PWS). *Pediatric Research, 23* (suppl), 207A (abstract).

Zachmann, M., Fernandez, F., Tassinari, D., Thakker, R., & Prader, A. (1980). Anthropometric measurements in patients with growth hormone deficiency before treatment with human growth hormone. *European Journal of Pediatrics, 133,* 277–282.

Zappulla, F., Salardi, S., Tassinari, D., Villa, M.P., Fréjavile, E., Ventura, D., & Montanari, P. (1981). Studio dell'asse ipotalamo-ipofisi-gonadi nella sindrome di Prader-Labhart-Willi. *Minerva Pediatrica, 33,* 201–204.

Zárate, A., Soria, J., Canales, E.S., Kastin, A.J., Schally, A.V., & Guzmßn Toledano, R. (1973/74). Pituitary response to synthetic luteinizing hormone-releasing hormone in Prader-Willi syndrome, prepubertal and pubertal children. *Neuroendocrinology, 13,* 321–326.

Zellweger, H., & Schneider, H.J. (1968). Syndrome of hypotonia-hypomentia-hypogonadism-obesity (HHHO) or Prader-Willi-syndrome. *AJDC, 115,* 588–599.

Zipf, W.B., O'Dorisio, T.M., Cataland, S., & Dixon, K. (1983). Pancreatic polypeptide responses to protein meal challenges in obese but otherwise normal children and obese children with Prader-Willi syndrome. *Journal of Clinical Endocrinology and Metabolism, 57,* 1074–1080.

Zipf, W.B., O'Dorisio, T.M., & Berntson, G.G. (1990). Short-term infusion of pancreatic polypeptide: Effect on children with Prader-Willi syndrome. *American Journal of Clinical Nutrition, 51,* 162–166.

Part II
The Interdisciplinary Process: Health Aspects

No one who has ever worked with D had ever even seen a PW person before (school, activity center, workshop, doctors, no one). We have found that people, even professionals who work with retarded people, do not understand his drive for food. They think it is a matter of training or discipline or an emotional problem. He has never fit into any program, even for the retarded, because of this drive to get food. He is ingenious at getting it and it causes all kinds of problems. It is all he really cares about. We wonder if all PW adults are like he is—or if many of his behavior problems have been caused because we didn't know what was the matter with him until he was 21. And even since then, professional people who have worked with him haven't really been able to accept and believe the extent of his handicap.

4
A Team Approach to
Case Management

Vanja A. Holm

Prader–Willi syndrome (PWS) is a disorder that produces a variety of symptoms affecting all aspects of the life of persons with the syndrome and their families. Meeting their needs requires that the knowledge and skills of professionals who can serve them be delivered through an efficient interdisciplinary system that implies that health, educational, and social service specialists share information and work together. Ideally, this approach encourages collaborative development of appropriate assessment and management strategies.

Holm and McCartin (1978) pointed out that successful interdisciplinary teams depend on a comprehensive approach to serving the developmentally disabled and understand that team effectiveness depends on participation by competent professionals who have the ability to interrelate. Philosophically, this means that the members of such a team are capable of developing holistic interventions that optimize maximum growth based on a developmental model that targets normalization in the least restrictive setting. The developmental process model proposes that where services are appropriate, developmentally disabled individuals can continue to learn and grow throughout their lives. Normalization, in its broadest sense, refers to providing the handicapped with opportunities to live and work in environments as close as possible to typical community patterns (Wolfensberger, 1972). The concept of "least restrictive environment" supports the rights of the developmentally disabled to live as independently as possible, limited only by their individual capacity to make decisions.

The implementation of the team approach as a strategy for delivery of services to the developmentally disabled has been recognized by the public sector some 40 years. Outpatient clinical services for children with developmental disabilities first appeared as community clinics for the mentally retarded. From the beginning it was recognized that the professional composition of such services needed to consist of several disciplines

(Hormuth, 1957). Federal funding [Mental Retardation Facilities and Community Mental Health Centers Construction act of 1963 (PL 88-164); Education for All Handicapped Children Act of 1975 (PL 94-142)] provided for interdisciplinary training, research, and delivery of services. In 1978, the federal government clearly defined "developmental disability" and established eligibility criteria [Developmental Disabilities Act Amendments of 1978 (PL 95-602)]. This legislation mandates that training and service delivery in the field of developmental disabilities be interdisciplinary. Subsequent amendments emphasize consumer orientation with family-directed services and parental involvement as an essential part of the team process. There are about 30 University Affiliated Programs across the United States that implement integrated services to the developmentally disabled far beyond the capacities of any one health or education discipline. The rights of this population to receive public funding and services are discussed in depth in Chapters 14 and 15.

Having discussed team intervention in general terms and acknowledged that there is formalized support of this service delivery model, the question arises, "Is a team approach appropriate in management of PWS?" The answer to this query is a firm "Yes." A team approach is sensible simply because PWS presents a constellation of symptoms that requires the expertise of many disciplines for management. It is a realistic way to provide on-going assessment of multifaceted issues that continue over time because needs shift as the child grows older and family circumstances change. Diagnostic, medical, nursing, and nutritional issues predominate early in life, and all but the diagnosis remain constant concerns throughout life. Language, education, motor therapies, and social services become greater issues as the child grows older. Behavioral and social problems become a major source of family stress; vocational guidance and appropriate living arrangements become the cornerstone of adaptation to adulthood.

The specific disciplinary composition of the team is not as important as the skills each team member provides, which should be complementary. Gaps have to be avoided at all costs. Teams need to concentrate on identified tasks. If available team members cannot perform specialized services, consultants need to be identified and temporarily incorporated onto the team process. For example, to assess the need for alternative communication in the rare nonverbal child with PWS may require outside intervention. Overlaps in professional skills are of less concern when the team functions well together. On such teams, turf conflicts between disciplines do not interfere. Team members respect the competence of each other and encourage all contributions to the team process. They learn from one another and transdisciplinary (cross-discipline) actions are welcome. Family conflict over the management of a child with PWS is an example of an important issue that should be of concern to all team members regardless of discipline.

An interdisciplinary team has to be guided by a common philosophy of child development, whether articulated or not. Most accepted disciplinary teachings in child development are complementary, but some are less so. Psychoanalytical and strict behavior modification views about child development are often difficult to reconcile. Professionals in the child development field have to be open to new ideas. However, in this area, as in other chronic conditions, alternative treatments may be proposed. A knowledgeable, sensitive team must be aware of the dangers of dissention when an enthusiastic, single-minded member proposes a far-out cure, whether it is a diet, drug, or physical manipulation.

Early interventions focus on therapy for hypotonia, nutritional guidelines, and nursing and medical management of failure to thrive. Later the potential for obesity becomes an overriding concern. Historically, physicians thought that death from obesity at early age was inevitable (Steffes, Holm, Sulzbacher, 1981). Now a combination of nutritional and behavioral management in childhood can avoid this outcome (Chapter 1). With modern cytogenetics and molecular genetic techniques, a highly probable diagnosis can be established if the attending physician(s) consider the possibility of PWS early in infancy. Children fortunate enough to be identified early in life require an interdisciplinary team that can explain the diagnosis and its implications. The child is likely to still be in the failure to thrive state where parents tend to be overwhelmed. The physician is the logical person to discuss the diagnosis; the nutritionist can provide dietary advice; the nurse offers the family not only practical help about how to handle the fragile infant, but also support as the family tries to adapt. In some settings social workers serve the latter role. Depending on available resources, the team's occupational/physical therapist may assist in locating a suitable professional for the family and suggest appropriate interventions. One team goal is to guide the family to someone familiar with resources in the home community to access appropriate birth-to-five services.

Educational issues need to be addressed by the team, beginning with early intervention and concluding with options for vocational training. With the advent of pre-school years, the task of the team increases. Medical and nutritional intervention shifts to dealing with growth and weight. Decelerating linear growth may need endocrine assessment. Excessive weight gain requires dietary intervention. Although parents may be resigned to the diagnosis, they begin to question exactly where their child fits on the spectrum of the intellectual function associated with PWS. The team psychologist might either test the child or interpret school testing. At this stage questions about the need for special services arise. Should physical/occupational therapy be continued? What speech and language services are required?

During school years, nutritional and medical concerns continue (weight control, scoliosis, endocrinone abnormalities). School-related issues need increasing attention, particularly management of behaviors. The team of skilled, interested professionals can provide guidelines. Its task is to assist schools and parents to problem solve in areas of foraging for food, handling tantrums, and administering discipline to a child with a condition such as PWS, with its lack of internal control. Educational mainstreaming becomes an issue and the educational expert on the team should become actively involved, with the team of school personnel that includes school principals, cafeteria employees, maintenance workers, teachers, aides, and the school psychologist. Intervention for speech therapy begins in the preschool years and may need to be continued. It is essential that the team share information and recommendations in a collegial manner with school personnel and the family.

By late adolescence and adulthood, additional concerns arise such as establishment of vocational goals and the training needed to attain them. Financial planning by families and investigation of residential options become paramount. Considerable knowledge and skills are required to assist persons with PWS and their families to cope with these issues. A consultation by a legal expert may be necessary to assist the family and the team.

Despite the complexity of PWS, affected persons reportedly live into their sixties. And, over the years, in addition to a consulting child development team, they require the service of medical, educational, mental health, and social service providers. The Prader–Willi Syndrome Association (USA) has accumulated a vast amount of information over the years that is invaluable.

While detailed information about interdisciplinary teams in the field of child development is beyond the scope of this discussion, clearly, by virtue of impaired cognition and the presence of limited functional capacity, individuals with PWS fall well within the guidelines established by law and are eligible for a broad range of professional services. Each of the succeeding chapters describes sharply defined specialist procedures that, at the same time, represent the integral components of a comprehensive, interdisciplinary team approach to case management.

References

Developmental Disabilities Act Amendments of 1978. (1982). 42 USC Section 6000–6081.

Education for All Handicapped Children Act of 1975. (1982). 20 USC Section 1400–1420.

Holm, V.A., & McCartin, RE. (1978). Interdisciplinary child development team: Team issues and training in interdisciplinariness. In K.E. Allen, V.A. Holm, & R.L. Schiefelbusch (Eds.), *Early intervention–A team approach* (pp. 97–122). Baltimore: University Park Press.

Hormuth, R.P. (1957). Community clinics for the mentally retarded. *Children, 9,* 181–185.

Mental Retardation Facilities and Community Mental Health Centers Construction Act of 1963. (1982). 42 USC Section 6000–6081.

Steffes, M.J., Holm, V.A., & Sulzbacher, S. (1981). The Prader-Willi syndrome: Historical perspective. In V.A. Holm, S.J. Sulzbacher, & P.P. Pipes, (Eds.), *The Prader-Willi syndrome* (pp. 1–15). Baltimore: University Park Press.

Wolfensberger, W. (1972). *Normalization: The principle of normalization in human services*. Toronto: National Institute on Mental Retardation.

5
Medical and Nursing Interventions

RANDELL C. ALEXANDER and LOUISE R. GREENSWAG

Historically, physicians have been perceived as diagnosing, treating, and, if possible, curing disease states. Nurses have been viewed as providing holistic case assessment and patient care and education. However, in recent years there has been a blurring of traditional physician/nurse roles in response to the need for ongoing interventions for individuals with chronic disabling conditions. Nowhere is the importance of such a physician/nurse primary health team effort more apparent than in the delivery of care to individuals with Prader–Willi syndrome (PWS).

This chapter indicates the respective responsibilities of the physician and nurse and focuses on the potential for collaborative efforts in case management that ensure optimal growth and development for this population.

Medical Intervention

The initial problem for a physician on a primary health care team is the establishment of a correct diagnosis of PWS. Criteria for diagnosis have recently been developed (Holm, Cassidy, Butler, et al., 1993) but must be carefully distinguished from similar conditions (Chapter 1). Frequently a referral will be made to a genetics (or sometimes an endocrinology) clinic before a firm diagnosis is made. Typically, a single symptom (e.g., severe neonatal hypotonia, hypogenitalism, developmental delay, or gross obesity) is the rationale for initial evaluation from a primary physician or pediatric nurse-practitioner. Frequently the syndrome goes unrecognized for some time. However, once the proper diagnosis has been established it is critical that the presenting symptoms of PWS be understood as a developmental disability, to provide appropriate management.

The age at which individuals are diagnosed varies considerably (Greenswag & Alexander, 1990). Medical management of PWS requires a clear understanding of the characteristic signs and symptoms of PWS

66

and awareness of the syndrome's traditional delineation as a two-phase clinical course is important (Table 5.1) (Zellweger, 1988). Although this two-phase conceptualization is a convenient clinical guide, it should be kept in mind that not all characteristics of the syndrome show a two-phase progression. For example, changes do not occur in the level of cognitive impairments or structural features.

Developmental Stages of PWS

The developmental course of specific signs and symptoms should be considered in order to better assess their impact on both the child and family. This also aids the physician in evaluating the prognosis for specific symptoms and determining appropriate interventions. Many of the characteristics of PWS, their individual developmental courses, and current management concepts are indicated in Table 5.2.

Although there may be substantial variations, most individuals follow a characteristic course of development that can be divided into fetal, neonatal/infancy, early childhood, late childhood, adolescence, and adulthood periods. Child development within this conceptual framework represents a "cross section" of the changing and interwoven strands of development in much the same way that knowledge of a cross section of the spinal cord complements the knowledge gained about individual longitudinal neural pathways. In practice, the physician uses both strategies to provide anticipatory guidance and plan for future management.

Fetal

Mothers have frequently reported a decrease in fetal activity when compared to other pregnancies. This may reflect the very early onset of both

TABLE 5.1. The two clinical phases of Prader–Willi syndrome.[a]

Phase I	Moderate to severe neonatal hypotonia
	Poor suck
	Difficult feeding
	Hypogonadism
	Marked delay in motor milestones
Phase II	Much less hypotonia
	Short stature
	Hyperphagia
	Increasing obesity
	Labile emotions, stubbornness
	Cognitive limitations

[a] Adapted from H. Zellweger, (1988).

TABLE 5.2. Characteristics, developmental sequence, and intervention for Prader–Willi syndrome.

Characteristic	Developmental Sequence	Intervention
A. Structural		
1. Facial: almond-shaped eyes, triangular-shaped mouth ("fish-mouth"), narrow bifrontal diameter.	Present at birth but more noticeable by several years of age. Nonprogressive and persistent.	Cosmetic surgery not necessary since appearance is not distinctively "abnormal"; contraindicated because of diminished intellectual understanding.
2. Small hands and feet.	Most noticeable by 3–4 years of age. Persists, but nonprogressive.	No problems finding shoes or gloves. No orthopedic shoes.
3. Central fat distribution. Obesity most prominent around stomach, hips, and thighs.	Begins at 18–36 months with noticeable hyperphagia. Prominence depends partly on weight control.	Diet. To a mild extent, will have this abnormal fat distribution even when weight is "normalized."
4. Hypogonadism. Males: cryptorchidism, small testes; short, underdeveloped penis and scrotum. Females: flattened, hypoplastic labia.	Present at birth. Nonprogressive but a more marked contrast with normal individuals during teenage years and beyond.	(See Chapter 3)
5. Short stature. Average adult height: males, 5′0″; females, 4′8″.	May be slightly smaller at birth but more noticeable during elementary school age. Very noticeable during teen years and beyond (no potential "growth spurt").	(See Chapter 3 and Appendix B)
6. Eye problems. More likely to have myopia, strabismus.	May be present at any age. Course similar to that of normal peer group.	Index of suspicion. Should have preschool vision screening and periodic school screening. Surveillance.
B. Regulatory/functional		
1. Hypotonia.	Decreased fetal movements may be severe at birth. Often low Apgars. Poor suck. May need gavage feeding in first 1–2 months. Failure to thrive concern diminishes with age; feeding improves by 12–18 months. Hypotonia persists to mild degree even as adult.	Relationship to possible articulation problems, scoliosis, and respiratory problems likely. Child abuse may be alleged in early failure to thrive stage. May lead to misdiagnosis in infancy (e.g., muscular distrophy), but obesity and lessening of the hypotonia with age rule out neuromuscular diagnoses. Symptomatic treatment.

TABLE 5.2. *Continued*

Characteristic	Developmental Sequence	Intervention
2. Decreased motor skills. Probably combination of hypotonia, decreased cognitive abilities, and deficits in motor planning.	Delayed motor milestones even for mental age. May not walk until 2–3 years. Gross motor skills tend to be more affected than fine motor skills. Tend to "catch up" somewhat during elementary school years, but always remain behind the norm.	Special physical education adaptations useful. Anticipatory guidance for safety issues where motor skills are a factor, such as bicycle riding (see Chapter 8).
3. Thermoregulation. Poor temperature control, usually hypothermia. May have cool hands or feet at times. Poor ability to compensate for heat stress reported anecdotally.	Most troublesome in neonatal period. Less problematic after several months of age; can have high fevers when ill.	Symptomatic treatment. Isolette to maintain temperature is common for newborns.
4. Hyperphagia. The feeding drive often appears insatiable; affected individuals describe it as "hunger."	Not clinically evident for first 18–24 months (possibly masked by the increased hypotonia at earlier ages?). Develops during 18–36 months of age in most cases. Persistent, but nonprogressive beyond mid-childhood.	Diet and external behavioral controls (see Chapters 7 and 9 and Appendix E.1). Weigh weekly (school nurse may help with this). Medications to control appetite have not proven useful to date. Gastric bypass has rarely been successful. Watch for ingestions (poisoning). Locks on refrigerator and cupboards may be necessary. Keep child from eating garbage, dog food, and other atypical "foods." Stealing food may occur and sometimes leads to legal problems.
5. Higher vomiting threshold (less likely to vomit). May not vomit when ill or overeating at the point when others will. However, at least 36% vomit at some point in their life.	May be somewhat more likely to spit up as an infant than later. About two-thirds of those who vomit first do so under 6 years of age.	Ipecac works about 50% of the time—use with caution and watch for toxicity. Consider gastric lavage as alternative.
6. Rumination (at least 10–17%).	No age relationship known.	Behavior management. Overly strict weight control may induce or aggravate rumination.

(Continued)

TABLE 5.2. *Continued*

Characteristic	Developmental Sequence	Intervention
7. Hypoactivity. Physical activities are slow and without wasted efforts.	Begins with decreased fetal activity. Decreased activity at all ages.	Calories not consumed as quickly. Diet must contain fewer calories (see Chapter 7). Exercise program less effective for weight regulation and cardiovascular fitness (see Chapter 8).
8. Decreased sex hormones. No pubertal growth spurt. Sterility. Little or no menstrual flow in female teens and adults. (About Tanner Stage 2.)	Decreased at all ages, although most noticeable difference when teenage and older (essentially no pubertal development).	Affects psychosexuality. Exogenous hormones may affect activity level and/or behavior in unpredictable ways (see Chapters 3 and 13).
9. Sleep/respiratory disturbances. May fall asleep in classrooms (especially in afternoons). Sleep apnea, Pickwickian-like syndrome, and respiratory failure have been observed where weight is not controlled. Snoring may have multiple etiologies (sleep apnea, hypotonia).	Daytime sleepiness more apparent in school-age patient. May increase with age and/or weight.	Weight control may help. Small changes may lead to large effects on day and night disturbances (more so than a "Pickwickian" basis alone). Awareness of sleepiness as a feature of the syndrome is very helpful. Watch for scoliosis leading to respiratory compromise. Sleep apnea testing, CPAP, or tracheostomy may be warranted in extreme cases (Appendix A).
10. Decreased pain responsiveness. Not known if this is a decreased sensitivity to pain, a decreased affect toward pain, or some combination of both.	Apparently constant throughout life.	Expect more minor accidental injuries (bruises, burns), especially given the poorer gross motor skills. In light of decreased cognitive skills, safety issues must be discussed with the care providers.
11. Skin picking. Very frequent; arms, hands, and feet most commonly affected. Stimulus unknown, but decreased pain responsiveness may be an associated factor.	Rare before 5 years of age. Tends to persist at same frequency in a given individual.	Self-injurious behavior modification programs can help. Cut fingernails short and often. Watch for secondary infections.
C. Cognitive		
1. Decreased intelligence. Most often mildly retarded. Parental intelligence may have at least some effect on the levels.	Nonprogressive, but may be difficult to assess at early ages when confounded with poor motor skills and hypotonia.	Appropriate educational programming (see Chapters 9 and 11). Early referral helpful.

TABLE 5.2. *Continued*

Characteristic	Developmental Sequence	Intervention
2. Speech/lanugage deficits. Controversial: language problems may be a symptom of decreased intelligence. Speech may be affected by structural and/or hypotonic abnormalities.	Speech delays typical because of decreased intelligence. Speech/ language problems are apparent at early ages. Variable causes.	Appropriate speech/language programming (see Chapter 10). Early referral helpful.
3. Behavior problems. Stubborness, emotional lability, food-seeking-related behaviors. Often major family stressor.	Unusual before 3 years of age. Tend to intensify over time and then plateau as an adult. Considerable individual variations.	Coupled with the constant food seeking, problem behaviors frequently are the reasons teenagers and young adults go to a supervisored group home. Anticipatory guidance regarding residential care. However, behaviors seldom ceases entirely and goals must be modest. Psychology referral (see Chapter 9).

D. Probable secondary effects

Characteristic	Developmental Sequence	Intervention
1. Poor dentrition. Cause frequently controversial; many believe there are enamel deficits, xerostomia, differences or decreases in saliva. Decreased IQ, poor eating habits, possible rumination, and poor brushing secondary to poor motor skills may contribute.	Multiple caries during early childhood. Progressive.	Floride supplementation as indicated. Watch for rumination. Early referral to dentist (see Chapter 6).
2. Sciolosis. Occasional. Probably a result of hypotonia.	Cases seen in late childhood but most as teenagers. Follows typical pattern and course of idiopathic scoliosis in normals.	Yearly exam from 10 years of age until skeletal growth stops (often early 20's). X-rays if significantly obese or any question. Orthopedic referral if detected.
3. Undescended testes universal in males. Likely due to lack of neonatal/postnatal sex hormones.	Present at birth. Do not spontaneously descend.	Surgery at 4–5 years of age may be considered. No known cases of cancer with untreated cases (see Chapter 3).
4. Diabetes (Type II). Rare; undoubtably due to obesity.	With significant obesity. More likely at older ages, as with normal persons.	Urine screening for all patients beyond 5 years old on a yearly basis. Weight management. Standard diabetic treatment (Chapters 3 and 7).

(Continued)

TABLE 5.2. *Continued*

Characteristic	Developmental Sequence	Intervention
5. Occasionally, heart disease/respiratory compromise. Usually due to morbid obesity, although severe scoliosis may contribute.	In the past, teenagers and young adults died of this. Still more frequent in these ages and beyond.	Weight management. Orthopedic management if appropriate. Symptomatic treatment.
6. Increased bruisability. Often pale skin, poor gross motor skills, decreased, poor muscular fitness, and decreased pain responsiveness may all contribute to increased bruising. Coagulation studies are normal. Bruisability most likely at extreme end of "normal range," not pathological.	Seen with the ambulatory child. May increase when placed in unstructured environments.	Heals normally. Anticipatory guidance regarding safety issues. May complicate any child abuse concerns.

hypotonia and decreased activity levels. The index of suspicion for the presence of PWS is quite low at this time and it is only through incidental amniotic or chorionic chromosomal analysis that the 15th chromosome deletion might be detected. Should a fetus have this chromosomal deletion, there is no known treatment, but genetic counseling is advised (see Chapter 2). It has been estimated that 10–40% of PWS births are breech, which may indicate decreased motor and cognitive abilities. Polyhydramnios is often present. Although the length of gestation is normal, birth weight may be slightly less than average. The birth process itself is relatively unremarkable, with no known reports of an increased rate of fetal distress or delivery complications.

Neonatal/Infancy

The neonate usually manifests severe hypotonia at birth and Apgars tend to be low. Thermoregulation may be a significant problem in the newborn with PWS, and use of an isolette is frequently necessary. Initially, poor suck, "floppiness," and consequent failure to thrive may suggest a variety of diagnostic possibilities. Gavage feeding may be required for the first several weeks of life. Gradually the infant develops sufficient muscle tone to suck efficiently, although increased feeding time and limited consumption may necessitate smaller and more frequent feeds. Occasionally, child abuse (failure to thrive) has been suspected. However, recognition of the hypotonia, which affects the infant's feeding, and may continue into the second 6 months of life usually alters concerns about abuse. Unfortunately given the feeding difficulties, it is possible that a care provider might neglect to feed the child adequately. Confounding physiologic complications like gastroesophageal reflux and iron-deficiency anemia should always be considered and appropriate therapeutic interventions made. Aughton and Cassidy (1990) conducted a retrospective study to identify physical features of neonates with Prader–Willi syndrome. Proper nutrition and specific feeding methods should be reviewed frequently. Regular immunization should begin, but no special indication exists for influenza or pneumococcal vaccines during infancy or childhood.

Early Childhood

By 18 months to 3 years of age feeding difficulties have been replaced by hyperphagia (Greenswag & Alexander, 1990). Initially this increased appetite is welcomed by parents, physicians, and nurses, who vividly recall earlier feeding problems. Unfortunately, this sense of relief may delay the recognition of the emerging problem of obesity. The combination of short stature, hyperphagia, and obesity usually results in a referral to medical specialists able to diagnose PWS. As the hypotonia diminishes, these children increase their motor skills and learn to walk between the age of 2 and 3 years. This also is the time when consideration may be given to surgery for undescended testes in preschool males. Dental problems often begin to appear that may be related to poor brushing skills (due to decreased cognition and fine motor skills), intrinsic defects, the type and amount of consumed food, and, in some instances, the ability to ruminate (Alexander, Greenswag, & Nowak, 1987) (see Chapter 6).

Early educational intervention is important because cognitive and motor delays, and possible speech/language difficulties should be addressed. Most children begin to display stubbornness and other aberrant behavior by 3–5 years of age (Greenswag & Alexander, 1990). Anticipatory guidance should include education of the providers about potential obesity and behavioral issues. Appropriate referral for nutritional counseling should be made. Marked dietary restrictions necessitate supplemental vitamins and minerals; cases of iron-deficiency anemia have been seen in balanced diets that are very limited in quantity. Because persons with PWS are less active, sufficient calcium and vitamin D are essential to reduce the possibility of osteoporosis later in life (see also Chapters 3 and 7). Questions about administration of growth hormone to increase stature begin to arise during this period (see Chapter 3).

Late Childhood

Without careful management, there will be excessive weight gain. In a study of children with PWS in the United States and Canada between 7 and 11 years of age, 83% were reported as massively obese (greater than

2 standard deviations above the 95th percentile of weight for height) and 8% were obse (Greenswag & Alexander, 1990). Some children get up at night to forage for food, and as their motor skills increase, they are more able to climb and defeat simple attempts at restricting access to food. Close observation sometimes works, but by this age many families must resort to chains or locks on refrigerators and cupboards. Motion detectors or other electronic devices may be helpful and are a much better alternative than locking the child in his room.

Behaviors such as stubbornness and temper outbursts begin to intensify. School becomes a prime focus of activity in late childhood, and appropriate classroom placement is essential (usually special education). Placement may be confounded by problems such as verbal or physical aggressiveness. Often children with PWS are given food by their peers or find some other way to obtain it. Such behavior can alter social settings such as the school lunchroom. Short stature, poor gross motor skills, obesity, mental retardation, and underdeveloped genitalia can result in painful teasing by other children, causing further isolation and stigmatization. Skin picking and falling asleep in the classroom may be noted. Anticipatory guidance should include appropriate counseling of parents and school personnel. The school psychologist frequently will need to coordinate behavior management at school and home (see Chapters 9 and 11).

Obese children should have periodic urinalyses to check for proteinuria or glucosuria and blood pressure should be monitored. Weekly weight checks are appropriate and any significant deviations should be reported. Weight-for-height curves are particularly useful, and successful weight management results in a child who is within at least the upper-normal percentiles.

The presence of a child with PWS on overall family functioning, particularly in regard to other siblings, may be detrimental. Family counseling, support groups, or help from PWSA chapters can avert more serious difficulties (see Chapter 12).

Adolescence

Attention to secondary effects of obesity continues into adolescence. Scoliosis may be observed, and usually follows the same course of "idiopathic" scoliosis as in normal teenagers. It is uncertain whether the typical mild hypotonia or osteoporosis seen with PWS contributes additional risks (see Chapter 3). There may be a somewhat longer period of risk because skeletal maturation may not be complete until the early to mid-20s.

Teenagers with PWS do not have the "growth spurt" or surge of sex hormones as non-PWS developmentally disabled or normal peers. Without exogenous hormone intervention, males and females usually do not progress beyond physical and public hair development consistent with a Tanner Stage 2. Females may have occasional spotting but true menstrual periods do not occur. The obvious physical differences between PWS and normal teenagers can cause emotional distress. For boys, testosterone supplementation may reduce the appearance of immature genitalia and increase the growth of body hair, although problems with short stature remain. The lack of reproductive capacity for both sexes is discussed in Chapter 3. Although this simplifies parental concerns about birth control for this mentally handicapped population, sex education is still important. While pregnancy is not an issue, education about the risk of sexually transmitted diseases is vital. Such education should be developmentally appropriate with the focus on interpersonal skills and relationships and incorporation of parental values (see Chapter 13).

School concerns, both academic and behavioral, continue (see Chapters 9 and 11) and vocational training is important (see Chapter 16). As teenagers become physically larger and often more frustrated, they may intimidate other family members or prove more difficult to control. Many parents begin to acknowledge the need for out-of-home placement (see Chapter 15). Anticipatory guidance should emphasize the need to make legal preparations such as wills and assignment of guardianship prior to the age of majority (see Chapter 14).

Adulthood

In the past, complications of morbid obesity (e.g., diabetes, cardiac or respiratory complications) doomed nearly all affected individuals to die young. Increased awareness of the syndrome and more aggressive attention to its management have significantly reduced the likelihood of early death. It is no longer inevitable that adults with PWS will be obese and information about this stage of life is beginning to accumulate. It is now known that skin picking, behavior problems, and food seeking persist. When seeking food, the adult-aged person with PWS may steal money and/or food. To avoid court adjudication, it is necessary to explain to proper authorities the "addictive" nature of the eating disorder, the cognitive limitations, and the inappropriateness of incarceration to remediate these behaviors Greenswag (1984, 1987), in a survey of 232 individuals with PWS ages 16 years and beyond, found that those few who attempted to live independently were significantly more obese than those living in a more restrictive setting. In most instances the persistent food-seeking behaviors, the need for peer stimulation and work, and the stress to the family usually lead to an out-of-home placement. Just as with any other developmentally disabled adult, psychosexual adaptation, interpersonal relationships, and vocational training are important. Meaningful opportunities to contribute to society should be encouraged.

The elderly adult with PWS is not well understood. The impact of the lifelong fight with obesity, the hypotonia, the difficulty in attaining cardiovascular fitness, and the natural history of the syndrome itself will become more apparent in the decades to come. Although one woman with PWS lived to be 65, life expectancy probably is shorter than normal, as is true for other cognitively limited populations. It is possible that specific medical problems may emerge in the elderly PWS population (e.g., osteoporosis, respiratory difficulties, circulatory problems).

Nursing Interventions

As professional who "care for" and "teach," nurses incorporate concepts of physical and emotional growth and development, family, environments, and society into intervention strategies. Whether in a tertiary, community, or school setting, pediatric nurse-practitioners (PNPs), school nurses, or community health nurses, with their holistic perspective on health care, are in an optimum position to aid in coordination of case management. They may also function as a source for information and support.

Once the initial diagnosis of PWS is made, attention should be directed not only to current symptomatology and medical treatment, but also to the development and maintenance of the optimum health and enhancement of family stability. Nursing interventions that best meet these goals are based on the following:

1. Documentation of the child's physical and behavioral condition.
2. Recognition that the developmental processes of children with PWS differ significantly from the majority of children.
3. Ongoing assessment of health needs throughout the life span.
4. An understanding of the degree to which the physical and emotional/behavioral dimensions of PWS impact on the family system. Evaluation of family dynamics and potential problem areas.
5. An awareness that in addition to alterations in lifestyle, problems with social interactions, spousal difficulties, and indifferent public attitudes, the presence of PWS imposes considerable financial burdens.
6. An awareness that many disciplines are involved in providing care, that confusion can occur, about delivery of services and that the nurse can help "make sense of it all."

Strategies for nursing interventions begin with compilation of a nursing history. This process, initiated during the first visit, includes a review of the diagnosis of PWS and a baseline health assessment that takes into account growth parameters, a physical examination, and a review of laboratory studies. Observation should incorporate photographing the child; this provides a permanent record that is useful in future consultation and retrospective review. Next, data collection should focus on feeding problems and interventions, since weight/height information is critical to nutritional planning. Personal hygiene, grooming, skin care, and any indication of self-injurious behaviors (skin picking or hair pulling) should be noted along with assessment of the child's capacity for self-health care. Careful evaluation of adaptive function is necessary since emotional ability, inappropriate behaviors, alterations in thought processes, and poor social skills are frequently observed and provide important background for psychological management.

Assessment of patient/care provider knowledge and perceptions about PWS in critical and requires that the nurse evaluate parenting skills. Safety factors in the living environment and evaluation of the child's cognitive capacity for judgement in hazardous situations require ongoing review. Certainly, availability of food is a major issue that affects the child's health status and the family's ability to cope. Nursing diagnosis, interventions, and indications of positive outcomes to presenting problems are described in Table 5.3.

Counseling and anticipatory guidance for health-related matters are essential nursing interventions. This includes teaching about routine health issues such as feeding, toilet training, accident prevention (particularly since there is evidence that many children with PWS have decreased response to pain), personal hygiene, skin care, and emotional ability. Teaching guidelines are listed in Table 5.4.

Family stability and parental coping mechanisms require sensitive management. Pediatric nurse practitioners who are members of tertiary clinic teams, choral and community nurses should look for opportunities to organize and facilitate parent discussion groups. Follow-up visits should be encouraged to collect interval health history information, monitor growth and development, assess current status, and detect any new health problems. Any family problems and/or new concerns should result in appropriate referral to other medical and allied disciplines.

The Physician/Nurse Primary Health Care Team

Delivery of primary health care to individuals with PWS is the responsibility of the physician and nurse team, and the multidimensional aspects of the syndrome call for a holistic approach based on the collaborative efforts of both disciplines. Integration of the expertise and skills of both professions is the keystone to achieving workable case management strategies. Examples of teamwork include comparing physical assessment data, exchanging historical information, discussing laboratory results, and identifying the need for other interdisciplinary services. Whether focusing on a specific symptom over time or a set of symptoms at a given age, the physician/nurse team can aid the patient and family by supplying information, guarding against fads or "cures" (e.g., eliminating sugar in the diet

TABLE 5.3. Nursing diagnoses, interventions, and indications of positive outcomes for individuals with Prader–Willi syndrome.[a]

Nursing diagnoses	Nursing interventions	Indications of positive outcomes
Alteration in nutrition: caloric intake greater than body requirements	Teach parents/caregivers to lock refrigerators, freezers, and any cabinets where food is stored Search for hidden edibles Weigh daily until weight goals are reached, then twice weekly Supervise and observe frequently Collaborate with dietary specialists Instruct caregivers for newborns in methods of administering nasogastric feedings or use of other feeding aids Assist in teaching prescribed diet to caregivers Stress importance of maintaining diet and of reporting inability to maintain appropriate weight Teach integration of exercise into overall care plan	Maintains established weight within a range of up to two standard deviations above norms of each individual's weight for height
Impairment of skin integrity, both actual and potential	Provide skin care Encourage personal hygiene Discourage self-injurious behaviors, such as skin-picking and tearing at healing wounds by adequate covering of affected areas and protective clothing	Wounds heal completely Good hygiene is maintained Patient demonstrates decreased self-injury
Disturbance in self-concept: body image and self-esteem	Encourage self-care and responsibility Offer positive reinforcement for successful behaviors	Verbalizes improved feelings of self-worth Shows pride in self-care Demonstrates ability to cope with limitations of highest level of functional ability Family participates in socialization experiences Patient participates in socialization experiences Patient participates in developmentally appropriate activities with others

TABLE 5.3. *Continued*

Nursing diagnoses	Nursing interventions	Indications of positive outcomes
Alteration in thought processes	Reduce confusing stimuli Set limits Provide a safe environment Structure daily living activities	Behaviors are appropriate for identified levels of cognitive function Remains free of harm to self, others, and property of others Demonstrates social behavior and positive coping mechanisms expected for intellectual and emotional age

[a] From *J. Ped. Health Care*, 4(1), 36 (1990). Adapted with permission from *Endocrine and Metabolic Systems* by Anderson, Bosmaas, Boykin, et al., 1986, in J.M. Thompson et al., *Clinical Nursing* (p. 922), St. Louis: C.V. Mosby. Reprinted by permission of the Prader-Willi Syndrome Association, St. Louis Park, Minnesota.

to control behavior), supporting other family members, and intervening at the early stages of specific symptoms. It should also be noted that the primary health care team process need not be limited to tertiary clinic settings. Physicians and nurses at the community level should plan to network their services.

In summary, the importance of a physician/nurse primary health team cannot be understated. The professional tasks of each discipline comple-

TABLE 5.4. Teaching guidelines for nurses who care for individuals with Prader–Willi syndrome.[a]

Instruct care providers for newborns in methods of administering nasogastric feedings or use of other feeding aids
Assist in teaching prescribed diet to care providers
Stress importance of maintaining diet and reporting of signs and symptoms of exacerbation of weight
Instruct care providers in maintaining skin integrity and daily hygiene.
Teach integration of exercise into overall care program.
Stress importance of the following and assist in planning for
    Continual supervision and observation
    Educational and environmental stimulation
    Setting of behavioral expectations and limits
Inform care providers about and econourage use of support and counseling groups
Ensure that care providers know about community resources available to assist with compliance

[a] From Endocrine and Metabolic Systems by Anderson, Bosmaas, Boykin et al., 1986, in J.M. Thompson et al., *Clinical nursing* (p. 922), St. Louis: C.V. Mosby. Adapted by permission.

ment one another and collaboration provides the basis for optimal case management.

References

Alexander, R.C., Greenswag, L.R., & Nowak, A. (1987). Rumination and vomiting in Prader-Willi syndrome. *American Journal of Medical Genetics*, *28*, 889–895.

Anderson, L., Bosmaas, C., Boykin, P., Choate, T., DiGiorgi, D., Drass, J., Hench, K., Long, J., McAtee, A., Robbins, P., Solomon, R., & Wells, M. (1986). Endocrine and metabolic systems. In J. Thompson, G. McFarland, J. Hirsch, S. Tucker, & A. Bowers (Eds.), *Clinical nursing* (pp. 823–942). St. Louis: C.V. Mosby.

Aughton, D.J., & Cassidy, S.B. (1990). Physical features of Prader-Willi syndrome in neonates. *AJDC*, *144*, 1251–1254.

Greenswag, L.R. (1984). *The adult with Prader-Willi syndrome: A descriptive investigation*. Doctoral thesis, University of Iowa. (DA 056952, University Microfilms International, Ann Arbor, MI.)

Greenswag, L.R. (1987). Adults with Prader-Willi syndrome: A survey of 232 cases. *Developmental Medicine and Child Neurology*, *29*, 145–152.

Greenswag, L.R., & Alexander, R.C. (1990). Early diagnosis in Prader-Willi syndrome: Implications for managing weight and behavior. *Dysmorphology and Clinical Genetics*, *4*(1), 8–12.

Holm, V.A., Cassidy, S.B., Butler, M.G., Hanchett, J.M., Greenswag, L.R., Whitman, B.Y., & Greenberg, F. (1993). Prader-Willi syndrome: Consensus diagnostic criteria. *Pediatrics*, *19*, 398–402.

Zellweger, H. (1988). Differential diagnosis in Prader-Willi syndrome. In L.R. Greenswag & R.C. Alexander (Eds.), *Management of Prader-Willi syndrome* (pp. 15–22). New York: Springer-Verlag.

6
Dental Manifestations and Management

ARTHUR J. NOWAK

Dentists and their staffs should be active members of all interdisciplinary heath teams serving Prader–Willi syndrome (PWS). Interaction with the patient and family should begin no later than the time of the eruption of the first tooth. Only then can the benefits of a comprehensive dental health program be fully enjoyed and the effects of oral disease reduced or even eliminated. The major role of the dental team is to provide early preventative counseling, indicated treatment, and periodic follow-up. Too frequently the dental team is called upon to interact with the patient only after complaints of oral discomfort or just prior to entering the educational system, when an oral examination is requested.

As an active member of the health team, the dentist provides comprehensive evaluation of the oral–facial system. Because this system is associated with many important physiological processes it important that it be maintained in an excellent state of health and, if already ravaged by disease, restored to health. The patient must be evaluated during the initial team interaction, not as a secondary examination. The results of the dental examination then become part of the initial assessment of the patient and can be included in the individualized plan and prioritized.

Compromising conditions and limitations imposed by the presence of PWS increase the risk of dental disease. The syndrome requires modification of diet and may have direct oral manifestations. Medical therapy may alter expected growth and development, and required dental care may be delayed or withheld because of social and financial considerations.

Dental interaction continues throughout the patient's involvement with the team. Because dental disease is a continuing risk that varies with age and medical status, PWS patients require evaluation and continuing supervision that are best monitored by the dentist during periodic visits.

Dental–Oral Characteristics of PWS

The dental literature is void of any comprehensive studies of the dental characteristics of the PWS patient. The few references (Foster, 1971; Hart, 1994; Krautmann, Barenie, & Myers, 1981) available are primarily case studies. The most frequently reported findings are delayed eruption, hypoplastic enamel, rampant caries, and abnormal saliva. Secondary findings include micrognathia (small jaw), high arched palate, microdontia (small teeth), and xerostomia (dry mouth). Fourteen patients with the diagnosis of PWS are currently being followed at the dental clinic of The University of Iowa. They consist of seven males and seven females, ranging in age from 3 to 24 years. Ten of the 14 patients reside in communities with optimally fluoridated water. The most common oral finding is generalized marginal gingivitis secondary to poor oral hygiene (Figure 6.1). Dental caries is a minor problem, with most patients having decay rates similar to non-PWS patients. However, one male had all of his teeth removed and dentures inserted at 19 years of age, as a result of caries and fractured teeth (Figure 6.1). Other common findings in this group have been crowding, malocclusions, enamel attrition, and grinding.

Rumination and vomiting have recently been reported as a finding in patients with PWS (Alexander, Greenswag, & Nowak, 1987). In these cases enamel decalcification and erosion may have placed the teeth at greater risks for caries. Additionally, with loss of enamel tooth sensitivity has been reported, especially to acidic foods and cold liquids. Nonoral/dental characteristics of PWS may affect the oral health and management of the patient, both in and out of the office. The characteristic constant eating by PWS patients greatly increases the availability of fermentable carbohydrates necessary to the development of dental caries. Increased dietary intake coupled with crowded dental arches results in food retention and increased plaque formation, leading to gingival irritation and inflammation.

Developmental delay and/or mental retardation in PWS compromise management. The patient may not be able to comprehend how to practice daily oral hygiene, manual dexterity necessary to manipulate the toothbrush and dental floss may be minimal, and modification of dietary practices may be impossible—all of which increase the risk for oral disease.

Assessment

Assessing the dental health status of the PWS patient requires an oral examination, since no laboratory or diagnostic tests are available. Only through evaluation of the hard and soft tissues will it be possible to determine the presence or absence of disease.

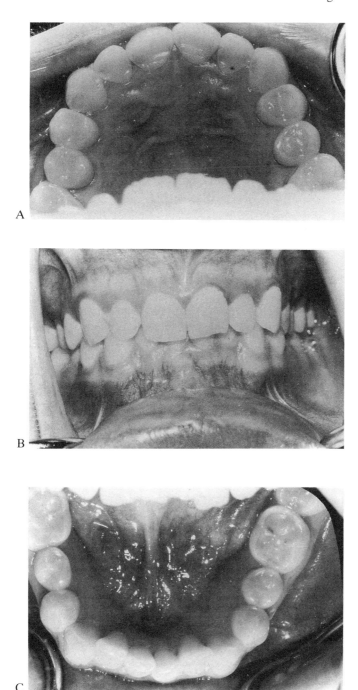

FIGURE 6.1. (A–C) Oral manifestations of Prader Willi Syndrome in a teenage patient. Note areas of marginal gingivitis and enamel erosion.

It has been suggested that certain populations are at higher risk for dental disease. Although PWS patients have many high-risk characteristics, the literature remains inconclusive as to their actual oral problems. The one major PWS characteristic, overeating, undoubtedly is the major risk factor.

A thorough history is important. Information on the eruption dates and sequencing of the erupting teeth is helpful. History of trauma to the face and mouth should be obtained. Dietary habits, especially eating frequencies and types of foods consumed, are important. Fluoride intake, either from the community water or through supplements, should be reviewed, as should oral hygiene practices, including the number of times each day brushing takes place, the kind of brush, the type of dentifrice, and whether it is supervised or performed by a parent. Question whether the patient has any sucking, chewing, or swallowing problems. Are some foods more difficult than others? Does the patient appear to have or complain of a dry mouth? Does the patient demonstrate habits such as nonnutritive sucking or tooth grinding (day, night, or both)? Does the patient complain of facial muscle pain or discomfort in the area anterior to the ear? Is there a history of repeated vomiting and holding food in the mouth? A family dental history, including siblings and parents, is important.

If the first oral examination happens to occur at or around the time of eruption of the first primary tooth, the examination is relatively short and will be a pleasant experience for the infant. If the diagnosis is not made until after all the teeth erupt, and if the patient has had some unpleasant experiences in the health delivery setting, the oral examination may be more difficult.

The developmental and mental status of the patient will thus influence the examination process. Some patients may be combative or resistant. The length of appointments may have to be decreased because of short attention spans and overactivity. Obesity may make it difficult for patients to be comfortable in the dental chair, and because of the reported micrognathia, small oral opening, and the increase in adipose tissue around the face, oral examination may be compromised. Nevertheless, PWS patients should be able to be managed with minimal difficulty by a knowledgeable team, regardless of age. The older patients (school age) are more inquisitive and require additional explanations, a little more time, and considerable positive reinforcement. For patients with extensive needs, management may consist of treatment in the dental office with local anesthesia and/or conscious sedation management. Finding the necessary landmarks for the administration of local anesthesia may be difficult because of the limited oral openings and the excessive oral tissues. Treatment with general anesthesia in the hospital or ambulatory surgical center may be necessary.

As with all patients, a dental team familiar with PWS will make the visit pleasant, efficient, and productive. Parents/guardians should inform the clinic or office coordinator of the child's diagnosis, the developmental level, whether the patient has ever had an oral examination (and if so, where and when), if the patient is presently in any oral pain, and if there are any additional medical problems present. This information allows the dental staff to prepare for the visit, and, if the patient was examined previously, contact the previous office for past history and radiographs.

When examining infants, the knee-to-knee position (between the dentist and parent), with the patient straddled in the cradle developed by the upper legs, is ideal. The parent will have an excellent view of the examination as well as be able to participate in the exam. With increasing age, positioning the patient in a dental chair is appropriate. It may be difficult for obese patients with PWS to lie in a supine position because of the weight and pressure on the upper body; reclining the chair slowly, allowing the patient to adjust, may help. It may be necessary to keep the chair at a 45° angle to the floor rather than the traditional 180°. With time, most patients gain confidence and adjust very nicely to the traditional position.

If the oral opening is limited, and if the excessive tissues intrude into the mouth, additional time will be necessary to complete an examination. If radiographs are indicated, the age-appropriate size of film may not be able to be used. Use the next smallest film size instead.

Treatment and Follow-up

After completion of the examination, an individualized treatment plan is developed. A comprehensive preventative program is initiated, including use of optimal systemic and topical fluorides and daily oral hygiene by the patient and/or parent/guardian. Because dietary intake and frequency are major findings that affect not only the patient's general medical status but oral health as well, discussion with the rest of the members of the team is indicated. Dietary guidelines must be developed that will respond to both the medical and dental concerns (Kriz & Cloninger, 1981).

If dental treatment is indicated, the patient's behavior needs to be anticipated. The use of local anesthesia, mouthprops, and a rubber dam will assist the team to isolate the areas to be treated and help the patient keep his or her mouth open. If administration of the local anesthetic, especially the inferior alveolar and the posterior alveolar nerve blocks, is difficult, consideration should be given to alternatives, including the periodontal ligament injection. As indicated earlier, for extensive treatment and/or the apprehensive or uncontrollable patient, consideration should be given to a general anesthetic.

Follow-up should be scheduled as per the individual needs of the patient, but at least semiannually. Because poor oral hygiene is widespread, parents/guardians must be involved with the patient daily in preventing it. They should participate actively in *cleaning* the teeth, not just in passively observing that the patient is brushing. In addition to the use of the toothbrush, dental floss, and a dentrifice, consideration should be given to other plaque-reducing methods. Oral rinses with bactericidal properties are now available that may be indicated as a supplement to daily oral hygiene. If the patient has a history of vomiting and rumination, extra attention should be paid at home to additional cleaning and frequent rinsing to rid the mouth of stomach acids and partially digested foods. If decalcification is noted, topically applied fluoride should be considered on a daily schedule. If the decalcified areas progress to cavitation, full coverage with stainless steel crowns (in the primary dentition) may be indicted. Periodic follow-ups should be scheduled no less than every 6 months, and more frequently if other risk factors are identified, such as hypoplastic enamel, rumination, vomiting, or poor oral hygiene.

If the health care of the patient is managed by a team, communication between members is facilitated by the usual reporting process. If treatment is performed independently, changes in history or any treatments should be reported to the primary health care provider, who must keep the dental team informed of the patient's systemic conditions as well as of major changes taking place in medications and diet.

Summary

It has been reported that dental caries is generally decreasing in school-age children in the United States, due largely to fluoridation and increased awareness of the importance of oral health. PWS patients can enjoy the same benefits if modifications in oral management can be recommended and carried out. It is important for the dentist, as a member of the health team, to be able to make appropriate recommendations. Early intervention, initiation of a comprehensive preventative program, and scheduled follow-up may ensure that PWS patients can enjoy optimal oral health.

References

Alexander, R.C., Greenswag, L., & Nowak, A. (1987). Rumination and vomiting in Prader-Willi syndrome. *American Journal of Medical Genetics, 28*, 889–895.

Foster, S. (1971). Prader-Willi syndrome: Report of cases. *Journal of the American Dental Association, 83*, 634–638.

Hart, S. (1994). The oral manifestations of Prader-Willi syndrome: A review of the literature and results of a parent-reported questionnaire. *Prader-Willi Perspectives, 2*, 7–10.

Krautmann, P.J., Barenie, J.T., & Myers, D.R. (1981). Clinical manifestations of Prader-Willi syndrome. *Journal of Pedodontics*, *5*, 256–261.

Kriz, S., & Cloninger, B.J. (1981). Management of a patient with Prader-Willi syndrome by a dental-dietary team. *Special Care in Dentistry*, *1*, 179–182.

7
Nutritional Management

Diane D. Stadler

Two extremes of inappropriate growth impact on the nutritional management of individuals with Prader–Willi syndrome (PWS): failure to thrive and morbid obesity. Infants with PWS present as hypotonic, with insufficient suck and swallow reflexes, and failing to thrive. Sometime after 1 year of age, short stature, hyperphagia, and obesity become evident as well as an insatiable, nonselective appetite. Left untreated, adolescents and adults with PWS become morbidly obese and at increased risk of diabetes mellitus, hypertension, cardiopulmonary disease, respiratory distress, cyanosis, and sleep apnea. The severity of the associated health problems is directly associated with the degree of obesity and these problems resolve when the individual returns to an ideal weight range. Because of these obesity-associated health problems, individuals with PWS, at any age, require nutritional intervention. The nutritionist, as a member of a multidisciplinary health care team, assesses the nutritional status of individuals with PWS, develops dietary recommendations that promote appropriate linear growth and weight gain, educates care providers so they may successfully implement dietary recommendations, and provides ongoing support.

Typical Findings

Infants with PWS usually experience feeding difficulties throughout the first year of life. They often fail to awaken for feeding sessions, and when finally aroused are listless and demonstrate poor rooting reflex, weak suck at breast or bottle, and poor head and neck control. Alone, or in any combination, these characteristics place the infant with PWS at risk for consuming insufficient energy and nutrients, which results in poor weight gain. Adequate energy intake may be facilitated by early transition from breast to bottle feeding of either expressed breast milk or commercial infant formula. Latex nipples should be used and the openings enlarged. Short frequent feedings, concentrated formula, and/or supplementation of expressed breast milk is suggested. If necessary, short-term nasogastric or orogastric tube feedings may be initiated.

Between 1 and 2 years of age the severe hypotonia of early infancy resolves and affected children gradually develop the musculature, coordination, and stamina to complete feeding sessions and to consume sufficient energy to promote adequate weight gain. Once weight gain commences, care providers (usually parents) become pleased and relieved with the ease and success of feedings, and mealtimes become positive experiences for the family. Unfortunately, if the strategies described above to promote weight gain during the initial hypotonic phase of the disorder continue into the second phase of the disorder, morbid obesity results within months.

Obesity is the most prominent physical characteristic of PWS and occurs in 94% of all affected individuals (Butler, 1990). Of those affected, one-third or 33% weigh more than 200% of their estimated ideal body weight (Schoeller, Levitcky, Bandini, et al., 1988). Obesity results from a combination of events. In instances where the diagnosis of PWS is not established early, traditional dietary guidelines are recommended. These recommendations, along with the parents' emotional need to follow a regimented feeding schedule, the child's limited capacity for physical activity, lack of satiety, and ability to gain weight on significantly fewer calories promote excessive fat deposition and weight gain. In addition, any one or a combination of the following inappropriate behaviors contribute to excessive weight gain: creative food seeking, stealing, foraging, hoarding, gorging, and the consumption of nonfood items (Pica). Environments or work conditions that tempt individuals with PWS to these aberrant behaviors must be avoided.

Causes of Obesity—Decreased Energy Expenditure

Obesity is typically defined as being overweight with respect to height and body frame size and results when more energy is consumed than expended. Energy is consumed in the form of food and beverages and is expended by physical exercise and physiological functions such as maintaining heart rate and breathing, and digesting and absorbing food. The components of energy intake and expenditure have been explored, albeit in relatively few studies, to help elucidate the cause of obesity in individuals with PWS. Understanding the causes of obesity in this syndrome helps multidisciplinary team members target treatment strategies to specific problem areas.

Basal Metabolic Rate

When energy consumed equals energy expended then body weight is maintained. When energy consumed exceeds energy expended then weight gain occurs. Basal metabolic rate (BMR), the amount of energy used to maintain physiological function while resting, is normal among individuals with PWS when expressed per unit of body surface area, a function of weight and height (Nelson, Anderson, Gastineau, et al., 1973). BMR is reduced among individuals with PWS by 20% when expressed per unit of height, and reduced by 50% when expressed per unit of weight (Widhalm, Veltt, & Irsigle, 1981). BMR measured in 36 children with PWS and 31 unaffected children (20 normal weight, 11 obese) was significantly lower among PWS adolesscents than either the unaffected normal weight or obese children: 44, 59, and 70 kcal/hr, respectively. The lower BMR of children with PWS was attributed in part to decreased fat-free body mass (FFM), the metabolically active tissue responsible for resting energy expenditure. Adipose tissue does not contribute significantly to energy expenditure. Comparable results were reported by Schoeller et al. (1988), who observed similar BMR/kg FFM but lower FFM/kg body weight among individuals with PWS than obese individuals.

Thermogenic Response to Food

Thermogenic response to food- or diet-induced thermogenesis is the energy expended with the digestion and absorption of food. Thermogenic response to food has not been assessed in the PWS population, however, it has been assessed in the obese population. Segal, Gutin, Albu et al. (1987) compared the thermogenic response to food among lean (12.8% body fat) and obese (29.6% body fat) individuals of similar FFM, age, and height. BMR, determined by indirect calorimetry, was similar between the lean and obese groups. Thermogenic response to food, however, was lower among the obese individuals. It was noted that exercise performed prior to a meal accentuated the energy expended by digestion and metabolism of food among the obese individuals. In contrast, exercise following the meal potentiated the thermogenic response to food among the lean individuals. Because FFM was similar in this study the authors suggest that the differences in thermogenic response to food may be due to the difference in the amount of body fat. Insulin sensitivity may also contribute to the observed differences. These findings may have significance for the PWS population because exercise in relation to meal time impacts on total energy expenditure, and subsequent weight gain.

Physical Activity

The contribution of physical activity to total energy expenditure was considered in two studies. Energy expended by individuals with PWS performing a step-test was normal suggesting normal work efficiency (Nelson, Anderson, Gastineau, et al., 1973). However, in a report by

Nardella, Sulzbacher, and Worthington-Roberts (1983) activity levels among individuals with PWS were very low to normal. Subjects in the latter study participated in a summer camp program during which they consumed a diet providing 1,000 kcal/day (23% fat, 23% protein, and 54% carbohydrate) for 1 to 2 weeks. All participants either lost or maintained weight. The heaviest individuals tended to lose the most weight and more weight was lost during the first week than the second week of the program. Those who lost the most weight were not necessarily the most active as assessed by pedometer and acrometer readings suggesting that factors other than physical activity affected weight loss. Two issues complicated this study. The effect of caloric intake on weight loss was not controlled and individuals with severe scoliosis requiring Harrington rod placement, or other means of bracing that inhibits activity, were not excluded. These two studies suggest that, as a group, individuals with PWS are somewhat inactive but that their physical activity is as energy consuming as physical activity performed by those unaffected.

Body Composition

Body composition of individuals with PWS has been determined by various methods including skinfold thickness, total body water, and bioelectrical impedance analysis (BIA). Hill, Kaler, Spetalnick, et al. (1990) determined body composition by BIA and by sum of skinfold thickness measurements (triceps, subscapular, and suprailiac). The correlation coefficient of the two methods was 0.80, 0.91, and 0.74 for lean and obese unaffected individuals and for individuals with PWS, respectively, suggesting that skinfold analysis is an appropriate way to estimate percentage of body fat in obese individuals with or without PWS. Body composition, expressed as FFM/kg body weight, was similar in obese individuals and subjects with PWS, both of which were different from lean subjects. The authors also report increased FFM with increased body weight and suggest that at any given body weight, individuals with PWS are not fatter than unaffected obese individuals. These results differ from those of Schoeller et al. (1988) who determined total body water by the deuterium dilution method. Body fat was between 27 and 42% among individuals with PWS who were within 117–142% of their ideal body weight for height–age and FFM decreased as body weight increased suggesting that individuals with PWS are fatter than their weight-matched non-affected peers. The difference in results seen in these two studies may be due to differences in age and percent body fat of the subjects, definition of ideal body weight, and methodology. Using yet another technique, Meaney and Butler (1989) estimated percent of body fat in adults (>18 years) with PWS by TSF measurements. The average percent body fat in affected adults was 29% (5 males, 4 females). When determined by gender, the average percent body fat was 22.3% for males and 37.5% for females. Percent body fat of children 8–18 years of age based on TSF and mid-calf skinfold thickness was 47% [12 males (50.8%), 8 females (41.5%)]. When the adults and children were considered together, the average percent body fat was 41.5% [17 males (42.4%), 12 females (40.2%)]. The authors concluded that the skinfold measurements were abnormally high and that the calf skinfold measurements deviated the most from the norm, suggesting that excess fat is deposited in the distal limbs as well as the truncal region. They also observed greater fat deposition by males than females with PWS on all measurements, which is the opposite of the pattern of fat deposition in unaffected individuals. In general, males with PWS deposit approximately three times as much fat as unaffected males whereas females with PWS deposit approximately two times as much fat as unaffected females. The differences in fat deposition between males and females with PWS were most pronounced in the limbs and least apparent in the truncal region. The average percent body fat of 41.5% observed by Meaney and Butler (1989) was considerably lower than the 52% body fat of PWS individuals reported by Nelson, Huse, Holman et al. (1981). Meaney and Butler (1989) suspect that percent body fat was underestimated by their choice of skinfold measurement sites. Underestimation of percent body fat by skinfold measurement is supported by Schoeller et al. (1988), who report that determination of body fat by skinfold thickness measurement underestimates the actual value by 16%.

Body fat distribution in PWS has been described as atypical, unusual, and resembling the distribution of adipose tissue in females (Holm, Sulzbacher, & Pipes, 1981). Although body fat in individuals with PWS appears to be distributed in the truncal region, few studies have actually measured body fat at various sites. Early descriptions of individuals with PWS suggested that fat is deposited primarily in the trunk, buttocks, and proximal limb regions. Zellweger and Soper (1979) included in their description of abnormal fat distribution the forearms and lower leg. Meaney and Butler (1987) assessed fat distribution by skinfold thickness in 40 individuals with PWS (23 males, 7 females; 2 to 39 years of age). Sites of measurement included the triceps, forearm, subscapular abdomen, suprailiac, thigh, and mid-calf. Skinfold measurements were converted to Z-score values to control the effects of age and gender and data were compared between males and females and between individuals with and without the 15q11–13 deletion. Percent body fat was calculated using triceps skinfold thickness in adults and triceps skinfold and calf skinfold thickness in adolescents and children. After 3 years of age, TSF is almost always above the 90th percentile, except when an individual is maintained under very strict dietary management. Similar patterns were seen with the subscapular, suprailiac, forearm, and calf skinfold measurements. No differences were detected between the deletion and nondeletion groups. Significant differences in fat distribution existed between the males and females in that skinfold measurements were larger at each site in males than females. The largest differences were at limb sites and the smallest differences were at truncal sites. There is no tendency for weight or skinfold Z-scores to change with age, suggesting that degree of obesity does not change with age. Measurement of circumference at various sites suggested a similar pattern of fat distribution between males and females.

Meaney and Butler (1989) suggest that increased fat stores are present before the child with PWS becomes overweight. Obesity, defined as triceps skinfold measurements (TSF) greater than the 85th percentile, was present in a female toddler with PWS during the first year of life as her weight for age increased from the 5th to 50th percentile. A similar trend was noted in a 3-year-old boy whose TSF was above the 95th percentile while his weight for age was less than the 50th percentile. Butler, Butler, & Meaney (1988) reported the first prospective longitudinal study of weight, height, and skinfold thickness among four individuals with PWS from birth to the onset of obesity. Birth weight, length, and weight for length ratios were within the 5th to 50th percentile for all four individuals. Between birth and 36 months of age most of the growth parameters were below the 50th percentile. TSF and subscapular skinfold measurements were at or above the 85th percentile, suggesting that excessive body fat was present prior to the onset of rapid weight gain. The authors suggest restricting energy intake to 60% of the recommended energy requirement based on age to prevent the early onset of obesity.

The effect of caloric restriction and macronutrient intake on body composition has not been reported for individuals with PWS. However, changes in these parameters have been assessed in unaffected obese and lean individuals. Yang and Van Itallie (1976) examined the effect of short-term (10 day) starvation, 800 kcal ketogenic, or 800 kcal mixed diets on weight loss in a randomized cross-over design with 6 men, 19 to 58 years of age, who were 135–239% of their estimated desirable body weight. Each of the treatment diets was separated by a 1,200 kcal mixed diet. Average rate of weight loss was different during the three treatments: 751, 467, and 278 g/day for the starvation, ketogenic, and mixed diets, respectively. Weight loss ceased during the 1,200 kcal diets following the starvation and ketogenic diet treatments but continued at a lower rate (163 g/day) following the mixed diet treatment. Nitrogen loss was 8.18, 2.9, and 1.6 g/day for the starvation, ketogenic, and mixed diet, respectively.

Throughout the study, energy balance was negative; energy expenditure of 2,400 kcal/day remained the same. Ketone production was 9 and 3 g/day during the starvation and ketogenic diets and absent during the 1,200 and 800 kcal/day mixed diets. Protein deficit was not significantly different between the mixed and ketogenic diets (9.5 and 17.9 g/day, respectively), however, significantly greater losses occurred with the starvation diet (50.4 g/day). Fat loss was greater during the starvation diet (234 g/day) than either the mixed or ketogenic diet (165 g/day). Although the ketogenic diet resulted in faster weight loss, presumably by increased water loss, than the mixed diet, there was no difference in the protein sparing quality of the two diets. Although the starvation diet resulted in an increased loss of fat by 50% it also produced 2.5 to 5.0 times the protein loss of either the mixed or ketogenic diet. To apply the results of this study to the PWS population, it may be concluded that weight loss in which fat is utilized and protein is spared may be induced by either the mixed or the ketogenic diets. However, because of its more varied macronutrient composition, the mixed diet may be more easily prepared and better accepted by the individuals and their families.

Nutritional Intervention

Nutritional intervention for infants, children, and adults with PWS should include complete nutritional assessment (Figure 7.1). It is the

---

Name: _____   Present Address _____

Date of Birth: _____   _____

Date of Evaluation: _____   Telephone (___) _____

Age: _____

Height Age: _____

Diagnosis: _____

ANTHROPOMETRICS:

Weight: ____ kg, ____ %ile; increase/decrease of ____ g in ____ days.

Length (Height): ____ cm, ____ %ile; increase of ____ mm in ____ days.

WT/LT (Height): ____ %ile.

% IBW/LT (Height) ____.

Rt. Arm Circumference: _____ cm   _____ % ile.

Rt. Triceps Skinfold: _____ mm   _____ % ile.

Rt. Subscapular Skinfold: _____ mm   _____ % ile.

Arm Muscle Area*:   _____ mm^2 _____ % ile.

Arm Fat Area*:   _____ mm^2 _____ % ile.

Estimated energy requirement: _____ kcal/cm.

Estimated protein requirement (RDA): _____ g.

Estimated Caloric Intake: _____ Kcal _____ Kcal/cm.

Estimated Protein Intake: _____ g/day.

Multivitamin/mineral Supplement: _____   _____
                                                          (brand/dose)   frequency

*Calculated as:

$$\text{Upper Arm Area (mm}^2) = \left(\frac{\text{Arm Circumference (mm)}}{3.14}\right)^2 \times 0.79$$

$$\text{Arm Muscle Area(mm}^2) = \frac{[\text{Arm Circumference(mm)} - 3.14(\text{Triceps Skinfold(mm)})]^2}{12.57}$$

Arm Fat Area (mm^2) = Upper Arm Area—Arm Muscle Area

FIGURE 7.1. Nutritional assessment sheet.

HOME ENVIRONMENT:

Which meals are eaten at home?
Are meals eaten as a family? Y/N _____
Are serving bowls placed on the table? Y/N _____
What size serving is offered?   Meat _____, Starch _____
                                  Vegetable _____, Fruit _____
                                  Dairy _____, Other _____

How many servings are offered? _____
How long does it take child to complete meal? _____
Is food available at other times of the day? Y/N _____
Are cabinets/refrigerator/freezer locked? Y/N _____
Do you have a garbage disposal? Y/N _____
Do you own a pet? Y/N _____. If so, how is pet food stored? _____
Do you own a home scale? Y/N _____ What type? _____
Do you weigh your child? Y/N _____ How often? _____

Does child participate in school lunch program? hot _____, cold _____
Is the lunch room supervised? Y/N _____
Is a salad bar available at school lunch? Y/N _____
Are snacks available at school? Y/N _____

School Nurse (name) and telephone number: _____
School Dietitian (name) and telephone number: _____

PROBLEM BEHAVIORS:

　　Food preferences _____
　　Food foraging _____
　　Food Stealing _____
　　Rapid Consumption _____
　　Pica (non-edibles)_____
　　Non-discriminatory _____
　　School Concerns _____
　　Other _____

PHYSICAL CONCERNS:

　　Constipation/diarrhea _____
　　Vomiting, gagging, choking _____
　　Sleep Apnea _____
　　Drowsiness _____

ACTIVITY: (note time spent on activity per day and number of days per week)

Walking _____ Swimming _____ Bicycling _____ Dancing _____
Other _____

INVOLVEMENT OF LOCAL SERVICES: (list names of therapists)

_____ WIC   _____
_____ Visiting Nurse Association _____
_____ Area Education Agency   _____
_____ Other (please specify)   _____

FIGURE 7.1. (*continued*).

responsibility of the nutritionist to (1) design appropriate diets that include calculation of average intakes of energy, protein, fluid, and macronutrients from diet records, (2) keep accurate records that document anthropometric measurements and nutritional status, (3) provide nutritional education to care providers, and (4) be an on-going resource for support and information relative to nutritional issues.

Assessment

Nutritional status of individuals with PWS should be based on measurements of weight, height, skinfold thickness, and body circumference and nutrient analysis of food intake records. This information allows the nutritionist to determine the effect of changes in the diet on linear growth, weight gain, and body fat stores. Food intake records are used to evaluate the adequacy of diet as well as the appropriateness of food choices. Weight and height measurements are used to determine the recommendation for caloric intake, therefore accuracy in taking these measurements cannot be overstated. Infants should be weighed on a pan-type infant scale without clothing or diaper when the child is calm and still. Children and young adults should be weighed on a calibrated single beam scale while wearing undergarments and paper gowns. Height or length measurements should be performed using calibrated vertical stadiometers or length boards. Weight and height measurements should be recorded and plotted with respect to age on standardized growth charts (Hamill, Drizd, Johnson, et al., 1979). Weight-for-height ratio and height–age should also be determined. Although adolescents and adults with PWS are not expected to follow the linear growth patterns of unaffected individuals, these charts may be used to monitor individual growth patterns. PWS-specific growth charts have been designed to describe linear growth during childhood, adolescence, and early adulthood in affected individuals (Holm & Nugent, 1982). These charts take into account the lack of, or diminished, adolescent growth spurt and provide a means to detect inappropriate linear growth among individuals with PWS (see Appendix B).

Longitudinal skinfold thickness and circumference measurements provide information about the regional deposition and utilization of somatic protein stores and subcutaneous fat stores during periods of weight gain and weight loss. Like weight and height measurements, skinfold and circumference measurements may be compared to normal values established for unaffected children (Frisancho, 1981). Ideally, skinfold measurements should be taken with a calibrated skinfold caliper at multiple sites, including the triceps, biceps, subscapular, suprailiac, midaxillary, abdominal, thigh, knee, and calf sites. Circumference should be measured with a metal or nonstretch flexible fiberglass tape measure and taken on the right side of the body while the patient stands tall and relaxed with weight evenly distributed between the feet. Common sites for circumference measurements include chest, waist, hips, mid-thigh, mid-calf, ankle, upper arm, and wrist. Figure 7.2 provides a recording sheet that may help organize growth and nutritional information in an easily retrievable fashion.

Dietary Guidelines

In general, the dietary management of infants and young children with PWS should follow the recommendations developed by the Committee on Nutrition of the American Academy of Pediatrics. Breast milk or infant formula should remain the primary source of nutrition during the first 6 months of life. Beikost (any food product other than breast milk or infant formula) should be introduced between 5 and 6 months of age or when

Name: _____	Diet Prescription:
Date of Birth _____	Kcal/cm _____
Diagnosis _____	Kcal/day _____
	Protein (gm/day) _____

Date:								
Age: Weight (kg)								
Height (cm)								
IBW/HT (kg)								
%IBW								
Energy								
kcal/day								
kcal/cm								
kcal/kg IBW								
Protein (g)								
g/kg IBW								
% kcal								
Carbohydrate (g)								
% kcal								
Fat (g)								
%kcal								

FIGURE 7.2. Nutritional management record sheet.

the child is able to sit without support and has good head and neck control. Introduction of strained foods should progress from iron-fortified cereals to fruits, vegetables, and meats. Desserts and high-calorie solids should be avoided because of excessive caloric concentration. Once the child begins to crawl and pull to a stand, foods with higher texture (Stage Three baby foods) may be added to the diet. Cow's milk is not recommended for infants less than 1 year of age because of its high salt and protein content. Once introduced, low fat (1%) or skim milk should be used unless otherwise directed.

During the first 2 years of life energy intake should be adjusted to promote growth within the 25th to 75th percentile weight for height. Once weight gain or excessive fat deposition becomes a problem, the goal of dietary intervention is to restrict energy intake so that weight remains at or below the 75th percentile weight for height. A realistic goal is to achieve weight maintenance and allow the children to "grow into their weight." When children present as morbidly obese at a very young age, weight loss programs need to be initiated as soon as possible. The severe energy restriction required for this intensive loss of weight should be conducted only under the supervision of a qualified nutritionist or medical personnel.

Attempts to manage the weight of individuals with PWS include energy restriction with behavior management (Kriz & Cloninger, 1981), hypocaloric diets (Evans, 1964; Jancar, 1971; Juul & DuPont, 1967; Holm & Pipes, 1976), hypocaloric–protein sparing diet (Bistrian, Blackburn, & Stanbury, 1977), 1,000 calorie-ketogenic diet (Nardella, Sulzbacher, & Worthington-Roberts, 1983), and a balanced macronutrient diet devoid of simple sugar (Coplin, Hine, & Gormican, 1976; MacReynolds, personal communication referenced in Coplin, Hine, & Gormican, 1976). Each dietary regimen required frequent professional intervention over a long period of time and, unfortunately, resulted in only limited ability to maintain weight goals.

Two studies (Coplin, Hine, & Gormican, 1976; Holm & Pipes, 1976) attempt to explain the difficulties encountered by this population in achieving weight loss. They indicate that individuals with PWS require 1/3 to 3/4 less energy to maintain weight compared to unaffected individuals. In addition, Bray, Dahms, Swerdloff, et al. (1983) described the characteristic drive to consume massive amounts of food and reported that, left unsupervised, the *ad libitum* energy intake of individuals with PWS reached 5,167 ± 503 kcal/day. The ease with which individuals with PWS gain weight and their drive to eat makes weight management a frustrating battle requiring continuous supervision by parents or other care providers.

Determination of Recommended Energy Intake

The energy requirement of healthy individuals may be assumed to be met when gains in length and weight proceed within a normal range specific for age and gender. Because individuals with PWS demonstrate abnormal patterns of growth the adequacy of their energy intake cannot be judged from monitoring growth. Height and chronological age, do however, provide indices for estimating the energy needs of an individual with PWS.

Holm and Pipes (1976) first described the estimated energy needs of individuals with PWS in terms of kilocalories per centimeter of height (kcal/cm). Table 7.1 provides a compilation of the results of weight management attempts of individuals with PWS with respect to age, kcal/cm, percent weight loss, and length of dietary intervention. Individuals with PWS at any age can lose weight on a energy-restricted diet of 7 kcal/cm/day (18 kcal/inch). Significant weight loss, up to 43% of total body weight, over a 13-month period has been documented (Marshall, Elder, O'Bosky, et al., 1979). Weight maintenance has been reported with diets that provide 8–11 kcal/cm/day (20 to 28 kcal/inch). Using these recommendations, daily energy intakes range from 600 to 800 kcal among young children and from 800 to 1,300 kcal among older children and adults.

Table 7.2 was adapted from a chart that identifies energy (caloric) intake recommendations for children with PWS between the ages of 3 and 9 years of age that indicate a slightly different range of suggested energy intakes (Borgie, 1994).

When weight is gained on an appropriately designed diet it is likely that food is available from sources such as school cafeterias, snack machines, fast food restaurants, convenience stores, neighbors, or stealing. Management strategies that restrict food accessibility should include locking refrigerators, freezers, cabinets, and pantries, disposing of leftover foods immediately, making pet food and garbage cans inaccessible, and, when possible, locking the kitchen door. Additional suggestions are presented in Table 7.3.

Macronutrient Composition of the Diet

The macronutrient composition of the diet should approximate 25% protein, 50% carbohydrate, and 25% fat. If 1,000 kcal/day is recommended, 27.7 g fat, 62.5 g protein and 125 g carbohydrate should be included (27.7 g of fat is the amount in 2½ Tbsp. of margarine). Protein intake should meet the Recommended Dietary Allowance (RDA) and be of high biological value (contain all of the essential amino acids), carbohydrates should be complex, and fat should be limited to that found naturally in lean foods (Figure 7.3). Because prolonged and severe energy restriction predisposes an individual to insufficient intake of many vitamins and minerals, a multiple vitamin and mineral supplement is essential. Table 7.4 provides information on available multivitamin and mineral preparations and their nutrient compositions.

TABLE 7.1. Energy intake of individuals with Prader–Willi syndrome of various ages.

Age (years)	Diet prescription (kcal)	Energy intake			Weight change (percentage)	Time interval (weeks)
		Actual intake (kcal)	kcal/kg	kcal/cm		
$1^{8/12 a}$	775	800	—	9	(−0.6 kg)	3
2^a	—	815	—	9	(−1.4 kg)	12
2^b	—	800	—	8	0	—
3^b	—	950	—	10	0	—
$3^{4/12 c}$	—	715	53	—	0	24
$4^{3/12 c}$	—	863	28	—	+1	24
4^b	—	990	—	10	0	—
$4^{9/12 c}$	—	560	24	—	+1	24
4^a	—	880	—	9	(−1.6 kg)	12
4^b	—	880	—	10	0	—
$5^{1/12 c}$	—	890	32	—	+1	24
6^a	—	980	—	9	(−3.6 kg)	12
6^a	—	690	—	6	(−4.8 kg)	Approximately 1
$6^{5/12 c}$	—	1060	43	—	−10	24
$6^{5/12 c}$	—	755	26	—	−11	12
6^d	1000	—	18	18	(−5.6 kg)	—
7^b	—	1020	—	9	0	—
7^b	—	1280	—	11	0	—
7^d	1.5 protein/kg Protein sparing fast Restricted fluid	—	—	—	(−6.8 kg)	0.1 yr
7^d	Protein sparing fast	1200	—	—	(−22 kg)	—
8^d	—	1200	20	10	—	—
9^b	—	1180	—	10	0	—
$9^{3/12 c}$	—	938	23	—	−11	24
$10^{8/12 c}$	—	600	6	—	−26	24
11^b	—	1990	—	15	0	—
11^e	1000	—	17	7	−4	2
12^e	1000	—	36	8	0	1

12[e]	1000	—	28	7	-2	2
12[e]	1000	—	22	22	-2	1
12[f]	1.4 g protein/kg Protein sparing fast	—	—	—	—	—
12[d]	1.5 g protein/kg	—	—	—	—	—
13[e]	1000	—	22	7	-1	1
13[e]	1000	—	16	7	-4	2
14[e]	1000	—	16	7	-3	2
15[e]	1000	—	19	7	-3	1
17[e]	1000	—	15	7	-3	2
17[f]	1.5 g protein/kg Protein sparing fast	900	8	6	-53	40
18[e]	1000	—	18	7	-2	2
18[e]	1000	—	15	7	-5	2
19[f]	1.9 g protein/kg Protein sparing fast	1100+	9	7	-36	112
20[g]	1000		11	7	-37	72
21[g]	1000		13	7	-40	52
21[g]	1000		12	7	-43	52
22[e]	1000		8	7	-3	2
24[f]	1000 kcal, 2.1 g protein/kg Protein sparing fast		10	7	-32	44
26[g]	1700	—	16	12	-58	52
20[h]	900	—	—	—	(-7.7 kg)	32
					(-12.7 kg)	72

[a] Pipes and Holm (1973).
[b] Holm and Pipes (1976).
[c] Coplin, Hine, & Gormican (1976).
[d] Bye, Vines, & Fronzek (1983).
[e] Nardella, Sulzbacher, & Worthington-Roberts (1983).
[f] Bistrain, Blackburn, & Stanbury (1979).
[g] Marshall et al. (1979).
[h] Kriz and Cloninger (1981).

TABLE 7.2. Energy intake recommendations for children with PWS for weight maintenance or weight loss[a]

Age (years)	Gender and height	Suggested Energy Intake for weight maintenance (20–28 kcal/inch) (7.87–11.0 kcal/cm)	Suggested Energy Intake for weight loss (18 kcal/inch) (7.0 kcal/cm)
3	Girls 35″	700–980	630
	Boys 37″	740–1036	660
5	Girls 40″	800–1120	720
	Boys 42″	840–1176	760
7	Girls 44″	880–1232	790
	Boys 47″	940–1316	845
9	Girls 48″	960–1344	864
	Boys 53″	1060–1484	954

[a] Adapted from Borgie (1994).

Nutrition Education

As soon as the diagnosis of PWS is made, care providers must be taught to complete accurate records of food intake that include meal time and type, amount, and energy content of the foods consumed (Figure 7.4). Solid food intake is best described using common household measurements (e.g., cups, teaspoons, fluid ounces), or standard (ounces) or metric (grams) weights. To familiarize care providers with standard portion sizes, and to increase awareness of the energy content of various foods, the first 2 months of nutritional intervention should begin with encouraging the care provider to weigh or measure and record all foods provided. Care providers should be given instructions and appropriate resources to design meals that meet the child's nutritional needs while complying with the necessary energy restriction. The choice of instructional model is dependent upon the care provider's understanding of the individualized guidelines and the ability to follow recommendations.

One commonly used model for diet planning is the exchange system used by diabetics. This system divides foods into six groups: milk, meat, fruit, vegetable, bread, and fat. Portion sizes assigned to foods in each group provide equal amounts of protein, carbohydrate, fat, and calories (Table 7.5). Using this model, foods within a group may be substituted or "exchanged" freely. Exchanges are allocated into a specific meal plan to meet the needs of the child while attempting to conform to the family's lifestyle. An example of a 1-week meal pattern based on the food exchange system and a sample menu is presented in Appendix C. Verbal and written instructions for using the exchange system must be provided and menus should be designed with the nutritionist as an on-going

TABLE 7.3. Weight reduction and dieting tips

1. Establish a consistent meal pattern immediately. Do not deviate from the meal pattern. The calorically restricted diet should become a way of life rather than a burden or punishment for the individual.
2. Provide three meals daily. If food is inappropriately consumed between meals, subtract an equal amount of calories from the next meal.
3. Smaller portion sizes of the family meal may often be provided to the individual with PWS. Discretion must be used and alternatives provided when necessary.
4. Measure average portion sizes of food to be served; divide in half and serve the second half as a second portion. If the second portion is not requested, do not offer the remaining food.
5. Serve food on smaller plates (8 inch vs. 10 inch) and beverages in smaller (6 oz.) glasses.
6. Serve food in the kitchen, away from the table, and leave remaining food in kitchen. Do not set serving dishes on the eating area.
7. Cut meat and vegetables into small pieces.
8. Dilute fruit juices. An increased volume may be offered if this is done. Use only *unsweetened* juices.
9. Purchase frozen fruit juice bars or make your own as a substitute for ice cream.
10. Bake, broil, steam, or microwave foods instead of frying in oil or margarine. Take advantage of "Lite" or "nonfat" food alternatives. Keep in mind that nonfat does not mean no calories. Read labels carefully. Also use products sweetened with nonnutritive sweeteners (aspartame, saccharine) instead of sugar, sucrose, fructose, high-fructose corn syrup.
11. Snack suggestions: Provide a variety of fresh fruits and vegetables or use canned fruits and vegetables *packed in their own juice*. Prepare large quantities of tossed salads to have available for immediate consumption after school, or as an evening or night-time snack. Always provide a salad with the evening meal and at lunch if possible. Lettuce takes up space on the plate and in the stomach but has few calories.
12. Family members may want to consume a larger meal at lunch-time while at work or while the individual with PWS is at a workshop. A lighter family meal may then be served in the evening.
13. Send a sack lunch to school, day care, or workshop to avoid excessive or unintended caloric consumption. Make sure that appropriate supervision is provided during each meal.
14. Set restrictions on the types of foods purchased (do not purchase ice cream, peanut butter, cookies, or candy if these foods are inappropriately consumed).
15. Limit the use of food as a reward. Instead use a book, record, TV time, or activity as positive reinforcement for appropriate behavior (see Appendix C).
16. Include the individual with PWS in family activities, however, be prepared to provide appropriate supervision.

resource. Intermittent nutritional assessment provides the opportunity to modify dietary recommendations as age increases, activity levels change, or as new issues arise.

Follow-up

Nutritional follow-up plans should be discussed and presented in writing to care providers based on the individualized needs of the child and family. Initially, daily food intake should be recorded and sent with

1. Estimated energy need based on age and _____ kcal/cm
   height (Tables 7.1 and 7.2)   _____ kcal/day

2. Protein Requirement (RDA): _____ g.
   Energy from protein: _____ kcal.
   Percent of total kcal: _____.

3. Energy from carbohydrates (approximately 50% total kcal: _____ kcal.
   Grams of carbohydrate: _____

4. Energy from fat [total kcal—(kcal from protein and carbohydrate)]: _____ kcal.
   Grams of fat: _____. Percent of total kcal: _____.

5. Multivitamin/mineral supplement: _____ (brand/dose).

6. Allocation of energy into food groups (see Table 7.5) for macronutrient
   values):

FOOD GROUP	No. of Exchanges	Energy (kcal)	PRO (g)	CHO (g)	FAT (g)
Bread					
Fruit					
Vegetable					
Meat					
Dairy					
Total	_____	_____	____	____	___
% Energy					

7. Distribution of food exchanges into meal pattern:
   Breakfast _____
             _____
             _____

   Lunch   _____
             _____
             _____

   Dinner   _____
             _____
             _____
             _____

   Snacks: _____
             _____
             _____

FIGURE 7.3. Diet prescription worksheet.

weight measurements to the nutritionist on a weekly basis. When care
providers are able to follow the recommendations and weight loss or
maintenance is established, 3-day food records and weekly weight measurements should continue for 2 more weeks. If, after 4 weeks weight and

dietary goals are met, a 3-day food record and weekly weight measurements should be submitted monthly. When all the above goals are met, formal nutritional consultation should take place every 4–6 months. When compliance with dietary recommendations is good, but the weight goal is not met, the diet should be reevaluated. If the weight goal is not met because of inability to comply with the recommendations, additional nutritional counseling is necessary. This may include a home visit to evaluate if the environment is appropriate. If necessary, referral may be made to a primary health care agency to provide more frequent support.

A Case Study

The following information illustrates successful dietary management of a young child with PWS.

TR carries the medical diagnosis of PWS. She weighed 3.96 kg (95th percentile) and was 53.3 cm in length (95th percentile) at birth (50th percentile weight for length. (Figures 7.5 and 7.6). She tracked along the 50th percentile weight for age between 1 and 3 months of age, and along the 25th percentile weight for age between 3 and 6 months. She demonstrated accelerated weight gain between 6 and 21 months, during which time she crossed from the 25th percentile to much above the 95th percentile. Her linear growth progressed along the 90th percentile until 3 months of age, was below the 25th percentile at 7.5 months of age, and tracked within the 25th to 75th percentile between 8 and 21 months.

TR was referred to the Division for Developmental Disabilities by her local pediatrician at 21 months of age. At that time she weighed 14.6 kg (>95th percentile) and was 82.4 cm in length (25th to 50th percentile). Her food intake included soft mashed table food, diluted juices, and whole milk and she consumed three meals and three to four snacks a day. Computer nutrient analysis of her reported food intake suggested that TR consumed approximately 785 kcal (9.5 kcal/cm) and 34.4 g of protein per day (RDA for protein = 23 g). The completeness of this report was questioned as her total energy intake seemed low. The following micronutrients did not meet 66% of the RDA/age: vitamin D, vitamin E, vitamin C, zinc, iodine, niacin, and iron. By report, TR did not demonstrate hunger or satiety but consumed all foods provided to her.

Dietary intervention was initiated at 21 months of age and was designed to restrict energy intake while providing adequate nutrition for optimal linear growth. Intake was restricted to 575–600 kcal/day (7–8 kcal/cm) to initiate gradual weight loss. Specific dietary recommendations included providing food in three meals and two snacks daily, limiting the size of portions and the number of servings, diluting fruit juices with water in a 1:4 ratio, providing skim milk and cheeses made of skim or low-fat milk,

TABLE 7.4. Multivitamin and mineral supplements and their contents.

Product[a]	A (IU)	D (IU)	E (IU)	B1 (mg)	B2 (mg)	B3 (mg)	B5 (mg)	B6 (mg)	B12 (µg)	C (mg)	Fe (mg)	FA[a] (mg)	Biotin (µg)	Other (mg)
RDA[b] for children 1–3 years of age	400[c] (µg RE)	400	6	0.7	0.8	9	3	1	0.7	40	10	0.050	20	
Poly-Vi-Sol® (1 ml)	1,500	400	5	0.5	0.6	8		0.4	2	35				
Poly-Vi-Sol® with iron (1 ml)	1,500	400	5	0.5	0.6	8		0.4	2	35	10			
Tri-Vi-Sol® with iron (1 ml)	1,500	400								35	10			
Vi-Daylin® drops (1 ml)	1,500	400	5	0.5	0.6	8		0.4	1.5	35				
Vi-Daylin® plus iron ADC (1 ml)	1,500	400								35	10			
Vi-Daylin® plus iron (1 ml)	1,500	400	5	0.5	0.6	8		0.4		35	10			
RDA for children 4–6 years of age	2,500 (µg RE)	400	7	0.9	1.1	12	3–4	1.1	1	45	10	0.075		
Bugs Bunny™ plus iron	2,500	400	15	1.1	1.2	13.5		1.1	4.5	60	15	0.3		
Bugs Bunny™ with extra C	2,500	400	15	1.1	1.2	13.5		1.1	4.5	250		0.3		
Flintstones® chewables	2,500	400	15	1.1	1.2	13.5		1.1	4.5	60		0.3		
Flintstones® plus iron	2,500	400	15	1.1	1.2	13.5		1.1	4.5	60	15	0.3		
Flintstones® with extra C	2,500	400	15	1.1	1.2	13.5		1.1	4.5	250		0.3		
Flintstones® plus calcium	2,500	400	15	1.1	1.2	13.5		1.1	4.5	60		0.3		Ca (200)
Vi-Daylin® liquid (1 ml)	2,500	400	15	1	1.2	13.5		1	4.5	60				
Poly-Vi-Sol® chewable	2,500	400	15	1	1.2	13.5		1	4.5	60		0.3		
Poly-Vi-Sol® with iron chewable	2,500	400	15	1	1.2	13.5		1	4.5	60	12	0.3		
Sunkist® chewable multivitamin	2,500	400	15	1.1	1.2	13.5		1.1	4.5	60		0.3		Vit K (0.005)

Sunkist® chewable multivitamin plus extra C	2,500	400	15	1.1	1.2	13.5		1.1	4.5	250	15	0.3		Vit K (0.005)
Sunkist® chewable multivitamin plus iron	2,500	400	15	1.1	1.2	13.5		1.1	4.5	60	15	0.3		Vit K (0.005)
Vi-Daylin® chewable Bugs Bunny™ complete	2,500	400	15	1.1	1.2	13.5		1	4.6	60	18	0.3		
	5,000	400	30	1.5	1.7	20	10	2	6	60	18	0.4	40	Ca (100), P (100), I (0.15), Mg (20), Zn (15), Cu (2)
Flintstones® complete	5,000	400	30	1.5	1.7	20	10	2	6	60	18	0.4	40	Ca (100), P (100), Mn (2.5), Zn (15), Cu (2), Mg (20), 1 (0.15)
Centrum® high potency	5,000	400	30	1.5	1.7	20	10	2	6	60	18	0.4	30	Ca (162), P (109), Mg (100), Zn (15), I (0.15), Cut(2) Mn (2.5), K (4.0), Vit K (0.025), K (40), Cl (36.3), Cr (0.025), Mo (0.025), Se (0.02)
Centrum, Jr.® plus iron	5,000	400	30	1.5	1.7	20	10	2	6	60	18	0.4	45	Ca (108), P (50), Mg (40), Zn (15), I (0.15), Cu (2), Mn (1), K (1.6), Vit K (0.01), Mo (0.02), Cr (0.02)
Centrum Jr.® plus extra C	5,000	400	30	1.5	1.7	20	10	2	6	300	18	0.4	45	(as above)
Centrum Jr.® plus extra calcium	5,000	400	30	1.5	1.7	20	10	2	6	60	18	0.4	45	Ca (160), others as above
One-A-Day®	5,000	400	30	1.5	1.7	20	10	2	6	60	18	0.4		
One-A-Day® maximum multivitamin/mineral supplement	5,000	400	30	1.5	1.7	20	10	2	6	60	18	0.4	30	Ca (130), P (100), Cl (34), Cr (0.01), Zn (15), I (0.15), Mg (100) Cu (2), Se (0.01), Mo (0.01), Mn (2.5), K (34)

(Continued)

TABLE 7.4. *Continued*

Product[a]	A (IU)	D (IU)	E (IU)	B₁ (mg)	B₂ (mg)	B₃ (mg)	B₅ (mg)	B₆ (mg)	B₁₂ (µg)	C (mg)	Fe (mg)	FA[a] (mg)	Biotin (µg)	Other (mg)
One-A-Day® men's multivitamin supplement	5,000	400	45	2.25	2.55	20	10	3	9	200		0.4		
One-A-Day® women's multivitamin supplement	5,000	400	30	1.5	1.7	20	10	2	6	60	27	0.4		Ca (450), Zn (15)
Sunkist® chewable multivitamin complete	5,000	400	30	1.5	1.7	20	10	2	6	60	18	0.4	40	Vit K (0.01), Ca (100), P (78), Zn (10), Mg (20), Cu (2), Mn (1), I (0.15)
Theragran® tablets advanced tablets	5,000	400	30	3	3.4	20	10	3	9	90		0.4	30	
Theragran® liquid with niacin and vitamin C (5 ml)	5,000	400		10	10	100	21.4	4.1	5	200				
Theragran® stress formula			30	15	15	100	20	25	12	600	27	0.4	45	
Theragran® tablets	5,000	400	30	3	3.4	20	10	3	9	90		0.4	30	
Theragran-M® tablets	5,000	400	30	3	3.4	20	10	3	9	90	27	0.4	30	Cu (2), I (0.15), Mg (100), Mn (0.005), Zn (15), Ca (40), P (31), Cr (0.15), Mo (0.015), Se (0.01), Cl (7.5), K (7.5)

[a] Information compiled from the *Physician's desk reference for nonprescription drugs*, 15th ed. Montvale, NJ: Medical Economics Data Production Co., 1994.

[b] *Recommended Dietary Allowances*, 10th ed. National Research Council. Washington, D.C.: National Academy Press, 1989.

[c] RDA for vitamin A is listed in µg retinol equivalents (RE). Vitamin A content in vitamin supplements is listed in international units (IU). One microgram RE is defined as 6 µg all-*trans*-β-carotene or 1 µg all-*trans*-retinol. One IU is defined as 0.3 µg all-*trans*-retinol or 0.6 µg all-*trans*-β-carotene. Vitamin A in vitamin supplements is derived from retinyl acetate and β-carotene; the amount of each is not specified, so, conversion to RE cannot be performed.

Name: _____
Date: _____
Weight: _____ lb.

Meal/Time of day	Food offered	Amount consumed	Energy (kcal)	PRO (g)	CHO (g)	FAT (g)
				(parents leave blank)		

Was this a typical day? _____ If no, please comment _____

Did you observe any of the following events? (if so, please indicate and comment):

_____ Food foraging
_____ Consumption of nonfood items
_____ Consumption of unauthorized food
_____ Other, please describe

FIGURE 7.4. Twenty-four hour food intake record.

substituting bite-sized pieces of fresh fruit for dried fruit, and providing a multivitamin and mineral supplement. Written information on the energy contents of foods was provided to enable accurate calculation of total energy (caloric) intake by the parents. Arrangements were made to have TR weighed at her local pediatrician's office and a 72-hr food intake record was to be completed and returned for analysis. Telephone contact was made following receipt and analysis of the record to provide additional recommendations. Thereafter, records and weight measurements requested on a monthly basis and frequent telephone contact was made to discuss any needed changes.

At 26 months of age, 5 months after dietary intervention, TR weighed 13.6 kg (75th to 90th percentile) and was 85.8 cm in length (25th per-

TABLE 7.5. Energy and macronutrient content for standard portion sizes of foods in each food group.

Food group	Calories (kcal)	Protein (g)	Carbohydrate (g)	Fat (g)
Dairy (non fat)	80	8	12	—
Fruit	40	—	10	—
Vegetable	25	2	5	—
Starchy vegetable	70	2	15	—
Bread/cereal	70	2	15	—
Meat (lean)	55	7	—	3

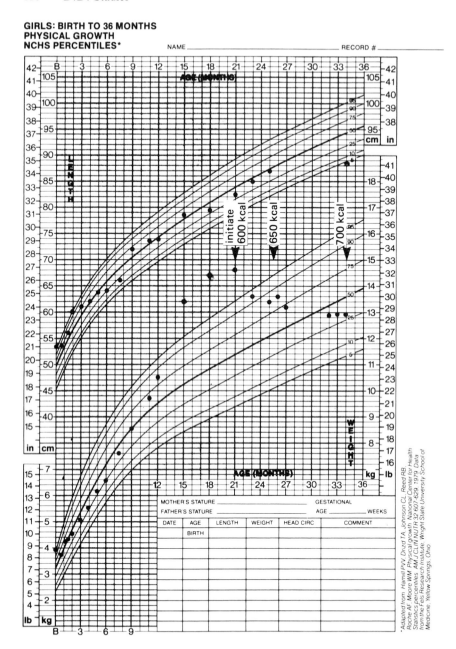

GIRLS: BIRTH TO 36 MONTHS
PHYSICAL GROWTH
NCHS PERCENTILES*

FIGURE 7.5. Linear growth (*top curve*) and weight gain (*bottom curve*) plotted over time for TR. Dietary energy intake indicated on weight gain curve by arrowheads. Chart reprinted by permission of Ross Biomedical Publications.

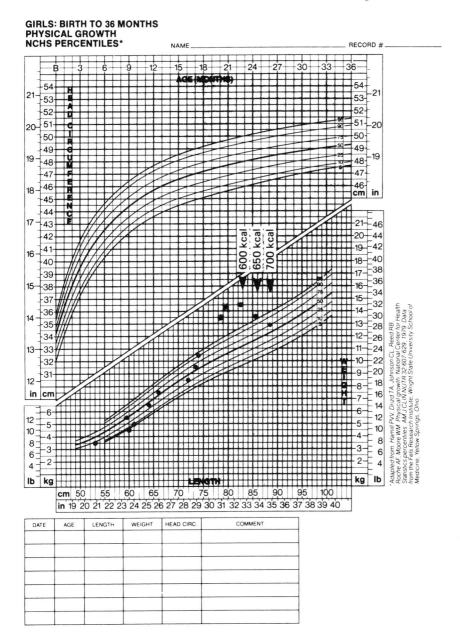

FIGURE 7.6. Weight for length measurements plotted over time for TR. Dietary energy intake indicated by arrowheads. Chart reprinted by permission of Ross Biomedical Publications.

centile). Her desirable body weight estimated at the 75th percentile weight for height was 12.5 kg. Her mother reported that TR consumed 100% of the foods offered and that she did not demonstrate hunger or satiety nor inappropriate food-seeking or food consumption behaviors. Her energy intake was adjusted to 650 kcal (7.6 kcal/cm) per day. Food intake records and monthly weight measurements were continued.

At 34 months of age, 13 months after her initial evaluation, TR weighed 12.9 kg (25th to 50th percentile) and was 88.5 cm in length (<5th percentile). Her weight-for-length ratio was at the 75th percentile, her desired body weight. Triceps and subscapular skinfold thicknesses (50th to 75th percentile and 90th to 95th percentile, respectively) and mid-arm circumference were measured. Arm muscle area (90th to 95th percentile) and arm fat area (50th to 75th percentile) were calculated. She had been maintained on a diet of 650 kcal (7.3 kcal/cm) and had lost an average of 80 g/month (0.18 lb/month). Her protein intake exceeded the RDA and a multivitamin and mineral supplement was provided to meet micronutrient needs. TR's caloric intake was increased to 700 kcal/day (7.9 kcal/cm) by increasing the amount of meat and dairy products consumed. Her weight and length will be measured monthly, and caloric intake will be adjusted as necessary to promote appropriate growth. Formal evaluation, including anthropometric assessment, will take place every 6 months.

Summary

Nutritional intervention for individuals with PWS is indicated at any age and continues throughout life. Left untreated, infants with PWS fail to thrive, and children, adolescents, and adults become morbidly obese. Older children and adults with PWS require significantly less energy to maintain weight than unaffected individuals. This, in combination with an uncontrollable hunger, results in morbid obesity. Weight management of this population is difficult and requires continuous supervision. The nutritionist works with the multidiciplinary team and the primary care providers to assess and monitor nutritional status, to develop appropriate dietary guidelines and teach providers how best to implement them, and to provide follow-up assistance. Each person with PWS is unique and requires individualized nutritional intervention. Similarly, because each child's family unit is also a distinctive entity, the content, the approach, and the extent of nutritional counseling must be sensitive to the family's dynamics and culture. Effective communication skills and a willingness to offer on-going support are essential if the nutritional needs of children with PWS are to be met.

References

Bistrian, B.R., Blackburn, G.L., & Stanbury, J.B. (1977). Metabolic aspects of protein-sparing modified fast in the dietary management of Prader Willi obesity. *New England Journal of Medicine*, *296*, 774–779.

Borgie, K.H. (1994). *Nutrition care for children with Prader-Willi syndrome. Prader-Willi California Foundation.*

Bray, G.A., Dahms, W.T., Swerdloff, R.S., Fisher, R.H., Atkinson, R.L., & Carrel, R.E. (1983). The Prader-Willi syndrome: A study of 40 patients and a review of the literature. *Medicine*, *62*, 59–80.

Butler, M.G. (1990). Prader-Willi syndrome. Current understanding of cause and diagnosis. *American Journal of Medical Genetics*, *35*, 319–332.

Butler, M.G., Butler, R.I., & Meaney, F.J. (1988). The use of skinfold measurements to judge obesity during the early phase of Prader-Labhart-Willi syndrome. *International Journal of Obesity*, *12*, 417–422.

Bye, A.M., Vines, R., & Fronzek, K. (1983). The obesity hypoventilation syndrome and the Prader Willi syndrome. *Australian Paediatric Journal*, 19, 251–255.

Coplin, S.S., Hine, J., & Gormican, A. (1976). Out-patient dietary management in the Prader-Willi syndrome. *Journal of the American Dietetic Association*, *68*, 330–334.

Evans, P.R. (1964). Hypogenital dystrophy with diabetic tendency. *Guys Hospital Reports*, *113*, 207–222.

Food and Nutrition Board, National Academy of Sciences-National Research Council (1989). *Recommended Dietary Allowances* (10th ed.).

Frisancho, A.R. (1981). New norms of upper limb fat and muscle areas for assessment of nutritional status. *American Journal of Clinical Nutrition*, *34*, 2540–2545.

Hamill, P., Drizd, T., Johnson, C., Reed, R., Roche, A., & Moore, W. (1979). Physical growth: NCHS percentiles. *American Journal of Clinical Nutrition*, *32*, 607–629.

Hill, J.D., Kaler, M., Spetalnick, B., Reed, G., & Butler, M.G. (1990). Resting metabolic rate in Prader-Willi syndrome. *Dysmorphology and Clinical Genetics*, *4*, 27–32.

Holm, V.A., & Pipes, P.L. (1976). Food and children with Prader-Willi syndrome. *American Journal of Diseases of Children*, *130*, 1063–1067.

Holm, V.A., Sulzbacher, S.J., & Pipes, P.L. (Eds.). (1981). *The Prader-Willi syndrome*. Baltimore: University Park Press.

Holm, V.A., & Nugent J.K. (1982). Growth in the Prader-Willi syndrome. *Birth Defects: Original Articles Series*, *18*, 93–100.

Jancar, J. (1971). Prader-Willi syndrome. *Journal of Mental Deficiency Research*, *15*, 10–29.

Juul, J., & DuPont, A. (1967). Prader Willi syndrome. *Journal of Mental Deficiency Research*, *11*, 12–20.

Kriz, S.J., & Cloninger, B.J. (1981). Management of a patient with Prader-Willi syndrome by a dental-dietary team. *Special Care in Dentistry*, *1*, 179–182.

Marshall, B.D., Elder, J., O'Bosky, D. Wallace, C., & Liberman, R. (1979). Behavioral treatment of Prader-Willi syndrome. *Behavior Therapy*, *2*, 22.

Meaney, F.J., & Butler, M.G. (1987). Assessment of body composition in Prader-Willi-Labhart syndrome. *Clinical Genetics*, *35*, 300–309.

Meaney, F.J., & Butler, M.G. (1989). Characterization of obesity in the Prader-Labhart-Willi syndrome: Fatness patterning. *Medical Antropology Quarterly*, *3*, 294–305.

Nardella, M.T., Sulzbacher, S.I., & Worthington-Roberts, B.S. (1983). Activity levels of persons with Prader-Willi syndrome. *American Journal of Mental Deficiency*, *87*, 498–505.

Nelson, R.A., Anderson, L.F., Gastineau, C.F., Hayles, A.B., & Stamnes, C.L. (1973). Physiology and natural history of obesity. *Journal of the American Medical Association*, *223*, 627–630.

Nelson, R.A., Huse, D.M., Holman, R.T., Kimbrough, B.O., Wahner, H.W., Calaway, C.W., & Hayler, A.B. (1981). Nutrition, metabolism, body composition, and response to the ketogenic diet in Prader-Willi syndrome. In V.A. Holm, S. Sulzbacher, & P.L. Pipes (Eds.), *Prader-Willi syndrome* (pp. 105–120). Baltimore: University Park Press.

Pipes, P.L., & Holm, V.A. (1973). Weight control of children with Prader-Willi syndrome. *Journal of the American Dietetic Association*, *62*, 520–524.

Schoeller, D.A., Levitcky, L.L., Bandini, L.G., Dietz, W.W., & Wolczak, A. (1988). Energy expenditure and body composition in Prader-Willi syndrome. *Metabolism*, *37*, 115–120.

Segal, K.R., Gutin, B., Albu, J., & Pi-Sunyer, F.X. (1987). Thermic effects of food and exercise in lean and obese men of similar lean body mass. *American Journal of Physiology*, *252*, E110–E117.

Widhalm, K., Veitl, V., & Irsigler, K. (1981). Evidence for decreased energy expenditure in Prader-Labhart-Willi syndrome: Assessment by means of the Vienna calorimeter. In *Proceedings of the International Congress of Nutrition XII* (p. 189). Abstract of papers; minisymposia and free communication, Aug. 16–21. New York: A.R. Liss.

Yang, M.U., & Van Itallie, T.B. (1976). Composition of weight loss during short-term weight reduction. *Journal of Clinical Investigation*, *58*, 722–730.

Zellweger, H., & Soper, R.T. (1979). The Prader-Willi syndrome. *Medical and Hygenics*, *37*, 3338–3345.

8
Physical and Occupational Therapy

ELIZABETH TRUE LLOYD and MARY ALICE DEUSTERHAUS-MINOR

Professional physical therapists and occupational therapists are significant members of interdisciplinary teams who work with the developmentally disabled. Each retains his or her professional responsibility to evaluate clients and recommend therapeutic interventions unique to his or her discipline and at the same time contributes to the team process by collaborating with other professionals to establish diagnoses and plan and implement appropriate management strategies. The "interrelatedness" of the role of both the physical and occupational therapist is reflected in the goals and concerns they share. These include recognizing that children change over time, promoting gross and fine motor development, fostering interest in activities that promote weight management, optimum health, and work potential, achieving independence in daily living by encouraging pursuits that enhance self-esteem and creativity, and training and supporting parents/care providers.

Individuals with Prader–Willi syndrome (PWS) require physical and occupational therapeutic interventions beginning early in life; the efforts of these professionals to promote optimal motor development throughout these children's growth and development is essential. It should be pointed out that it is not unusual for physical and/or occupational therapists to provide services to unidentified cases of PWS. The potential for these professionals to identify undiagnosed individuals should not be underestimated and, in many instances, they may be responsible for an initial referral for diagnostic clarification.

Typical Findings Associated with Physical Activity in PWS

Children with PWS typically are hypotonic. This low muscle tone interferes with normal progression through the developmental sequence of gross and fine motor skills. PWS children, although delayed in acquisition of normal motor milestones, may achieve independent ambulation, dressing, and self-care skills. In the infant and toddler state, feeding difficulties due to the hypotonia and oral motor involvement may present significant problems. Affected children are prone to develop significant scoliosis, even at a very young age. School performance is influenced by senso-rimotor integration or perceptual problems such as difficulties in motor planning, integrating the two sides of the body, and developing visual–perceptual skills. Poor overall gross motor performance and a preference for fine motor repetitive play are characteristic.

Therapeutic Interventions

Implications for Physical Therapists

Selection of physical therapy interventions for a PWS child is affected by the age of child and the presenting symptoms. Assessment should take into account cognitive and motor development, skeletal integrity, general and aerobic fitness, and sensory and perceptual function.

A variety of standardized assessments are available to evaluate and monitor development of gross and find motor skills. At least until skeletal maturity is achieved, postural–skeletal assessment is very important. Muscle tone and range of motion are monitored using traditional methods. Such tests as the revised Gesell (Knobloch, Stevens, & Malone, 1980) and the Bayley (1969) are appropriate for the younger child. The Bruininks–Oseretsky Test of Motor Proficiency (Bruininks, 1978) can be used with older children. Necessary information can be obtained using observations of the child during free and directed play. Where appropriate, a step test or stress test can be included. The child must be able to follow directions and attend to the task in order to yield meaningful data. Consideration must be given to the child's cognitive capacity, his or her behavioral adjustment in the testing setting, and observations and impres-sions of how care providers handle the child.

An infant or young child who has feeding difficulties, low tone, and developmental delay requires a developmental evaluation. Such assess-ment determines:

1. Level of gross motor development
2. Status of feeding skills
3. Level of muscle tone
4. Status of skeletal system
5. Activity level of the child
6. Equipment needs for positioning and mobility.

This information can be used to direct and instruct parents/care providers in how best to facilitate gross motor development, feeding skills, and activity levels. Feeding of infants in the hypotonic state of PWS can be enhanced by varying sensory stimulation, type of equipment used, and the consistency of the food. However, *eating and food-related issues must be carefully considered in light of the PWS child's predictable development of an insatiable hunger drive.* Monitoring the skeletal system for indication of the development of scoliosis or other orthopedic problems is essential. Suggestions about the use of baby equipment such as baby walkers and strollers for mobility as well as proper positioning and handling of the child are part of the teaching process (Harris, 1984).

In addition to standardized tests that are used to indicate level and rate of motor development, motor control and movement patterns must be monitored. Hypotonia prevents development of good stability/cocontraction. Hypermobilty of the joints may accompany low muscle tone. Hypermobile joints also make attainment of stability/cocontraction difficult. When stability/cocontraction is delayed, abnormal movement patterns often develop to compensate. The child needs to develop stability/ocontraction of the trunk, shoulder girdle, and pelvic girdle followed by weight-shifting and truck rotation in order to progress through the developmental sequences of gross and fine motor skills (Sullivan, Markos, & Minor, 1982). Motor control and movement patterns are assessed by observation and manipulation of the child to elicit stability/cocontraction, weight shifting, trunk rotation, and skilled activity (Minor & Minor, 1985).

Physical therapy assessment of preadolescents with PWS is important not only for parents/care providers but also to provide essential information to school personnel. Determination of the status of the skeletal system, girth measurements, aerobic and general fitness, activity levels, and gross motor development is critical to establishment of activities, goals, and expectations for performance. The PWS child who has any associated sensorimotor integration or perceptual problems such as difficulties in depth perception or kinesthesia requires careful management. If a child spends most free time in fine motor play, such as coloring, reading, or writing, decreased integration of the two sides of the body may prevent crossing of the midline. Care providers and teachers should encourage involvement in gross motor activities such as tricycle riding or playing with a ball. The child with perceptual motor problems may need more supervision when engaged in gross motor play and may have more difficulty with associated tasks. For example, depth perception difficulties may cause him or her to trip frequently. Negotiating playground equipment and/or games may be frustrating.

The school-age child with PWS should not be excluded from participation in physical education classes unless a valid health concern exists. In fact, physical education classes can reinforce the use of gross motor play for the development of skills, weight management, and wellness. The therapist is a resource person for the physical education and classroom teachers regarding activities that promote motor skills and wellness.

Games and sports that encourage motor and perceptual skill development are generally more beneficial than strengthening through progressive resistive exercise.

Suggestions for modification in the classroom include chairs that provide back support and are of appropriate height (hip and knee angle of 90° with feet resting on the floor). Desk or table tops should be at elbow height, keeping in mind that PWS children are typically very short. Often an easeled work surface is an easier and less fatiguing work space.

By late childhood regular exercise should be included in the child's weekly routine for general fitness and weight management (Carmen, 1981). Walking, tricycle or stationary bike riding, swimming, and low-impact aerobics classes are appropriate. It has been reported that the knee joints of individuals with PWS are not protected well enough to allow jumping or twisting exercises, jogging, or any other high-impact activities (M. Wett, personal communication, the Prader-Willi Syndrome Association, Edina, MN, 1987). Supervision is usually necessary, but with encouragement, PWS children can learn to take their own pulse readings.

Evaluation of adolescents and young adults with PWS is essentially the same as for preadolescents. The older individual may be able to complete the stress test and may be capable of assuming responsibility for selecting and carrying out exercise and activity programs. One important consideration in all such assessment is the cognitive capacity of the individual.

Implications for Occupational Therapists

Typical assessment and intervention procedures for occupational therapy for children with PWS are compiled on the basis of the degree of developmental delay evidenced. In initial evaluation, the subjective and objective tests used are determined by the child's age, developmental history, and presenting problems. Children with PWS might be expected to have difficulties in sensorimotor areas that include:

1. Low muscle tone
2. Diminished balance
3. Low energy postures and movement patterns
4. Deficits in use of arms for postural support
5. Deficits in endurance in antigravity postures
6. Poor trunk rotation and weight shifting with lack of differentiation of shoulder and hip girdles
7. Weak proximal musculature
8. Predominance of lower extremity external rotation and abduction
9. Scoliosis
10. Visual–motor deficits
11. Impaired fine motor dexterity and proficiency

12. Postural insecurity
13. Poor bilateral integration leading to decreased quality of bilateral hand use.

Developmental Assessment

Several standardized and nonstandardized developmental tools are used to establish age-equivalent scores and functional levels. The Peabody Developmental Motor Scales, fine motor subtest (Folio & Fewell, 1983) may be used for assessment of children ages 0–72 months, and is usually administered by an occupational therapist with a background in developmental pediatrics. The Beery Developmental Test of Visual-Motor Integration (1967), Goodenough Draw-A-Person (1927), and Motor Free Visual Perception (Colarusso & Hamill, 1972) tests are easily administered and reliable. An annotated list of these evaluation tools can be found in Appendix D, Section 1. Formal clinical observations provide valuable information and are generally included in any developmental assessment. Through comprehensive developmental evaluation each childs strengths and problem areas can be identified to further aid in planning home and school activities. For example, when the PWS child indicates interest, or is developmentally ready, strategies can be offered that promote independence in self-care activities such as dressing. Expecting a child to master donning and removing all clothing simultaneously may be unrealistic, but he or she may be able to learn to remove one piece at a time. Fastenings on apparel can be difficult to manage, and initially pull-on pants may be easier than those with zippers, buttons, or snaps. Use of large buttons before small ones is best; snaps may take a long time to master because of the pinch strength required (PWS children tend to have muscle weakness). Pull-on tops can be difficult for children with perceptual problems.

Recommendations for school activities are based on evaluation of fine and gross motor skills, sensorimotor development, visual perceptual and visual motor skill development, and speed, strength, and dexterity of hand/arm function. Following evaluation, appropriate activities are suggested to help the child adapt in the work–play environment. The focus of these activities is three-fold: first, to improve postural tone and cocontractions of the trunk, shoulder, and pelvic girdles; second, to improve joint stability; and third, to incorporate play and work activities that call for bilateral hand use. The school-age child's perceptual abilities influence educational progress, therefore compensatory strategies need to be incorporated into their activities. School physical education activities should focus on development of weight shifting and trunk rotation in prone, hands-knees, kneeling, sitting, and standing, and a developmentally sequenced sensorimotor program with movement into and out of a variety of postures should be encouraged. These play activities also enhance perceptual–motor integration and can be incorporated into home and school through noncompetitive games such as follow-the-leader.

Parents and teachers should be aware of the PWS child's tendency to gravitate to fine motor tasks (thus encouraging low-energy postures) as well as the tendency for perseveration and rote repetition. Fine motor play using puzzles and board games can be modified by varying the location of the activity in space. An example is to place the activity on the floor and have the child work from the all fours position, which is good for trunk, shoulder girdle, and hip stability. Encourage weight shifting by having the child reach for puzzle pieces or toss bean bags from a kneeling position. Movement-based interventions are essential and require ongoing supervision and monitoring by the occupational therapist. Teachers who carry out motor programs need to be aware of the importance of the quality of posture and postural control in order to facilitate normal movement patterns and avoid compensated postures. Several activity protocols are identified in Appendix D, Sections 2–6.

Prevocational Assessment and Planning

When a child with PWS reaches high school age, prevocational assessment can provide the foundation for vocational training for employment once the formal educational process is completed. A good resource for such an assessment is the occupational therapist, whose previous working relationship, experience, and familiarity with PWS will be very beneficial. Areas to consider in assessment of prevocational skills include posture and movement, hand/arm use (strength, speed, precision, coordination, and dexterity), positioning, and work habits.

Children with PWS have the postural and movement characteristics typical of children diagnosed as hypotonic, including poor stability of the pelvic and shoulder girdles, and diminished cocontractions of the trunk musculature. When assessing endurance for static activities, the presence of low trunk tone and reduced postural stability may contribute to early fatigue.

As with other types of hypotonia, individuals with PWS generally utilize low-energy postures and developmentally immature movement patterns of arms and hands. Underlying hypotonia with delayed development of trunk, hip, and shoulder stability as well as diminished trunk rotation and weight shift mean the lack of a solid base of support for precise hand and arm use. PWS children tend to utilize less efficient movement patterns that are not well differentiated. They prefer whole hand/arm patterns, which in turn tends to decrease the speed, precision, and dexterity necessary for fine motor manipulation tasks. Correct positioning for fine motor tasks is an important aspect of prevocational and vocational programming. For seated tasks, the chair height should permit the feet to rest flat on the floor with hips to the back of the chair. A chair with a low back might be preferred and the work surface should be at elbow height to permit ease of hand/arm movement. When standing, work surfaces should also be at elbow (waist) height. Proper attention to positioning will promote better posture and decrease postural fatigue.

Prevocational assessment may include measurement of upper extremity range of motion and strength as well as speed and precision of bilateral hand and arm use. A recommended test to assess upper extremity speed and dexterity is the Jebsen Developmental Test of Hand Function (Jebsen, Tayler, Treishmann, et al., 1969), which evaluates broad aspects of functions commonly used in everyday activities. The test is standardized and normed for ages 6 throught 19 years and may be administered in 20 to 30 min using readily available materials.

Earlier in this chapter, it was suggested that physical therapy assessment include the Bruininks–Oseretsky Test of Motor Proficiency (BOMP). This evaluation is also recommended for use by occupational therapists, particularly for fine motor assessment. Three subtests evaluate speed of motor response to a moving visual stimulus, visual motor control, and upper limb speed and dexterity. Although not as quickly or easily administered as the Jebsen, the BOMP does yield a composite score and percentile rank as well as age-equivalent scores. Both tests may be used to identify specific areas of strength and weakness.

Formal clinical observations are made during testing and may include:

1. Sitting posture
2. Ability to understand and follow instructions
3. Work habits
4. Precision of hand–arm use
5. Ability to cross the body midline
6. Analys is of movement patterns, including trunk rotation and weight shift
7. Control and grading of movement
8. Quality of movement
9. Postural control and stability during movement
10. Balance in sitting and standing.

In helping with work–study planning, the occupational therapist can provide invaluable assistance to teachers and vocational training personnel by evaluating the above motor functions, by developing work simplification techniques based on knowledge of fine motor strengths and weaknesses, and by consulting about optimal positioning and use of proper body mechanics.

Summary

Physical and occupational therapists may see children with PWS prior to their having been diagnosed. In these instances, they may be responsible for the initial referral for diagnostic clarification. Focus of concern about newborns and young children with PWS is on feeding problems and lack of progression through the normal developmental milestones. Therapeutic interventions incorporate strategies that promote motor development within the everyday routine of the child and his or her family (strategies are the same as those used with all hypotonic children). For older children, emphasis is placed on encouraging gross motor activity and independence in daily living. Individual therapeutic strategies and collaborative efforts can maximize the physical potential of individuals with PWS and enhance their capacity for integration into vocational programs.

References

Bayley, N. (1969). *Bayley Scales of Infant Development*. New York: Psychological Corporation.

Beery, K.E. (1967). *Developmental Test of Visual-Motor Integration: Administration and scoring manual*. Chicago: Follett Publishing Company.

Bruininks, R.H. (1978). *Bruininks-Oseretsky Test of Motor Proficiency*. Circle Pines, MN: American Guidance Service, Inc.

Carmen, P. (1981). Physical exercise for children and adults with Prader-Willi syndrome. In V.A. Holm, S.J. Hulzbacher, & P.L. Pipes (Eds.), *The Prader-Willi syndrome* (pp. 299–311). Baltimore: University Park Press.

Colarusso, R., & Hamill, D. (1972). *Motor Free Visual Perception Test*. Los Angeles: Western Psychological Service.

Folio, M.R., & Fewell, R.R (1983). *Peabody Developmental Motor Scales and Activity Cards*. In F. Needham (Ed.), Allen, Texas: DLM Teaching Resources.

Goodenough, F. (1927). *Children's drawings (measurement of intelligence by drawings)*. Downey, CA: Rancho Los Amigos Hospital.

Harris, S. (1984). Down syndrome (clinics in physical therapy). In S. Campbell (Ed.), *Pediatric neurological physical therapy* (pp. 169–204). New York: Churchill Livingstone.

Jebsen, R., Taylor, N., Trishmann, R., Trotter, M., & Howard, L. (1969). Objective and standardized test of hand function. *Archives of Physical Medicine and Rehabilitation, 50*, 311–319.

Knobloch, H., Stevens, F., & Malone, A. (1980). *Manual of developmental diagnosis: The administration and interpretation of the Revised Gesell and Armtruda Developmental and Neurological Examination*. Hagerstown, MD: Harper & Row.

Minor, M., & Minor, S.D. (1985). *Patient evaluation methods for the health professional*. Reston, VA: Reston Publishing Co.

Sullivan, P., Markos, P., & Minor, M.A. (1982). *An integrated approach to therapeutic exercise theory and clinical application*. Reston, VA: Reston Publishing Co.

Part III
The Interdisciplinary Process: Psychosocial Aspects

When J is feeling well, she is pleasant to get along with. But there is much of the time she is so listless. She doesn't want to do anything but eat and sleep. This makes life miserable not only for her but everyone around her.

If permitted, L would watch TV continually. She is difficult to motivate. Her disposition is usually good till someone tries to get her to change what she is doing or disagrees. Then she flares up.

At age 10 we were able to secure speech therapy. Until that time we were rebuffed due to his retardation. Today S can carry on a conversation quite well using many words.

Our main concern for P is that he will be able to function in a sheltered workshop. There is no one in the voc[ational] training program that understands that he can't be around food and that he will steal it.

9
Psychological and Behavioral Management

BARBARA Y. WHITMAN and LOUISE R. GREENSWAG

Mental health professionals who work with Prader–Willi syndrome (PWS) are constantly confronted with a complex set of challenging concerns associated with this developmental disability. Management strategies must reflect the unique aspects of the syndrome. In order to provide appropriate services, the cogniture, behavioral, and emotional dimensions of this syndrome must be clearly understood because the intense food seeking habits, emotional outbursts, and inappropriate behaviors can result in psychological and social problems for both individuals with PWS and their families.

This chapter proceeds from the point of view that understanding the relationship between the organic/neurological aspects of PWS, developmental processes, and associated behaviors provides a cornerstone for services. Observable personality characteristics, cognitive and emotional features, and psychosocial skills are described. Current research in brain function that documents the organicity of behaviors observed in PWS and issues associated with psychopharmacological interventions are discussed. Principles of psychological management are identified and suggested strategies for controlling the environment and behavior are linked to developmental eras. Timely information expands considerably beyond earlier reports and documents critical insights that have been gained over the last decade. It is hoped that this content will provide pragmatic information and guidelines for the reader.

An Overview: Fresh Approaches to Previous Concerns

Although persons with PWS demonstrate many individual mental and emotional characteristics, they also share many common traits. These commonalties are most likely the result of the organic brain defect in

PWS (see Chapter 1). Early in toddlerhood some atypical behaviors begin to emerge such as gorging on available food, breaking into locked food storage areas, foraging, and pica. Despite this mildly aberrant activity, most younger children are happy, personable, affectionate, compliant, and cooperative. However, by school age, behavior difficulties begin to emerge. Most clinicians acknowledge that somewhere around 8 years of age a shift from pliable, cheerful children to more rigid, irritable, emotionally labile young persons takes place. Adolescents and older persons are almost always described as extraordinarily stubborn, clever, manipulative, moody, and prone to temper outbursts. Descriptions also suggest that perseveration and egocentrism are often accompanied by self-stimulating behavior such as skin picking. Dishonesty in the form of lying is also common along with poor interpersonal skills, obsessions, and occasionally frank psychoses. Hoarding, pilfering of food and nonfood items, and verbal aggressiveness are reported; social skills appear to decline resulting in deteriorating peer relationships.

By the time persons with PWS reach chronological adolescence and adulthood, case management of the medical and behavioral issues of the syndrome are inextricably bound together. In fact, unless obesity is a complicating factor in this age group, the physical aspects of the syndrome appear to be subsumed by the behavioral issues. Indeed, unless obesity is life threatening, the aberrant behaviors that signify poor impulse control are the *prime* concern of care providers (Greenswag, 1987).

Initially, assistance for this population focused on aiding children and families who struggled to find out what was wrong. Even now, although the label of PWS may end parents confusion and bewilderment regarding the diagnosis, it is often only the beginning of a long journey of frustration, anger, ambivalence, and turmoil. The presence of persons with the syndrome has a profound effect on families, alters almost every facet of their lives, and takes its toll on family resources and energy. Parents/ caregivers struggling with their own personal growth and that of other nonaffected offspring need to recognize that management strategies simply do not work all the time. Depression, vulnerability, and exhaustion are normal responses to raising a child with PWS to say nothing of the fact that it is difficult for the person with PWS who must live differently from other family members and the rest of the world (Herrmann, 1981).

Currently new cases, often much younger children, are being identified by refined diagnostic criteria long before they are referred to a clinic (see Chapter 1). And, because more professionals are now knowledgeable about management, life expectancy has lengthened well into adulthood. Affected individuals and their families require support that extends beyond childhood and early adolescence; services must reach far beyond customary psychometric evaluation, advice about behavioral management, and episodic support of bewildered families. Those medical, educational, allied health, and residential providers unfamiliar with the syndrome require up-to-date, accurate information because, as a group, they tend to be understandably skeptical of family reporting (Sulzbacher, Crnic, & Snow, 1981). In fact, infrequent observers find parental anecdotes difficult to believe since most young children are affable and compliant and older persons *can* be articulate and socially appropriate. This "illusion" of normalcy is very misleading and professionals must be willing to teach whomever, whenever, and wherever necessary.

Guidelines for consistent management of disruptive and noncompliant behaviors, including supervision of food activities, should be instituted when the children are very young. Early infant and child stimulation programs should be the precursor to all educational programming and should include social skill training. These guidelines have significant impact on the degree to which persons with PWS adapt beyond their schooling to the time when out-of-home living, employment, and community participation become realities (see Chapters 7, 11, and 15). In addition to being members of a interdisciplinary team in a clinic setting (see Chapter 4) psychologists and other mental health professionals need to understand the organicity of PWS, be able to offer counseling to parents and families, and be available for consultation with primary providers.

Two aspects of PWS are of major importance. First, consideration must be given to the growing body of information that documents an organic basis for the syndrome (Chapter 1). Just as the observed lack of satiety is physiologically based, so too does this neurological flaw in the brain also affect cognition, emotions, and behaviors. Second, the significance of the presence of mental retardation cannot be underestimated.

Neuropsychological Issues

Cognition

All persons with PWS have some cognitive limitations. On closer examination, their cognitive profiles and functional capacity suggest severe learning and language disabilities often in addition to a global slowness. As a result, most affected persons present and perform as if mildly retarded even when IQ scores are higher.

In addition to the presence of mental retardation, studies of learning disabilities in PWS detail weaknesses in sequential processing and short term memory (Dykens, Hodapp, Walsh, et al., 1992a). Long-term memory, rote skills, and bits of information appear to be strengths along with simultaneous processing, i.e., the ability to see or hear a whole pattern of information.

The impact of this pattern of learning disabilities on behavior (independent of IQ) cannot be minimized because when sequential processing deficits are present, intake, processing, and production of a response to information are affected. Such deficits lead to difficulties in reading comprehension, interpretation and integration of multistep directions, and mastery of multiplication tables. Problems learning to tell time, confusion over time concepts and temporal meanings such as "before," "after," "until," and delayed grasp of experiential sequences (days of the week, months of the year) are common. No less important, this deficit results in diffculties in performing complex sequential motor tasks and sound sequencing of speech. Narrative organization and a limited capacity to sequence ideas in oral restatement and writing are reported. In short, persons with PWS often have trouble following a schedule, remembering what to do, when to do it, and in what order the elements of the task should advance. Since most life tasks require the ability to say "first I do this, then I do that," persons with this type of mental processing dilemma are often overwhelmed and lost. Everyday life patterns appear confusing and may result in anxiety, frustration, and acting out.

The presence of sequential learning problems not only limits language processing (see Chapter 10) but also the use of problem-solving strategies. Because of the inability to plan then alter actions, there is a strong proclivity to excessive rigidity. This inflexibility, perceived as stubbornness, is one of the most commonly described behaviors. While this behavior is less of a problem in special education settings where such deficits are accommodated, a sudden shift in plans or activities can cause a major and often inappropriate reactions in interpersonal relationships and in the social arena. What appears to be "just common sense" in a given situation is often inappropriately perceived by the person with PWS.

Another aspect of this sequencing deficit is an accompanying deficiency in the capacity to self-monitor, a tendency to think concretely, and trouble dealing with abstractions and systems of symbols. Attempting to explain an issue to persons with PWS who have already an established mind set usually reveals concrete thinking, lack of capacity to abstract or follow a chain of logic, inability to learn from experience, inability to shift perspective, or alter a preset train of thought. Failure to learn from experience may explain why traditional behavior modification programs have only limited success.

Of note is the fact that some children do appear to learn some concepts and rules by rote memory but have difficulty understanding how and when to apply them. There is a tendency to apply a single rule to all situations or conversely, not generalize at all. The fit between a "rule" and the situation as interpreted by persons with PWS often appears self-serving and contrived. However, despite these identified learning limitations, they often demonstrate spatial and patterning strengths expressed as proficiency at working puzzles and word search exercises.

Emotionally, persons with PWS have been described as having, at best, enigmatic and trying personalities. However, when these descriptors are matched with the behavioral outcome patterns of learning disabilities, a different picture begins to emerge. For these individuals, the world is often unpredictable and confusing. Because of the need for constant food mangement by outside care-providers, they function in an arena where they have "no control." In an attempt to cope with their world, they tend to "lock onto" what they know (or think they know) to the exclusion of any contradictory information. When this fails them, they become anxious, agitated, and work even harder to acquire some sense of internal control. Emotional turmoil is often the order of the day and results in acting out behavior.

In 1987, Whitman and Accardo documented a high incidence of such symptoms as "obsessive type behaviors" that included fear of doing something bad and/or dying, worrying about possessions being stolen, and the inability to change plans. The need for tasks to be in the same order and done the same way and a strong desire for consistent routine were often noted. Symptoms of anxiety, frustration, "being high-strung," argumentativeness, and tantruming were noted a great percentage of the time.

Other studies (Curfs, Verhulst, & Fryns, 1992, Dykens, Hodapp, Walsh, et al., 1992b) also described argumentativeness, along with an inability to concentrate, clumsiness, disobedience, generalized confusion about tasks, obsessiveness about food and personal possessions, and a preference for being alone. This suggests that the behavioral components of PWS are similar to other organic brain disorders such as Attention Deficit Hyperactivity Disorder and Tourettes syndrome, which follow a direct pathway from a learning disability to a behavioral profile with no psychiatric overlay. It is imperative that great caution be taken not to misdiagnose neurobehavioral problems as psychiatric disorders because the management strategies are radically different.

The Issue of Mental Retardation

As in the past, cognitive assessment to determine a general level of intelligence should begin as early in life as possible and follow-up re-evaluation is essential. As with other developmental disorders, the cognitive potential in PWS is difficult to assess and even the best pre-dictors are not highly valid before 18 months of age. It usually can be determined only on the basis of other observable developmental delays. Testing after 18 months places the majority of affected children in the mild to moderate range of retardation.

It is hard enough for parents and families to deal with the physical limitations of PWS. The added fact that retardation is also present makes adaptation even more difficult. In fact, having to cope with mental limitations compounds anxieties about management. Certainly, very early on, the presence of mental retardation needs to be demystified and destigmatized.

Conceptualizing a Developmental Model

All human beings grow through a series of developmental eras or stages (Donaldson, Chu, Coote, et al., 1994). Understanding these stages provides a framework for care-providers and encourages establishment of realistic expectations for the actions and relationships that can help persons with PWS adapt and at the same time reduce some of their frustrations.

It has been well documented (Chin, Drew, & Logan, 1979) that when the normal developmental process is compounded by a birth defect, the expectations for the child to become independent, socially mature, and sexually active may not be met. Parental responsibilities do not decrease and issues such as finding services, providing educational opportunities, and adapting to community life continue. Furthermore, studies of other handicapped populations indicate that the same emotional drives affect individuals, regardless of IQ (Kolstoe & Frey, 1965). In other words, cognitive limitations and physical handicap do not negate the capacity for feelings but the discrepancy between chronological and mental age becomes more pronounced over time. Moreover, lacking the intellectual capacity to make decisions or the maturity to set goals makes the development of interpersonal skills necessary for social acceptance difficult. Due to the previously identified neurobehavioral limitations, persons with PWS are rarely able to comply with any kind of unsupervised weight or behavioral programs.

This framework acknowledges that the developmental levels achieved by persons with PWS rarely go beyond a prelatency level (6 to 10 yers of age). For example, persons with PWS want relationships and friends but transfer allegiances easily just as normal prelatency children do. As is appropriate for this developmental level, there is a strong tendency to egocentrism (self-centeredness) and a lack of objectivity, despite verbal abilities. However, *they are not being obstinate*, they merely think very simply and need to feel safe. They avoid trouble and, hopefully, punishment, by denying wrongdoing. It is difficult for parents/caregivers to understand, let alone accept that confrontations regarding inappropriate behaviors are a waste of time.

Examples of "cleverness" abound, confusing and misleading parents/caregivers who resist the reality associated with mental limitations. Parents, extended family, and caregivers have a strong need to *believe* that affected persons *do* understand and *are* competent. Instead of insisting, "I can explain this to him," the question should be "does this person *really* understand?" While a few parents/caregivers will do this, most will not.

Management Issues

How can understanding and applying developmental stages affect behavioral management? The "thought processes" of prelatency children and how they perform provide a reasonable rationale for how persons with PWS think and behave. They need love and verbal praise, future time tends to be endless for them, and they fantasize adult roles. Therefore, their daily life requires structure, guidelines that change infrequently, specific rules about what is negotiable and what is not, and making choices should be limited to two or three options. Perhaps because there seems to be some evidence of auditory processing problems (see Chapter 10), demonstrating tasks rather than giving verbal instructions seems to work better. Avoiding adult interpretations of verbal exchanges helps. Programming should focus on reality, reward flexibility, and take into account the relationship between behaviors, moods, and stamina when establishing developmentally appropriate positive reinforcements.

Behavioral Management or Behavioral Modification?

Most attempts to change behavior follow a fundamental behavior modification formula that assumes the capacity to learn from experiences. The basic formula is (1) when an unwanted behavior occurs, a negative consequence is forthcoming, and (2) when a wanted behavior occurs, it is followed by a positive reward. This formula reflects a developmental process of *learning from experience and acting according to that learning*.

Unfortunately, traditional behavioral modification techniques are rarely effective with persons with PWS. First, they cannot generalize despite learned associations and desire for concrete rewards. Second, for those few individuals who demonstrate some abstract thinking, the biological hunger drive, impulsivity, and emotional vulnerability override learning. Third, such interventions rely on reactive (often punitive) methods of behavior change at the expense of proactive, planned behavior management. Because internal controls assumed by behavior modification methods are lacking, management strategies must focus on preventing the opportunity for the expression of impulsivity.

Behavior management differs from behavior modification. Management procedures are initiated prior to the occurrence of the deviant behavior and remove or reduce conditions that provoke problems. Such procedures present or emphasize conditions that *increase* the likelihood of appropriate behavior, *decrease* the opportunity for inappropriate behavior, and *minimize* the duration and intensity of problem behaviors following their occurrence. Therefore, management includes environmental control, operating guidelines that specify rules, routines, times, consequences, choice and reward management, consistency, anticipatory planning, behavioral rehearsal, and rewarding flexibility.

Strategies for Management

The following guidelines may help families and can be successful when implemented initially in the home, then carried over to the educational environment, and later to out-of-home living, work, and community life. General strategies consist of environmental and behavioral management. Use of the adjunction management strategies of social skill training and use of psychotropic medication are discussed separately.

The Environment

The quality of life for the person with PWS depends on the ability of caregivers to provide an environment that is structured enough to allow maximum freedom of movement and expression while minimizing the conditions that encourage inappropriate behaviors and impulsivity. Regulating the environment is the key to successful management. Expectations for individuals with PWS to be capable of completely managing their own lives are very unrealistic. Responsible life decisions should be guided by a guardian. Issues associated with protection and advocacy are discussed in Chapter 14. A supervised and restricted setting should be initiated when the children are very young. Limiting access to food and to the possessions of others is essential and should set the stage for practical patterns of behavior over time. Many weight management and behavioral strategies have been inadvertently sabotaged by well meaning extended family, school personnel, workshop staff, and residential providers. Specific environmental guidelines for educational, residential, and vocational settings are discussed in Chapters 11, 15, and 16. Case studies of a weight/behavioral management approach (Appendix E.1) and a token economy/house guidelines program (Appendix E.2) are described.

Behavioral Approaches

Once a decision has been made about an approach to management, rules/guidelines and procedures need to be identified and implemented. These rules provide a framework for the negotiable and nonnegotiable aspects of daily life and should be delineated ahead of time to reduce power struggles. Along with general guidelines, individual behavioral goals must be recognized so rewards and honors can be acknowledged.

Positive reinforcement for individuals with PWS is very effective where realistic expectations are clearly understood. Rewards should be cognitively and emotionally appropriate rather than age appropriate. This is not always easy because competition causes frustration and inter-personal conflicts. Mastery should be measured in simple successes rather than pressing to attain an unreachable or unrealistic goal. While most other mentally retarded persons tend to maintain a level of competency once a task is learned, the capacity of persons with PWS to retain learning fluctuates. They may be very productive and cooperative for a time, only to "loose it." Therefore, less complicated, less stressful activities make the "relearning process" easier on the individual (although more frustrating for those who work with them). This is not to infer that the presence of the syndrome means lack of the ability to learn or grow, it merely means that task performance tends to be characteristically erratic. More than with other mentally disabling conditions, the maximum potential for this population is very difficult to gauge.

Behavioral tracking is best done on a daily as well as a weekly basis. Concrete rewards need to be earned more frequently than once a week. In addition to praise, a sticker/star "token system" seems to work well as long as the amount of tokens to be earned for a reward initially is small and the time element relatively short. Over time if a system seems to be motivating, it may become more sophisticated.

Rewards should be on view as a reminder. For example, keep a book, game, or special prize wrapped in clear plastic and visible. (Appendix E.3) Under no circumstances should rewards be withdrawn once earned. However, earnings may be used to restore or replace items "borrowed" or destroyed. Any reward system should be integrated into *all* activities. When all primary providers are "playing with the same set of rules", consistency is easier to maintain in all settings. Where feasible, incor-porating ideas from persons with PWS into the decision-making process is beneficial.

Since food seeking is an uncontrollable neurological drive, managing this behavior means establishing permanent restriction of access to food and predictable time for meals. This invariant structure is critical to the creation of some reasonable eating patterns. Admittedly, this presents problems for other family members whose social lives normally would include less rigid eating activities.

Because behavioral management is never static the future must be anticipated. Therefore, planning for each day can help providers manage a variety of situations. Two examples follow that may help in control of food and perseveration. A school outing can be successful where structure is provided, where very clear limits for behavior are established along with preplanned lunches, and time to be spent on activities. When change is necessary, trying to predict and plan for outcomes and rehearsing responses are helpful.

Perseveration is another disconcerting behavior that causes great concern to family members and caregivers and requires some form of intervention. These repetitive verbalizations usually occur after a request or inquiry by the person with PWS has been turned down. This behavior seems to increase with age, is unsettling, and keeps alive issues that the listener would like to drop. The problem of how to handle perseveration is not a minor one and management begins with understanding that this behavior is *not* obsessional or a deep seated emotional problem.

Perseveration is, however, a function of a nervous system where the "off– on" switch often gets stuck in the "on" position and allows words to keep pouring out despite efforts to shut off the switch. A more human analogy likens this behavior to the erratic motor behavior of a newborn infant whose arms and legs begin to flail at will. The solution for quieting the baby is to wrap the blanket tightly around so that the flailing stops and the nervous system calms down, a technique known as "bunting." A solution for repetitive verbalizations may be a spoken version of "bunting." If these repetitions are a failure of a neurological off–on switch, then it follows that the *content* of these verbalizations is not the major issue; no reasoning or countering with logical arguments will have an impact. Therefore, avoid getting trapped into arguing or explaining. Establish a routine of stating, "this discussion is now over—if you need to think about this subject some more, please go to your room until you are ready to discuss something else." For an older person with PWS who needs to participate in the decision to stop, a time limit can be set and choices presented within those limits, e.g., "you can have five more minutes now or we can talk about it again for five minutes after supper." More of the decision for stopping is offered after which it can be pointed out that "We will discuss this only five more minutes after which time I must do—." Be sure to indicate the current time and what the time will be when five minutes are up. At the end of the interval indicate that it is time to stop and end the discussion. If necessary, leave the room. Verbally and behaviorally, "bunting" can work.

Once decisions have been made about management strategies, establishing specific rules for desired behaviors can benefit children and care-providers alike. As a background for developing these rules, several caveats must be kept in mind. There has to be unanimity about *what* behavior is expected and *when*. Where parents disagree, it is critical that they compromise and find some middle ground because when individuals with PWS sense parental/caregiver conflict, there is a strong tendency to play one person against another. Disagreements regarding rules or behaviors should not be discussed when the child is present. Rules should be appropriate to developmental level, ability, and temperament and stated in positive terms, such as "Bedtime is 8:00" versus "Don't stay up after 8:00." For older individuals, rules may be written as contracts and should include consequences when they are broken. Rules need to be reviewed frequently because children, caregivers, and situations change over time. Finally, other adults, such as extended family and friends must be expected to adhere to established guidelines, regardless of the setting.

Preventing Misbehavior

It is hard to look at misbehavior objectively. When children are difficult to deal with, attitudes become negative. Caregivers should be aware of issues most likely to precipitate disruptive behaviors. These include:

1. The need for *attention*: often, not enough reinforcement is given for positive behavior; acting out to get attention occurs then ends up as a crisis.
2. Boredom/understimulation: A barren, unstimulating environment can also trigger acting out.
3. Overstimulation—excess noise: Teasing, constant loud TVs or radios, redundant activity, and a chaotic living environment can stimulate problems.
4. Stress in living situations: Lack of the consistency among caretakers is confusing and unsettling.
5. Lack of personal space and need for territoriality: Personal space is critical, be it a desk in school or a section of a shared room that allows for privacy. A place to retreat is essential along with an area for personal items.
6. A need to test limits/refusal to obey rules: Testing to see if rules will be enforced, loss of personal power/control can cause difficulties.
7. Conflicts with others but a need for affiliation: Poor coping skills and a desire to fit in with others in a group while avoiding competition and envy can cause conflict.
8. Changes/interruptions in routine: Abrupt changes in routines and environments can trigger outbursts, especially if changes are unexpected.
9. Conflicts with authority figures: Personality problems, false acceptance, and inconsistent interactions tend to create problems because of the need to keep control and separate from authority figures.
10. Disappointments: Not getting a specific service, meal, desired activity or anticipated item creates feelings of deprivation and generates disruptive behavior.

Encouraging Appropriate Behavior

While preventing behaviors from becoming totally disruptive is not easy, there are techniques that may prevent "molehills" from becoming "mountains" (Redel & Wineman, 1952).

1. Planned ignoring: This is merely the skill of knowing when and when not to interfere. Sometimes it is better to ignore attention-getting infractions.
2. Signal interference: Some behavior may be prevented by signaling with a gesture of disapproval. For example; waving a finger, or saying "No."
3. Proximity and touch control: Overexcitement or restlessness often may be calmed down by moving closer to those involved. A friendly hand on the shoulder or a touch on the arm also may be used. This must *not* be done in a threatening way.
4. Involvement: A youngster on the verge of misbehaving is often diverted by a question concerning some task at hand. A chance to explain to an interested adult usually revives interest in normal pursuits.
5. Hypodermic affection: Sometimes all that is needed for ego support in the face of anxiety is a sudden additional "quantity of affection."

More specific suggestions include orchestrating situations where appropriate behavior can be performed and rewarded. Heavily reinforce cooperation and teach special, exciting skills that tend to draw positive attention. Make only relevant demands and do not expect too much more. Improve the environment by providing occasions to engage in constructive activity and opportunities for appropriate socialization and social skills trainning. Recognize the need for regular physical exercise, particularly for release of tension (e.g., jogging, walks, swimming). Encourage functional communication of needs and/or feelings. Do not assume that everything said is understood. Beware of stressful periods during the day, i.e., getting ready for the school bus in the morning and avoid offering choices if they are not realistic. Further suggestions for rewards and behavioral programs are listed in Appendix E.2.

Social Skills Training

Another major area of behavioral management concerns the development of appropriate social skills for persons with PWS. Many demonstrate difficulty with both verbal and nonverbal interpersonal interactions and often appear unable to read, and suitably react in social situations. Mitchell (1988) indicates that even when placed in programs that successfully focus on weight management and other behavioral issues, these individuals often experience significant difficulties because their social skill deficits compound other problems, such as impulsivity and poor judgement.

Such basic components of social interactions as eye contact, appropriate interpersonal distance, listening, turn-taking, and even the simple process of shaking hands are frequently missing from their social repertoire. In supported work environments, these deficits tend to create problems for supervisors and co-workers accustomed to interacting with clients with other (non-PWS) developmental disabilities. So serious are these deficits that they often cause persons with PWS not merely to lose jobs, but also to be precluded from consideration from any work placement. Therefore, if individuals with PWS are to become more independent and personally responsible, social skills training should routinely be included in all management programs.

Mitchell (1988) identified a model to teach direct care staff how to assess and instruct persons with PWS in prosocial skills and to reduce social transgressions in controlled, closely supervised settings. Roffman (1981) developed a curriculum and course materials for learning-disabled young adults call *Threshold*. Other researchers and practitioners such as Baker, Brightman, Heifitz, et al. (1976) have created specific parent-training materials to help parents teach their developmentally disabled children with behavior problems appropriate skills.

Assessment of a group of persons with PWS by Mitchell (1988) revealed that conversational skills were most limiting, and within this category, the greatest deficits were in turn-taking and in learning to listen. Inappropriate behaviors had the second highest priority, with emotional outbursts, verbal assertiveness, and noncompliance rated as the three most troublesome. Interestingly, theft of food and property and stereotypes were given lower priorities. It was speculated that these behaviors, common among clients with PWS, were already under good control compared to other behavioral issues. Deficits in assertive behaviors were ranked as a third priority, with nonverbal communication ranked as the lowest category. Assertive behavior deficits requiring the most attention were a relatively poor ability to express annoyance, presence of irritability, and refusal to interact appropriately. Failure to maintain appropriate distance was the most problematic issue in nonverbal communication. Teaching activities indicated that role-playing and modeling were considered to be the most effective. Games were rated second, followed by coaching, labeling feelings, and finally relaxation and biofeedback.

Because conversational skills were identified as the highest training priority, activities from Roffman's social skills curriculum were adapted and made into games.

The Timing Game consists of topical situations, printed in large letters on cards that can be read aloud in turn. Each player has a response card used to indicate whether the situation read by the leader presents a good or bad time to initiate a conversation. The goal is to improve the timing skills of clients and to encourage group discussions on this topic.

The Open/Closed Questions Game is similar in format to the Timing Game. Questions printed in large letters are read aloud, one at a time. Cards are held indicating whether each person thinks the question is open-ended (requiring more than a one- or two-word answer and thus stimulating further conversation) or closed-ended (requiring a very brief answer, and presenting an awkward silence thereafter). The goal is to teach how to begin and maintain conversations

The Assertive Game provides definitions of assertive, aggressive, and nonassertive behaviors. A group leader then reads the descriptions of behavior and each participant decides whether that behavior is assertive, aggressive, or nonassertive. The goal is to help increase understanding and use of assertive behaviors.

The Book Method teaches how to give criticism tactfully. Originally called the Sandwich Recipe by Roffman, the name was changed because of the sensitivity of clients with PWS to food-related themes. This method encourages initiating criticism with a positive statement (front cover of the book). This is followed by the criticism itself, along with a rationale (the contents), and finally by a request for a change (back cover). Participants are asked to write a book. The goal is to encourage constructive, assertive criticism.

The Ungame, a commercially available board game (The Ungame Company, 1984) can be effective. It is adapted by preparing directions relevant for individuals with PWS as a structured way to encourage turn-taking and listening.

Parents can model and teach these skills, which should be reinforced through special education classes, day activity centers, and residential programs. As an in-service project, social skills training can be done on a very small budget and, certainly, the single workshop format is most cost-effective.

Use of Psychotropic Medications

Over time, use of psychotropic medications to manage moods and behaviors has had both a positive and a negative impact on persons with PWS. An effective treatment tool in the hands of qualified professionals, drug intervention has proven a godsend for specific cases. However, too frequently these medications are employed as end treatments to control behaviors; unruly patients become less troublesome and difficult, case management is less of a burden, and the work of caregivers easier.

As previously discussed, behavioral volatility and labile moods are a direct consequence of the presence of the syndrome itself rather than an outcome of poor management. Unlike their normal peers, persons with PWS are less able to develop compensating emotional responses and behavior to help them overcome their emotional vulnerabilities. Escalating bizarre and inappropriate behaviors inhibit psychosocial adaptation.

Reports concerning the use of psychotropic medication in individuals with PWS have been conflicting and anecdotal accounts suggest widespread misuse to control those behaviors that tend to mimic mental illness. While a small number may have some significant psychiatric difficulties, most do not. Misinterpretation of behavior components as "psychiatric" becomes the rationale for caregivers to suppress inappropriate conduct through medication rather than developing nondrug strategies to improve adaptation.

Recently a systematic collection of data was initiated to investigate use of these medications a tool to manage behaviors. (Whitman & Greenswag, 1992a). Reports included information about appetite suppressants, anxiolytic, seizure, antidepressants, and antipsychotic drugs in addition to medication to counteract possible side effects. The most striking finding was that few medications have *any* effect and those few that did were so toxic they rendered the persons unable to function. However, three serotonergic medications consistently emerged as the most useful. They were, in descending order of cognitive suppression, Haldol, Mellaril, and Prozac. A second generation of the Prozac family, Zoloft and Paxil, is currently being tried (Whitman & Greenswag, 1992b).

Currently, Haldol or Mellaril are administered when behavior and emotional control are critically impaired; both medications appear to stabilize mood and behavior. Once stabilized, a shift to Prozac has proven very effective; it appears to reduce irritability and ease rigidity. There seems to be more control, a sort of "mellowing out." Situations that previously might have triggered an outburst or rage attack are less frequent, and individuals seem more reasonable and able to stay controlled for a somewhat longer period of time. It is suggested that the mechanisms of these medications are analogous to that of Ritalin in attention disorders; each renders the patient more amenable to management strategies.

It is important to point out that some individuals in initial trials of these medications demonstrated idiosyncratic responses. Early reports about Prozac were very positive but its effect appeared to dissipate after about 3 weeks. The impression was that the suppressed behaviors were returning. This belief led to the decision to *increase* the dosage, which was even more detrimental. Subsequent protocols indicate that while the initial dose was appropriate, over time it reached toxic levels causing increased agitation and irritability. In most cases, reducing the dose was effective. Clearly, these dosage levels are person specific. When considering use of this drug, any titration protocol should take these idiosyncratic findings in account and calibrate dosage accordingly. According to Boyle (1994), "there are new medications appearing all the time now which may benefit Prader-Willi patients. The potential for improved quality of life for these people is enormous. However, Prader-Willi syndrome is a rare and complicated disorder" (p. 4). Therefore, all new medicinal interventions require careful supervision by qualified professionals.

Summary

The impact of the psychological aspects of Prader–Willi syndrome cannot be underestimated. The severity and the consequences of these characteristics dramatically influence the quality of life for affected individuals, their families, and caregivers. A growing body of knowledge of the organic/neurological elements has come to play an important role in understanding the cognitive and emotional features and plays a critical role in the development of appropriate strategies for managing behaviors.

References

Baker, B.L., Brightman, A.J., Heifitz, L.J., & Murphy, D.M. (1976). *Behavior problems*. Champagne, IL: Research Press.

Boyle, I.R. (1994). *Psychiatric Medication and Prader-Willi syndròme: Notes from the frontiers*. Prader-Willi Perspectives, vol. 2, no. 2, p. 4.

Bray, G.A., Dahms, W.T., Swerdloff, R.S., Fisher, R.H., Atkinson, R.L., & Carrel, R.E. (1983). The Prader-Willi syndrome: A study of 40 patients and a review of the literature. *Medicine, 62*, 59–80.

Chin, P.C., Drew, C.J., & Logan, D. (1979). *Mental Retardation, A Life Cycle Approach*. St. Louis, Mo: The C.V. Mosby Co.

Curfs, L.M.G., Verhulst, F.C., & Fryns, J.P. (1992). Behavioral and emotional problems in youngsters with Prader-Willi syndrome. *Gernetic Counseling, 2*(1), 33–41.

Donaldson, M., Chu, C., Cooke, A., Wilson, A., Greene, S., & Stephenson, J. (1994). The Prader-Willi syndrome. *Archives of Disease in Childhood, 70*, 58–63.

Dykens, E., Hodapp, R., Walsh, K., & Nash, L. (1992a). Profiles, correlates, and trajectories of intelligence in Prader-Willi syndrome. *Journal of the American Academy of Child and Adolescent Psychiatry, 31*(6), 1125–1130.

Dykens, E., Hodapp, R., Walsh, K., & Nash, L. (1992b). Adaptive and maladaptive behavior in Prader-Willi syndrome. *Journal of the American Academy of Child and Adolescent Psychiatry, 31*(6), 1131–1136.

Greenswag, L.R. (1987). Adults with Prader-Willi syndrome: A survey of 232 cases. *Developmental Medicine and Child Neurology, 29*, 145–152.

Herrmann, J. (1981). Implications of Prader-Willi Syndrome for the individual and the family. In V.A. Holm, S.J. Sulzbacher, & P. Pipes (Eds.), *Prader-Willi syndrome* (pp. 229–244). Baltimore: University Park Press.

Kolstoe, O.P., & Frey, R. (1965). *A high school work-study program for the mentally subnormal student*. Carbondale, IL: Southern Illinois University Press.

Mitchell, W (1988). Social skills training for Prader-Willi Syndrome. In L.R. Greenswag & R.C. Alexander (Eds). Management of Prader-Willi Syndrome. (165–170) New York; Springer-Verlag.

Redel, F., & Wineman, D. (1952) *Controls from within: Techniques for the treatment of the aggressive child*. Glencoe, IL: Free Press.

Roffman, A. (1981). *The effects of social skills training on the attitudes and behaviors of CETA trainees*. Unpublished doctoral dissertation, Boston College.

Sulzbacher, S., Crnic, K.A., & Snow, J. (1981). Behavioral and cognitive disabilities in Prader-Willi syndrome. In V.A. Holm, S.J. Sulzbacher, & P.L. Pipes (Eds.), *The Prader-Willi Syndrome* (pp. 147–160). Baltimore: University Park Press.

Whitman, B., & Accardo, P. (1987). Emotional symptoms in Prader-Willi syndrome adolescents. *American Journal of Medical Genetics*, *28*, 897–905.

Whitman, B., & Greenswag, L.R. (1992a). The use of psychotropic medications in persons with Prader-Willi syndrome. In S. Cassidy (Ed.), *Prader-Willi syndrome and other chromosome 15q deletion disorders* (pp. 223–231). New York: Springer Verlag.

Whitman, B., & Greenswag, L.R. (1992b). *A survey of mediation usage and effectiveness in persons with Prader-Willi syndrome.* Paper presented at the PWSA-USA National Conference, Scottsdale, Arizona, July.

10
Speech and Language Issues

Debora A. Downey and Claudia L. Knutson

Speech and language abilities are the major tools of communication and, for individuals with Prader–Willi syndrome (PWS), the development of these skills are frequently problematic (Branson, 1981). Because communication is an essential function of daily living, educational programming, and personal and social growth, any limitations significantly impact on the quality of life. Although parents and caregivers can provide some stimulation of these abilities, the speech and language pathologist, an important member of the interdisciplinary team, can help to maximize this area of development.

While common characteristics in speech and language development have been identified, the cognitive status and degree of hypotonia present in this population are responsible for the variation in communication profiles and most of the typical speech-language skills that require interventions (Kleppe, Katayama, Shipley, et al., 1990; Munson-Davis, 1988). This chapter explores the importance of early intervention and monitoring of speech and language abilities of preschool and school-age children in order to assess and enhance their communication skills. It defines speech and language characteristics, offers practical strategies for management, and addresses pragmatic issues that affect the communication skills of older individuals with PWS (Munson-Davis, 1988).

Speech and Language Characteristics

Hypotonia and cognition are responsible for most of the speech and language skills of persons with PWS. Because commonalties and variations require early intervention (Kleppe et al., 1990), baseline evaluation should begin as early as 1 year of age. Continued periodic monitoring of speech and language development from infancy through school age is essential because difficulties may become apparent due to changes in the degree of hypotonia and environmental factors over time (Munson-Davis, 1988). Assessment and monitoring should include examination of oral motor structures/function, voice, fluency, articulation, and overall language abilities.

Oral Motor Structures/Function

Although oral motor structures for production of speech are usually intact, their function is greatly influenced by the degree of underlying hypotonia that accounts not only for the devastating feeding difficulties during infancy, but also for the varying abilities in tongue tip elevation and oral musculature, and decreased abilities to sequence rapidly alternating speech movements (Kleppe et al., 1990; Munson-Davis, 1988). This muscle weakness noted in oral structures and function is characteristic of flaccid dysarthria (Kleppe et al., 1990).

Voice

The most common characteristic of deviant voice usage is hypernasality, a direct result of inadequate velopharyngeal closure of the nasal cavity via movement of the soft palate (Boone, 1983). Because of this, total removal of all adenoidal tissue in not recommended. Hypernasality is commonly observed in patients who exhibit flaccid dysarthria (Kleppe et al., 1990; Munson-Davis, 1988). Clinical observations support the notion of the abnormal vocal quality of hypernasality and the occasional appearance of weak, breathy phonation indicating difficulty with bilateral vocal fold adductors.

Speech effectiveness is directly related to the ability to achieve adequate glottal closure. If expiratory air flow is used inefficiently and reduced glottal resistance is present, the resulting phenomenon is a decreased intensity level and reduced phonatory time (Linebaugh, 1993). When inadequate intensity levels are present, misuse of vocal cord functioning may also occur (Boone, 1983); any one or a combination of these factors of hypernasality, inappropriate pitch and/or intensity level, as well as phonating time, impedes intelligibility of speech.

Fluency

Traditional fluency disorders of stuttering and cluttering do not appear to be present in most individuals with PWS. Kleppe et al. (1990) reported a high occurrence of rather simple dysfluencies, i.e., interjections, revisions, and word repetitions, but 66–99% appear to have fluent speech. This observation concurs with reports that persons with decreased cognitive abilities have the complicated patterns of avoidance behavior commonly noted in advanced stutterers with normal cognition (Van Ripper, 1982). Clinically, the dysfluencies noted in the PWS population tend to be more episodic with few word and phonemic fears (Kleppe et al., 1990); hesitant behavior may be due to the limitations in language development associated with their overall cognitive status.

Articulation

Articulation abilities, the process of actual sound/phoneme development, and oral production, are frequently problematic and also are markedly affected by both cognition and hypotonia (Dyson & Lombardino, 1989; Kleppe et al., 1990; Munson-Davis, 1988). There is a direct correlation between the extent to which cognitive capacity affects the pattern of development and the rate of phonemic development. Some children with PWS exhibit relatively "normal, but delayed" development (Dyson & Lombardino, 1989), while others may exhibit atypical patterns, such as developmental apraxia of speech or a phonological disorder (Munson-Davis, 1988). The degree of distortions, substitutions, and/or omissions varies. Phonemes, which are more motorically complex, i.e., /r, l, dʒ, s, z, ʃ/, usually are the most difficult (Kleppe et al., 1990). This is not surprising considering the previously identified flaccid dysarthria. Post-vocalic deletions can be the most obvious source for errors to occur (Dyson & Lombardino, 1989). It follows that intelligibility differences may occur between single word production and connected speech, with the latter requiring significantly more coordination during motorically complex movements of the tongue and oral structures (Munson-Davis, 1988). The phonetic environment also can play a part in how articulators function and may cause assimilation and metathesis or migration errors (Dyson & Lombardino, 1989). Clearly, the presence of a wide variety of misarticulations has a negative impact on speech intelligibility.

Language Abilities

Receptive language abilities (comprehension) and expressive language abilities (the act of expressing one's thoughts, wants, or ideas) are critical to successful communication. Typically, language is thought of as the "words" used to communicate, but can also include any symbols, such as pictures, gestures, signs, or sounds. Without these "meaningful" sets of symbols, "language" as communication cannot exist.

Both receptive and expressive language abilities may be significantly compromised in the presence of PWS (Branson, 1981; Kleppe et al.,

1990; Munson-Davis, 1988). Even with possible gains in intelligibility of speech, weaknesses continue in information processing that involves auditory stimuli, precision in articulation and pronunciation of words, higher problem-solving skills, and conceptualization (Cassidy, 1992). Again, variability in language functioning is directly linked to over-all cognitive development (Rice, 1983). Since cognitive levels in individuals with PWS vary, so too will language functioning. Clinically, because there is a need to understand language before it can be used successfully, receptive language appears more intact than expressive language.

Early in the process of language development, receptive understanding may appear to be more delayed than it actually is because the hypotonia limits effective expression of what is comprehended (Munson-Davis, 1988). It also limits the capacity for play and exploration that ultimately affects the ability to learn such things as vocabulary and basic concepts. Less mobile children may not be familiar with actions such as skip, hop, etc. nor have the physical ability to respond to parental direction such as "Please get me the toy next to the . . . ." Deficits may exist solely from lack of experiences (Munson-Davis, 1988).

Expressive language, however, is often more significantly impaired than receptive language in the population with PWS. Suggested casual factors of this discrepancy in the school-age child include articulation problems, word recall problems, voice differences, vocabulary delays, word usage problems, grammatical errors, and incomplete sentence structure. As further reported by Munson-Davis (1988), these speech–language problems may "continue into adulthood" and should be closely followed.

Verbalizations of children with PWS, while often understood, may lack structural completeness. Typical utterances consist primarily of noun and verb construction. Morphological development that includes use of irregular past tense, plurality, and passive markers also tends to be significantly delayed (Kleppe et al., 1990). Two reasons may cause this deficit. First, the need for morphologic markers may not be understood, and second, production of the physical sounds, i.e., articulation ability, may be limited. Therefore, when assessing language development, the *reason* for the lack of morphological usage becomes critical to the remediation process.

Some expressive language difficulties are related to the ability to use language already acquired: this is known as "pragmatics." Pragmatics refer to the capacity to understand and apply rules to communicate using appropriate and socially accepted "manners." Individuals with PWS tend to use their language inappropriately. Disruptions in their communication processes include difficulty in maintaining topic, proximity, turn-taking, and performing socially acceptable skills.

Clinical Management

Federal law mandates that children with disabilities between the ages of 3 and 21 be identified, diagnosed, educated, and provided appropriate special services in the least restrictive environment possible. This is the legal right of all children with disabilities (see Chapter 14). Speech–language services can be obtained through the educational agency of local school districts.

Remediation of communication and its clinical management require speech–language pathologists to think not only in terms of the syndrome but also about the unique individual whose communication is significantly compromised by hypotonia and cognitive functioning. Early intervention is the key to maximizing their potential (Blackman, 1990). This is necessary because children begin to attach meaning to words very early in life and select a form of communication, such as pointing and gesturing, as well as speech. Severely delayed speech usually accompanies delays in gross and fine motor development. However, this does not mean that the communication process must also be delayed. Alternative forms of nonverbal communication, such as sign language, are available as "transitional steps" toward the development of functional speech and language skills.

Preschool Years

Nonverbal transitional intervention should begin prior to starting school. Educational programming is more successful when children have benefited from early intervention to maximize their communication experiences. Nonverbal transitional steps are reasonable and possible for children with PWS after the first 2 years of life. However, as the demand for communication increases (vocabulary and length of utterance), fine motor movements are necessary if signing is to be the primary mode. If speech intelligibility continues to be limited, additional forms of communication may also be required such as implementing a "total communication approach," which consists of combining speech, signing, pictures, and augmentative devices (electronic speaking devices). These allow the use of *all* available and appropriate methods necessary to communicate basic needs. Picture boards can be very effective with appropriate augmentative devices phased in as needed. The ability to "make choices" can be enhanced by use of picture boards that focus on activities of daily living. For example, boards can display pictures of important items of clothing, leisure activities or toys, family members, bath time, and food (Appendix F.1). Communication boards that identify foods should include only items that are dietetically appropriate. These authors are of the opinion that food items *not* be incorporated into the therapy process, but rather left to the discretion of the family.

School-Age Years

Appropriate educational programs and on-going evaluations require the speech–language pathologist to establish optimum communication, language comprehension, and social skills. Hopefully, by adolescence many of the physical, mental, and behavioral patterns have been recognized, diagnosed, and evaluated via effective speech–language programming.

The Importance of Diagnostics

Persons with PWS benefit from on-going formal and informal diagnostic evaluations from an interdisciplinary team to determine strengths and weaknesses across all domains (Luiselli, Taylor, Caldwell, 1988; Steffes, Holm, & Sulzbacher, 1981; Taylor, 1988). Speech–language pathologists are part of this team working with parents, families, educators, and other significant persons and contributing well-defined and well-structured strategies. These techniques should impact on effective learning, retention of material, behavior management, communication skills, and interpersonal relationships with peers and adults.

According to Spekman (1983), "Diagnostic assessment of pragmatic and communicative skills necessitate changes in or additions to many clinical procedures." Informal assessments, documented reports, and close observations serve as the basis for implementation of many long-term social communication goals. It is not unusual in children with pragmatic deficits to function adequately within familiar settings but less well in unfamiliar/unknown settings. Therefore, assessing functional use of language in a meaningful context is an important means of controlling and varying activities, routines, interaction, and environments (work, home, school, and community). To maintain a prognostic profile of cognitive, behavioral, and communication progress, it is necessary to continually document performance and monitor behavior and changes across settings. Year-to-year management plans should emphasize the "essentials" of functional programming and life-skills training.

Communication differences in speech and language domains in PWS require intervention. However, remediation processes of articulation/ pronunciation of words and syntactical structure of sentences to enhance clarity and precision of speech are only a part of communicative competency. It cannot be assumed that the presence of sound production, organization of words, and meaningful vocabulary equate with effective communication. Subsequent social interactions such as initiation and maintenance of conversation, speaker–listener roles, taking turns, use of appropriate social rules, relevancy of topic, and the termination of topic cannot be taken for granted. Training and rehearsal in pragmatics, the appropriate *use* of language with others, is critical (Appendix F.2).

Pragmatics training focuses on an awareness of appropriate behavior and rehearsal within the context of communicative interactions. In other words, it is within the natural setting of daily routines, tasks, and activities that persons learn *when* to say something, *what* to say, and *how* to say it. Individuals with disabilities that specifically affect cognition, attention, perception, and/or memory may also display deficits in abstract thinking that involve symbolization, conceptualization, language performance, generalization, and inferences (Spekman, 1983; Wren, 1983).

Ongoing monitoring for effective programming is indeed the key to training and learning of new material. Teaching strategies are designed to fit each child's profile as an accountable part of the special education program. Communication skills need to be specifically addressed; it cannot be assumed that receptive and expressive language learning will just "happen" without direct intervention and planning. Nor should it be assumed that social skills and pragmatic use of language will be inherent in the developmental process of communication skills. These skills need consistent and ongoing training, rehearsal, cueing, and prompting for effective, continued use.

The Importance of Communication Training

Behavior management strategies and functional communication training should be part of the early school curriculum with provision for consistency in expectations between home and school settings. The goal is to integrate linguistic, cognitive, and social skills, as they are the foundation of the communication system using verbal and nonverbal language modalities. The basic intentions to communicate are exhibited in commenting, requesting, answering, acknowledging, and protesting by using words, phrases, and sentences. Signing and other forms of augmentative communication have been effective supplements where poor intelligibility of speech is an issue.

The goals of functional training programs are to enhance verbal and/or nonverbal expression of wants and needs, feelings and attiudes, knowledge and information, directives and commands, social greetings and interactions, questions, answers, and comments. The function of language should consist not only of the ability to express basic wants and needs but also to expand communication skills. Training of appropriate communicative acts should be part of any long-range plan that promotes quality personal relationships and enhances opportunities for meaningful job placement. "Independence and normalization" are new challenges for caretakers and educators of persons with disabilities, including the PWS population (Hussey, Goguen, & Newton, 1992). However, the traditional behavior profile of PWS is often the major barrier for the promotion of independence for a population with known difficulties. Therefore, a well-defined structure with frequent and meaningful opportunities to communicate choice-making is important to maintain in everyday tasks and routines. Successful communication training may be a positive predictor of adaptation to residential and community living.

The Importance of Social Development

Aberrant behaviors such as food-seeking, verbal aggression, compulsions, opposition, and perseveration potentially limit constructive interactions with others. They can significantly affect social interactions with peers, family, and community members and make individuals with PWS very vulnerable in society (Curfs, 1992). Other specific characteristics contributing to this vulnerability include cognitive impairment, speech and language deficits, and deficient social skills. Given the reported profiles of older children with PWS who exhibit emotional lability, weight control problems, skin-picking, sleep disturbances, and severe learning problems (Cassidy, 1992; Curfs, 1992), it is not surprising that initiation and maintenance of positive relationships with peers are limited (Lupi, 1988; Mitchell, 1998).

Levine, Wharton, and Fragala (1993) recommended that behavior and social development be addressed in the preschool years within the learning process. They state: "Most children (with PWS) will need help in learning to appropriately initiate social interactions with a peer, in sustaining social play and dramatic play with peers, and in reading others' subtle social cues." Integrated social experiences with peers from regular classrooms are being promoted in many schools. The concept that "children learn from their peers" is a strong argument for integrating children with special needs such as those with PWS so that appropriate social communication can be developed.

Dykens, Hodapp, Walsh, et al. (1992) reported on 21 adolescents and adults with PWS that were subjects of parental concern. Informal conversations and formal questionnaires from parents indicated that their children with PWS exhibited strengths in daily living skills but weaknesses in socialization skills. Recognized weaknesses in socialization skills of the PWS population are common and emphasize the need to have early programming and ongoing training in this area.

The Importance of Research and Data

Research remains limited in longitudinal studies in following children with PWS through adolescence and adulthood. The majority of information and data are reported from case studies, parent questionnaires, and other nonempirical sources. Low incidence rates of PWS since 1956 may be one limiting factor, as well as the now defined medical–cognitive–behavior traits that have been established in the literature. Although variations exist in nonmedical characteristics (degree of obesity, cognitive differences, maladaptive/food-related behaviors), most studies have relied on establishing an understanding of the diagnosis and etiology of the syndrome (Curfs, 1992). In contrast, longitudinal studies following the development of speech and language abilities in the PWS child have been basically neglected.

PWS has been reported in all racial groups (Cassidy, 1992; Lofterod, 1992). Of recent interest is a study comprised of 8 PWS characteristics compared among 33 Japanese and 83 American children and young adults (Hanchett, Matsuo, Nagai, et al., 1992). Results reported a higher incidence in the Americans in the amount of obesity, skin-picking, speech problems, and behavior problems (significant at the $p = 0.001$ level). No differences between the two races were found in early hypotonia, developmental delay, cryptorchidism, and short stature. Differences in cultural attitudes, structure, diets, and life-styles are suspect explanations for these reported differences in obesity, behavior problems, and skin-picking. In contrast, speech deviations found between the two languages may be more affected by differences in ease of production of words as a result of variance in tonal abilities, motorical complexities, and pragmatic demands of these two sound systems. Further investigation is suggested.

Summary

If the special needs populations are to lead productive lives outside of an institutionalized existence, then it becomes of greater importance to address the need to develop optimum skills that promote positive socialization and interpersonal relationships and interactions with persons in their environment. It is not assumed, however, that behavior strategies, functional communication training, and specialized therapies will provide a "cure" for the PWS syndrome. However, it is probable that early programming and ongoing training in functional communication with goals tailored to specific strengths and needs of each child with PWS will effectively promote opportunities for the development of his or her potential.

Case Studies

SS (Birthdate 3/26/89)

All developmental milestones were delayed with evidence of significant hypotonia. SS received a diagnosis of PWS at approximately 5 months of age. By 19 months he was receiving in-home services from a developmental preschool teacher. He had just began to walk but remained nonverbal. A comprehensive speech–language evaluation was completed.

Formal testing indicated age-appropriate receptive language skills while expressive language abilities and articulatory functioning remained at a 12 month level. It was recommended that home intervention services continue and communication status be monitored.

At 23 months SS's communication skills were reevaluated; his receptive language abilities continued to be age-appropriate; a 4 month gain was noted in expressive language development but no gain was made in articulatory functioning. Consultative speech–language service was recommended to assist the home intervention teacher to implement "sign language" with targeted signs that included "help, more, ball, and book."

SS continued to improve overall, although some truncal hypotonia persisted. At 37 months of age his receptive language skills remained within normal limits and his expressive language improved greatly. He was able to use 2-word combinations and display naming confrontation skills; however, overall intelligibility remained problematic because of minimal gains in articulation.

It was recommended that individual speech–language therapy begin in order to decrease his level of frustration and improve his functional communication. SS was enrolled in a developmental preschool program and started receiving the recommended services. Therapy focused on implementing a "total communication approach" at home and in the preschool setting.

At 4 years, 5 months of age, SS returned for a reevaluation of his communication abilities. SS's receptive language development continued to increase, and his skills were placed at a 40 month level. SS's expressive language abilities were placed at a 28 month level, with scattered abilities up to 32 months of age. He successfully used minicommunication boards outside of the home (picture boards to select food items in restaurants and at preschool), signed approximately 52 signs, and had an oral vocabulary of 28 words. It was recommended that this "total communication" approach be expanded to include the use of an augmentative device in his special education classroom setting in order to enhance his participation in group activities and increase his capacity to communicate and relate to his peers.

MM (Birthdate 10/16/84)

MM was initially evaluated at 18 months of age by her local Area Education Agency (AEA). At that time, she was just beginning to use single words but had not begun to walk. A comprehensive evaluation by the Early Childhood Team of the AEA indicated her cognitive function to be 10–12 months of age; her language function appeared commensurate with her mental age. Biweekly home visits by the Early Learning Team was begun to facilitate her overall development and motor skills. At age 3, she entered a preschool program 3 days a week. One year later she was enrolled in a preschool handicapped program for 5 half-day sessions per week where occupational and physical therapy services and consultative speech–language services were provided. Direct speech–languge therapy was initiated at age 5. Other characteristics documented by the psychologist included developmental delays in the areas of cognition (mild mental retardation), motor skills, communication skills, and daily living skills. Many aberrant behaviors were present including excessive crying.

MM was first seen by the PWS Team at the Division of Developmental Disabilities, The University of Iowa, in March 1990, at the age of 5 years, 5 months. At that time, her speech–language diagnosis indicated "severe speech articulation problem, apparent problems with speech coordination, phonologic delay, inappropriate social communication interactions, poorer receptive performance than expressive, and behavior characteristics of spitting, pinching and hitting as modes of communication." The Receptive Expressive Emergent Language Scale (REEL) provided information about her capacity to communicate. Her mother's report and direct observation using this scale indicated her receptive and expressive language abilities at the 27 month level with a scatter of performance to the 30 to 33 month level.

Play therapy was initiated in the fall of 1990, due to her limited use of spontaneous communication in speech–language therapy sessions and in the special education preschool classroom. Four months later, at her next appointment with the PWS Team in January, 1991, her diagnosis also included "severe articulation deficit, severe expressive language delay, moderate receptive language delay, and 'at risk' in the areas of communication, learning, motor development and health due to obesity." Her poor speech intelligibility was further complicated by mental retardation and oral motor limitations. Intelligible words, phrases, and short sentences could be distinguished only inconsistently.

The speech–language pathologist at her school networked with the PWS Team's speech–language pathologist concerning MM. The following communication goals, programming, and plans for monitoring her status for the remainder of the school year were formulated:

1. Observe her social language intent with peers and adults through play and cooperative work activities. Periodically videotape interactions to monitor changes that indicate growth or the need for modification of goals and strategies.
2. Observe and record her initiation of communication involving verbal and nonverbal behaviors. Describe events and persons involved during these initiation attempts within the framework of language-based activities.

3. Continue the "Whole Language" approach for experiential-based learning for the expansion of vocabulary, concepts, and academic learning with frequent checks for comprehension and retention of material.
4. Rehearsal and repetition should be parts of ongoing strategies that incorporate and reinforce all the sensory modalities. A variety of activities should be created to activate and focus her attention.
5. Encourage use of all appropriate communication modalities (gestures, vocalizations, pictures, signing, and intelligible words) as a means of decreasing frustration and aggressive behavior. Augmentative communication devices may be appropriate to increase social interaction with her peers.
6. Provide consistent reinforcement to use/imitate appropriate verbal and nonverbal behaviors both in the home and school settings. A highly structured behavior management program should be in place.

At MM's last evaluation by the PWS Team at 8 years, 5 months significant gains were noted in her capacity to communicate functionally, although her diagnosis continued to indicate that her receptive language ability was greater than her expressive skills. Her responses were one to three words in length, her speech was generally intelligible within context, and her behavior and compliance improved. The impressive gains in her ability to communicate her needs were considered to be a result of the speech–language services available to her during her preschool and school experiences, appropriate school programming, and parental support of speech and language goals focusing on functional communication training. A continued "team" approach was recommended in order to understand and address her strengths and needs over time since integration of behavioral, physical, medical, academic, life-skills training, and communication goals should be ongoing.

References

Blackman, J. (1990). *Medical aspects of developmental disabilities in children birth to three* (2nd ed.). Rockville, MS: Aspen Publishers.

Boone, D. (1983). *The voice and voice therapy* (3rd ed.). Englewood Cliffs, NJ: Prentice-Hall.

Branson, C. (1981). Speech and language characteristics of children with Prader-Willi syndrome. In V.A. Holm, S. Sulzbacher, & P. Pipes (Eds.), *The Prader-Willi syndrome* (pp. 179–183). Baltimore: University Park Press.

Cassidy, S.B. (1992). Introduction and review of Prader-Willi syndrome. In S.B. Cassidy (Ed.), *Prader-Willi syndrome and other chromosome 15q deletion disorders* (pp. 1–11). New York: Springer-Verlag.

Curfs, L.M.G. (1992). Psychological profile and behavioral characteristics in the Prader-Willi syndrome. In S.B. Cassidy (Ed.), *Prader-Willi syndrome and other chromosome 15q deletion disorders* (pp. 211–221). New York: Spring-Verlag.

Dykens, E.M., Hodapp, R.M., Walsh, K., & Nash, L.J. (1992). Adaptive and maladaptive behavior in Prader-Willi syndrome. *Journal of the American Academy of Child and Adolescent Psychiatry, 6*, 1131–1136.

Dyson, A.T., & Lombardino, L.J. (1989). Phonological abilities of a preschool child with Prader-Willi syndrome. *Journal of Speech and Hearing Disorders, 54*, 44–48.

Hanchett, J.M., Matsuo, N., Nagai, T., Niikawa, N., & Tonoki, H. (1992). A comparison of characteristics in 33 Japanese and 83 American patients with Prader-Willi syndrome. In S.B. Cassidy (Ed.), *Prader-Willi syndrome and other chromosome 15q deletion disorders* (pp. 147–151). New York: Springer-Verlag.

Hussey, H., Goguen, M., & Newton, K. (1992). Ethical and practical considerations in developing the normalization and independence of the Prader-Willi individual. *Prader-Willi Perspectives, 1*(1), 13–17.

Kleppe, S.A., Katayama, K.M., Shipley, K.G., & Foushee, D.R. (1990). The speech and language characteristics of children with Prader-Willi syndrome. *Journal of Speech and Hearing Disorders, 55*, 300–309.

Levine, K., Wharton, R., & Fragala, M. (1993). Educational considerations for children with Prader-Willi syndrome and their families. *Prader-Willi Perspectives, 1*(3), 3–9.

Linebaugh, C. (1983). Treatment of flaccid dysarthria. In W.H. Perkins (Ed.), *Current therapy of communication disorders: Dysarthria and apraxia* (pp. 59–68). New York: Thieme-Stratton.

Lofterod, B. (1992). Prader-Willi syndrome in Norway: an epidemiological and socimedical study. In S.B. Cassidy (Ed.), *Prader-Willi syndrome and other chromosome 15q deletion disorders* (pp. 131–136). New York: Springer-Verlag.

Luiselli, J.K., Taylor, R.L., & Caldwell, M.L. (1988). Issues in Prader-Willi syndrome: Diagnosis, characteristics and management. In M.L. Caldwell & R.L. Taylor (Eds.), *Prader-Willi syndrome: selected research and management issues* (pp. 1–10). New York: Springer-Verlag.

Lupi, M.H. (1988). Education of the child with Prader-Willi syndrome. In L.R. Greenswag & R.C. Alexander (Eds.), *Management of Prader-Willi syndrome* (pp. 113–123). New York: Springer-Verlag.

Mitchell, W. (1988). Social skills training for Prader-Willi syndrome. In L.R. Greenswag & R.C. Alexander (Eds.), *Management of Prader-Willi syndrome* (pp. 165–170). New York: Springer-Verlag.

Munson-Davis, J.A. (1988). Speech and language development. In L.R. Greenswag & R.C. Alexander (Eds.), *Management of Prader-Willi syndrome* (pp. 124–133). New York: Springer-Verlag.

Rice, M. (1983). Contemporary accounts of the cognitive/language relationship: Implications for speech–language clinicians. *Journal of Speech and Hearing Disorders, 48*, 347–359.

Spekman, N. (1983). Discourse and pragmatics. In C.T. Wren (Ed.), *Language learning disabilities* (pp. 157–215). Rockville, MD: Aspen Publication.

Steffes, M.J., Holm, V.A., & Sulzbacher, S. (1981). The Prader-Willi syndrome: historical perspective. In V.A. Holm, S.J. Sulzbacher, & P.L. Pipes (Eds.), *The Prader-Willi syndrome* (pp. 1–15). Baltimore: University Park Press.

Taylor, R.L. (1988). Cognitive and behavioral characteristics. In M.L. Caldwell & R.L. Taylor (Eds.), *Prader-Willi syndrome: selected research and management issues* (pp. 29–42). New York: Springer-Verlag.

Van Riper, C. (1982). *The nature of stuttering* (2nd ed.). Englewood Cliffs, NJ: Prentice-Hall.

Wren, C.T. (1983). Language and language disabilities. In C.T. Wren (Ed.), *Language learning disabilities* (pp. 1–38). Rockville, MD: Aspen Publication.

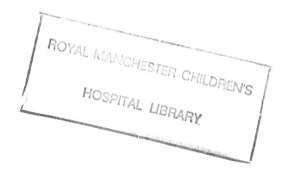

11
Educational Considerations

KAREN LEVINE and ROBERT H. WHARTON

Parents, teachers, and associated service providers need to be familiar with educational issues and options for children with Prader–Willi syndrome (PWS) and their families. This chapter provides comprehensive information associated with providing educational opportunities to these children. It delineates specific considerations associated with age and developmental milestones and offers pragmatic suggestions on how best to maximize the educational experience of students with PWS.

Education Legislation

Federal legislation requires that all children with a disability such as PWS have a written plan that describes how their educational needs will be met. For children less than 3 years of age, this plan is accomplished through an individualized family service plan (IFSP). This legislation, Part H of the Individuals with Disabilities Act (originally enacted as Public Law 99-457, The Education of the Handicapped Act Amendments), calls for statewide, comprehensive, interagency programs for all handicapped infants and their families and the establishment of developmental services to meet a handicapped infant's or toddler's developmental needs in any one or more of the following areas: physical development, cognitive development, speech and language development, psychosocial development, and self-help skills.

Public Law 94-142, the Education for All Handicapped Children Act, requires that children between ages 3 and 21 with disabilities are provided with identification, diagnosis, education, and related services in the form of an individualized education plan (IEP). The main difference between these laws relates to the role of the family. Whereas PL 99-457 focuses on supporting the family in their capacity to provide a nurturing environment for infants and toddlers and enhancing coordination of services required by both the child and family, PL 94-142 focuses on the role of schools to provide appropriate education in the least restrictive environment for

156

children with disabilities. Differences in the laws reflect responses to the needs of the children and parents at different points along the child's developmental continuum and an increased awareness of the importance of the family as part of the team.

To be eligible for services a child must have an identifiable condition that interferes with his or her educational process and normal school performance to the extent that special education services are required. Legislation requires that children be evaluated by an interdisciplinary team that designs an IEP, that children be educated in the least restrictive environment, that services be provided when deemed necessary by the evaluating team, and that child and parent rights to "due process" are protected.

As children grow older school systems assume increased responsibility for delivery of services. The rights of families to advocate for their children and participate in all educational planning has emerged as a cornerstone of the educational process across all ages. Chapter 14 discusses rights, due process, and protection and advocacy in depth.

Program Models

There are variations in classroom options for preschool and school age children with PWS. Which option is best depends on both the needs of the child and the support services school systems are able to provide in regular and specialized settings. Because children's needs change over time, placement and planning require periodic review. Any model must incorporate understanding and support for educational, emotional, and social development while normalizing all experiences as much as possible and optimizing the quality of life.

A recent development in educational planning is an "inclusion model" that involves including children in regular education settings while providing individualized accommodation and support as needed. Perhaps because it is new, this model is currently interpreted in different ways by different school systems. Where its interpretation is quite flexible and a broad array of educational and behavioral supports is available, it can be very effective. One advantage of this model is the implication that all children are included and valued regardless of ability level or capacity to accept on-going educational challenges. Another advantage is that children have an opportunity to develop friendships among classmates with whom they might not otherwise interact.

For children with PWS this model must incorporate implementation of support services when difficulties arise. For example, psychosocial/ behavioral consultation may be beneficial in situations such as managing frustration around transitions and facilitating development of friendships.

Computer instruction and extra use of a computer in class may be helpful accommodations as well. Other services (speech therapy, physical and occupational therapy) can either be incorporated into the classroom situation or be provided outside class. It is frequently necessary to have a classroom aide to assist with social, educational, and behavioral matters. Aides are most effective when they work with several children at once rather than just the child with PWS and encourage social interaction between the child with PWS and peers. This can be accomplished by having the child with PWS sit next to classmates during seated group activities, by prompting conversations about topics with which the child with PWS is familiar, and by becoming familiar enough with all the children to earn their trust and attention. When the inclusion model is not flexible or there are insufficent supports, children with PWS may be isolated from their peers and have fewer opportunities for academic, behavioral, and social development.

When practical limitations interfere with implementing an inclusion model, other formats may be pursed. For children with more significant learnign and/or behavioral problems who are placed in schools that have large classes and few supports, special class placement for most or all academic work may be beneficial. However, behavioral disturbed (BD) classrooms are *not* usually successful for children with PWS because their behaviors tend to be very different from those children typically placed in such an environment. When the classroom teacher needs to develop specific management strategies, consultation with a behvioral psychologist may be beneficial.

Regardless of the classroom model, social–emotional developmental benefits accrue from integrated experiences. Mainstreaming can be successful for structured activities such as hands-on science or art projects and story times but poses extra problems at meal times during the school day. The concept of reverse mainstreaming should be considered. That involves having a child without special needs join the special classroom to participate with the child with PWS in activities facilitated by the teacher. This child can subsequently "host" the child with PWS in the regular classroom.

Some children, especially older children, who are experiencing significant behavioral challenges, may benefit from placement in a residential school where predictable structure, a high staff-student ratio, and limited access to food creates an atmosphere that greatly reduces overall stress and stress-induced behavioral challenges. Clearly, even in this type of program, the family remains a vital, emotional core; close communication between the residential services and the home is essential. This residential model may provide "crisis intervention" until the circumstances surrounding initial placement stabilize. After a period of time, the child may either return home and attend regular school or remain in the program for a longer period of time. Periodic reevaluation of the child's needs is essential.

Whatever the program option, educators and all other school personnel must be taught about the food and behavior issues. Such education provides information on which to base management strategies associated with restricting access to food and will reduce frustrations. It is essential to help the school/community understand that children with PWS may, at times, display behaviors over which they have little control.

Medical Issues That Impact on the Educational Process

Educators should be aware of several of the medical features associated with PWS, particularly an altered level of arousal, pronounced appetite disturbance, and diminished muscle tone and motor planning skills. These features impact on both classroom performance and perceptions of the children by teachers and classmates.

Children with PWS frequently demonstrate a diminished level of arousal. Whereas some children with other medical conditions can be excessively active, the majority of children with PWS are underactive. This characteristic manifests itself as a general lack of dramatic affect, decreased initiation of activities, and a frequent lack of enthusiasm. Some children tend to fall asleep in sedentary or "boring" situations. Others demonstrate only minimum interest in classroom activities. This feature, sometimes misunderstood as an emotionally based lethargy or as inability to participate, actually is part of an altered level of arousal mediated by brain chemicals and is unrelated to intelligence.

Most disabling is the inability of children with PWS to control the drive to eat. Unlike arousal, however, this appetite disorder is one of excess rather than underactivity. This characteristic, while mild in some children and profound in others, is moderated by brain chemicals and beyond internal controls. The lack of capacity for control is *not* related to cognitive ability, disruptions in the home environment, or a need for comfort or emotional or physical nourishment.

Another physical feature associated with this syndrome is low muscle tone and a diminished ability to engage successfully in tasks requiring substantial motor planning skills. Children tend to appear quite weak and even simple motor tasks such as dressing can be challenging regardless of cognitive level or weight. Moving about the classroom, going through halls to change classes, especially where stairs are required, and engaging in exercise and/or athletic events may be arduous and trying. The inability to match the efforts of nonaffected peers in these areas must be understood on the basis of underlying problems of muscle strength and motor control.

Educational Issues Across Developmental Stages

Infancy and Toddlerhood

Infancy and toddlerhood, because these are periods of rapid development and learning, are crucial times for children with PWS. Infants with PWS, like other infants, develop strong attachments to parents, siblings, and other caregivers. Separation anxiety, happiness at greeting familiar people, and the particular smiles and eye contact for parents are all part of the special relationship that forms between the infant and his family. Aside from being a delightful quality, this strong social orientation is a vital strength to capitalize on in teaching and in interventions from the start. In the first few months, however, sleepiness and nonresponsiveness make nurturing and early attachment to caregivers a challenge. Low muscle tone and generalized weakness cause delay in reaching gross motor milestones such as sitting, crawling, and walking and there is also lag in development of fine motor skills.

Interventions

Because of developmental delays, infants can benefit from interventions beginning as early as 1 month of age. Feeding and oral motor skills, receptive and expressive communication achievements, and both gross and fine motor development should be assessed and addressed throughout infancy. Thereafter, programming should focus on physical stimulation, communication, and socialization. Regular "baby" play activities are important. Singing, nursery rhymes, books, mirror play, bubble, pictures, rough and tumble romping, and cuddling are vital developmental activities. However, adjustments are required to compensate for motor and speech limitations. In addition to directly assisting with motor development, the Physical and the Occupational therapists should be consulted regarding strategies to help the child compensate for limitations (see Chapter 8).

During these first years, due to the delays in the "output" systems of motor and speech, the "thinking" processes of these children tend to develop ahead of physical skills. That is, the capacity for thinking and understanding outdistances verbal expression. Expressive language (speech) generally lags behind receptive language (word understanding). Receptive language tends to correlate highly with cognitive development. The cause of this initial speech delay is poorly understood but is thought to be due, in part, to oral motor difficulty (see Chapter 10), and this delay frequently causes frustration for both the infant/toddler and the family. Indeed, limited expressive skills *and* motor skills make developmental assessment difficult, and can result in underestimation of cognitive abilities.

As soon as difficulties are noticed or diagnosis is suspected. Early Intervention Services should be ordered through the Department of Public Health by the pediatrician. Some early intervention programs offer speech and physical therapy and play groups while in other locales these therapies are not included and must be funded from other sources. Whatever the source, these specialized interventions should be taught to caregivers and incorporated into daily and weekly routines that encourage optimum adaptation over time. In addition to the special services just discussed, infants and toddlers can benefit from experiencing regular day care and play groups that provide rich opportunities for enhancing social, communicaton, and play skills, and offer families normalizing experiences.

Preschool (3 to 5 Years)

Toddlers, with or without PWS, begin to declare themselves as individuals as they progress through the developmental milestones of walking and talking. Personalities emerge as they learn to express themselves and struggle to gain control of their environment. Strong interests and preferences may be frequently "voiced" and adult directions may be met with opposition. During this era children know what they want and want immediate fulfillment of these "wants." When gratification of needs is not immediate or goals of others interfere, especially if verbal expression is limited, frustration turns to tantrums (the terrible two's!).

Although preschool children with PWS exhibit delayed motor and speech abilities, they still crave independence. Delays in achieving these milestones can contribute to resistance to physical activities, frustration at not being able to communicate, and tantrumming. Difficulties adapting to change, controlling frustration, and becoming calm once upset may occur: tantrums may also become more frequent and intense. Positive behavioral strategies, speech therapy, physical therapy, and a predictable environment are essential.

At the age of 3 years, children become eligible for comprehensive school programs and enter the public educational system through the process of evaluation by an educational team. This process involves evaluation of current cognitive, communicative, social, and behavioral skills, to guide educational approaches and goals. Supplying the child's team with educational information about PWS such as *Children* with *Prader–Willi syndrome: Information for School Staff* (Levine & Wharton, 1993) is beneficial.

Part of the process of determining educational needs and developing the IEP involves the use of standardized intelligence tests. Interpretation of test results requires an awareness of the broad spectrum and characteristic patterns of learning difficulties. Some children function in the average or borderline range with learning disabilities, others in the mild to moderate range of mental retardation, while a few are identified as severely impaired. The percentages of individuals in these categories are not known precisely and figures cited vary across studies (e.g., Gabel, Tarter, Gavaler, et al., 1986; Cassidy, 1984; Taylor, 1988; Warren & Hunt, 1981). However, taken together, the literature suggests that at least half of the children test in the average to borderline range. Recent studies suggest that there is no correlation between weight and intelligence and that intelligence remains stable throughout development (Dykens, Hodapp, Walsh, et al., 1992b). Regardless of IQ scores, children with PWS show substantial scatter in ability levels across domains. Moreover, since IQ scores are derived from averaging performances across skill areas and because these children usually have motor and speech delays, scores reported during these preschool years may underestimate cognitive levels.

Measures of receptive vocabulary such as the Peabody Picture Vocabulary Test–Revised (Dunn, 1981) are better predictors of cognitive development at this age. This test, using minimal motor and speech requirements, has good correlation with overall intelligence in the general population, but is not valid for children who have substantial attention difficulties. Intelligence test scores may become more meaningful for older school-aged children with PWS, whose speech and motor skills typically "catch-up" with other areas of development, and for whom there is less discrepancy in performance level across domains. However, when older children continue to show substantial "scatter" in skill levels across domains, the validity of the IQ scores remains questionable.

While IQ scores for preschoolers are not particularly useful for predictive purposes, the information from the testing still is quite helpful, providing guidance to teachers regarding learning strengths and styles. The specific test chosen (several are available) is less important than how test data are interpreted. Reports should discuss performance levels across areas of strengths and weaknesses, with particular attention to learning style and functional supports needed, and should be based on assessment by a psychologist or educator experienced with evaluating children with developmental disabilities.

Education Needs

Children with PWS who need specific educational and behavioral intervention may benefit substantially from a specialized preschool experience such as an integrated special needs language-based classroom. Others with fewer needs may benefit from enrollment in a regular preschool where, although less individualized attention is provided, there are substantial advantages gained from the socialization, language, play, and group experiences. A common successful approach is enrollment in a combination of special and regular programming, or in an integrated program with children, some of whom do not have special needs. Regardless of ability, most children with the syndrome are able to handle two programs as long as approaches and daily activities remain consistent.

Preschool IEPs should include a regular pre-academic curriculum in a developmentally appropriate context. Most children will continue to benefit from continuation of earlier assistance in speech and physical/ occupational therapies (see Chapters 8 and 10). These services are best delivered when therapists spend part of their time in individual and/or small group interventions and some time consulting with the classroom teacher about how best to incorporate therapy goals into the regular curriculum and classroom activities.

In addition to preacademic learning, preschool IEPs and programming should address behavioral and socialization needs, especially as social development tends to present difficulties as children get older (Dykens, Hodapp, Walsh, et al., 1992a). Early social skill training is crucial and can help children develop understanding of some of the more subtle aspects of socialization. These cues for social skills are best taught through teacher facilitation of child-to-child interactions and social and dramatic play.

Preschoolers sometimes display behaviors that can interfere with learning and acceptance in the classroom, particularly those that result in class disruption caused by schedule changes. These behaviors should be addressed through the IEP and anticipation is the first line of defense against outbursts. A predictable daily routine is important because there is a tendency to express distress and excessive anger in response to apparently minor alterations in planned activities. A picture schedule for daily routines and a wall calendar for upcoming events can help, and providing information about changes ahead of time may prevent or reduce upsets. Bringing some sort of anticipatory object such as a ball when going to physical therapy or a toy when going outside helps transitions. Providing predictable "change-in-routine" signals, such as singing certain songs, also helps anticipation and adjustment. Once upset, emotions are difficult to control. When tantrums do occur, it is best to remove the child from the situation, remain nearby, ignore the behavior, and avoid scolding or even trying to reason. For children who show decreased interest and lack of arousal, interspersing motor activity with sedentary projects and seating the child near the teacher can help. Whitman (1993) discusses "neurological bundling" as another option (see Chapter 9).

Perseveration is another behavior that challenges the patience of teachers and peers. It usually takes the form of repetitive questioning and/or repeated engagement in singular play (such as tearing paper or drawing circles). When repetitive play seems to be soothing it is beneficial to restrict the behavior to a certain place, perhaps a quiet area of the classroom, and to certain times that are predictably stressful, such as just before snack time, rather than attempting to totally eliminate it. Once a question has been answered, ignoring the redundancy and changing the subject are often sufficient for this age group.

Finally, at this age, children not only observe that eating is unrestricted for their peers but also note that food may be accessible. Several strategies can help manage this situation. During school hours, edibles can be kept outside the classroom in cubbies or in high cabinets. Snacks can be served in child-specific portions in front of each child rather than in large serving bowls. Supervision is necessary whenever food is available and children should not have to sit for long periods near others who are eating. This is a time for teachers and families to act as a team using structure and positive behavioral approaches that work at home and at school. When teachers are aware of potential difficulties, the environment can be structured to minimize problems.

School-Age Children (6–12 Years)

Developmental goals of school-age children include concepts of mastery of tasks and pride in achievements. There is a desire to acquire knowledge, skills, and control of their environment. Providing many opportunities for successes is vital to the development of healthy self-esteem during this period when awareness of differences emerge. Some children experience significant tantrumming during this period in response to unexpected changes, frustrations, and limited access to food. Social development continues as do social challenges, especially in the development of friendships.

Parents can benefit from learning about this stage of educational growth with the assistance of a developmental psychologist, an education specialist, and/or pediatrician knowledgeable about the syndrome, school options, and opportunities. Psychologists play a major role in the development of IEPs that link parents and school systems. Management of food-related concerns should be included in planning, and recommendations should stress close supervision. During this age period, feeling successful at some physical activity is important in shaping life-long attitudes toward exercise. If parents have concerns with the school evaluation or plan they have the right to obtain an independent evaluation paid for by the school.

Interventions

Younger school-age children with PWS usually do well in regular classrooms when provided with extra services. Another approach involves regular kindergarten classes in the mornings and a special language-based classroom in the afternoons that allows for individualized teaching. This format can be quite successful and may be continued through the elementary grades.

TABLE 11.1. Characteristic learning strengths.

Long-term memory for information
Receptive language
Visually based learning through pictures, illustrations, videos
Hands-on experiences
Reading

Meticulous attention must be given to the learning profiles of children with PWS as they begin their school experiences. Their learning profiles generally have characteristic strengths and weaknesses. Strengths, indicated in Table 11.1, are relative to their own abilities, not to peer performance. A particular strength in many children is long-term memory for information. This strength applies to academics as well as to events and names. While initially it may be more difficult to teach new material due to evidence of learning difficulties, it is worth the effort. Functional skills should be encouraged early in the curriculum using positive approaches such as compliments, showing high interest, and individualized attention. Classroom activities should move at a brisk pace with variety to maximize motivation.

Most children with PWS become skilled readers. Verbal information is best understood when presented in brief pieces and time is allowed to process it. Much can be learned through hands-on experiences. Absorbing visually presented information is also a common strength. Teachers should be aware that visual materials such as photos, illustrations, and videos are highly motivating, useful teaching aids.

Learning difficulties often present in children with PWS fall into distinct areas. (Table 11.2). One area of relative weakness is difficulty with short-term auditory memory (Fryns, 1991), which makes it a struggle to remember verbally presented information. Moreover, when a series of verbal directions or a list of steps or objects is presented, the demand for understanding and response is compounded by limited expressive ability. It may be that these children have difficulty transferring auditory information from short- to long-term memory. However, when given the opportunity to do this, through "rehearsal" and attaching meaning, information can be returned and recalled from long-term memory. The difficulty with being able to remember strings of verbally presented information can be misunderstood as disobedience because the child is

TABLE 11.2. Characteristic learning weaknesses.

Expressive language, especially in preschoolers
Short-term auditory memory
Fine motor skills, related to strength, tone, and motor planning
Interpreting subtle social cues—learning subtle social norms

unable to sequentially process "pieces" of the directions (see Chapter 9). It is not uncommon to find students very effective and productive for a given period of time. However, after a while, they appear to "loose it" and need to be "retaught," a very frustrating situation for educators. Performance can benefit from teaching rehearsal strategies, repeating directions, writing down lists or procedures, and having teachers and parents modify verbal instructions. The speech therapist will be helpful in working with the child as well as with the classroom teacher to teach these strategies.

Fine motor skills and motor planning tasks also present as relative difficulties although a few children are particularly good in this area. Most can improve over time. These difficulties cause problems in writing and drawing. Use of a computer should be taught in the classroom beginning as early as kindergarten. Minimizing writing demands as well as facilitating sufficient opportunities to practice new motor tasks can reduce frustration. Learning is more effective when the right answer can be checked from a multiple choice format rather than tracing or writing out the answer.

Physical education and therapy are useful for the development of strength, coordination, and balance as well as motor planning tasks. Gross motor activities able to be enjoyed include walking, swimming, soccer and low-impact aerobics. Scheduling physical activities at pre-dictable times several days each week can increase cooperation. Children should be encouraged to participate and keep personal records of their gross motor achievements for which they can earn rewards. Physical programming should enhance opportunities for socialization as well as the development of regular, healthy exercise patterns. However, comparisons or competition with others can be discouraging. The record keeping system should be designed to celebrate personal development and achievements with guaranteed successes.

While the behavioral and social challenges discussed in the previous section also apply to school-age children, perseveration may intensify. Management should include answering the question once, ignoring repetitions, and changing the subject. As children grow interested in writing and letters, writing down the answer to the perseverative question on a card to which the child can refer can be helpful. A child who repeatedly asks "Did I do a good job?" may proudly show an "answer card" that says "I did a terrific job today".

Home/school communication, with a notebook regarding activities, successes, and any special diet or behavior issues, can maximize continuity of the environments for the child.

Adolescence

Adolescence is traditionally a challenging time for children, having to cope with increased stress from several sources. For those with PWS, the increased awareness of the differences between themselves and their non-PWS peers occurs at the same time that being "just like" one's friends is so important. It may be difficult to develop and sustain friendships while normal siblings may be effortlessly acquiring concrete markers of independence such as a drivers license, a job, and girl/boyfriends. Issues of intimacy and sexuality can be particularly challenging (see Chapter 13) and individuals with PWS who observe changes in their peers but none in themselves are likely to demonstrate increased stress, which may create anger, resistance, and food-seeking behaviors that interfere with learning and adaptation.

Schools can benefit from parent conferences and outside consultation from a professional familiar with the syndrome. For some teenagers specific behavioral programs can assist with modulating excessive behaviors while others may require counseling or other forms of support. It should be remembered that out-of-control tantrumming behaviors reflect the inability to cope with stress and should be attended to promptly and comprehensively.

While challenges exist, there are positive aspects to this time of life for adolescents. Many develop effective verbal skills and become active participants and contributors to school activities. This is a time when vocational planning and work experiences should begin to be pursued, (see Chapter 16). Being a good reader helps and hobbies should be encouraged. While it is generally difficult for persons with this syndrome to cultivate friendships, supportive companionships are possible. Whereas adolescents without PWS strive to achieve emotional and physical independence, the adolescent with PWS may delay this drive to separate and continued dependency can produce several challenges. The question "Will our child ever be able to function independently?" frequently arises. Due to behavioral challenges—regardless of cognitive functioning—they are not ready for full autonomy and need continued supervision and protection. Both teachers and parents need to provide extra security in the school and home.

Intervention

School programs should capitalize on strengths; as with younger individuals, daily and weekly schedules should be as consistent as possible with a minimum number of transitions. In addition to the learning, behavioral, physical, and social considerations, prevocational teaching and planning become critical. Exposure to and participation in community-based work should be encouraged and choices of work in which individuals may be interested should be solicited through vocational assessment. While academic work clearly continues to be a part of school programs, emphasis should be placed on practical use of learning such as application of math skills to manage money, time, and use of public transportation. Skills necessary for community living should be part of any prework curriculum. Enhancement of social skills needs to continue (see Chapter 9), and educators should consider offering one of several excellent courses about sexuality that are designed specifically for persons with developmental disabilities (see Chapter 13).

Some adolescents may benefit from counseling in order to express feelings and work through frustrations associated with a desire for independence and conflicts surrounding the issue of "being different." A support group of other individuals who face similar challenges is usually very helpful.

Summary

Children and adolescents with PWS can achieve many successes in school and community-related activities. When educators understand each child as an individual with special strengths and needs, they then can determine how the attributes of PWS can contribute to successes and can assist families, educators, and, ultimately, the children to cope with the challenges associated with the presence of the syndrome and maximize their functioning, independence, and happiness.

References

Cassidy, S.B. (1984). Prader-Willi syndrome. *Current Problems in Pediatrics, 15,* 1–53.

Dunn, L.M. (1981). *Peabody Picture Vocabulary Test-Revised*. Circle Pines, MN: American Guidance Service.

Dykens, E.M., Hodapp, R.M., Walsh, K., & Nash, L.J. (1992a). Adaptive and maladaptive behavior in Prader-Willi syndrome. *Journal of the American Academy of Child and Adolescent Psychiatry, 31*(6), 1131–1136.

Dykens, E.M., Hodapp, R.M., Walsh, K., & Nash, L.J. (1992b). Profiles, correlates, and trajectories of intelligence in Prader-Willi syndrome. *Journal of the Academy of Child and Adolescent Psychiatry, 31*(6), 1131–1136.

Fryns, J.P. (1991). Strengths and weaknesses in the cognitive profile of youngsters with Prader-Willi syndrome. *Clinical Genetics, 40*(6), 430–434.

Gabel, S., Tarter, R.E., Gavaler, J., Golden, W.L., Hegedus, A.M., & Maier, B. (1986). Neuropsychological capacity of Prader-Willi children: General and specific aspects of impairment. *Applied Research in Mental Retardation, 7,* 459–466.

Individuals with Disabilities Education Act. Pub L No. 102–109, §303.128, 303.164, 303.321. Regulations published in *Federal Register*, October 27, 1992.

Levine, K., & Wharton, R.H. (1993). *Children with Prader-Willi syndrome: Information for school staff* (revised edition). New York: Visible Ink.

Taylor, R.L. (1988). Cognitive and behavioral characteristics. In M.L. Caldwell & R.L. Taylor (Eds.), *Prader-Willi syndrome: Selected research and management issues* (pp. 29–42). New York: Springer-Verlag.

Warren, J., & Hunt, E. (1981). Cognitive processing in children with Prader-Willi sydrome: In V. Holm, S.J. Sulzbacher, & P. Pipes (Eds.), *The Prader-Willi syndrome*. Baltimore: University Park Press, pp. 161–177.

Whitman, B.Y. (1993). Ask the professionals. *The Natursed View*, vol. XVIII, no. 1, Jan.–Feb., p. 9.

12
Social Work Intervention

BARBARA Y. WHITMAN and LORI A. HILMER

The health of the child is a function of the health of the family. . . .
The health of the family is a function of the health of the child.

Diagnosis of Prader–Willi syndrome (PWS) in a child redefines "the health of the child" and links the two truths in the statement above in a delicate balance. It is this inextricable and often fragile linkage that provides the entry point for social service intervention.

Individuals with PWS present with very unique needs to their families and communities. As a member of the interdisciplinary team, the social worker identifies the frustrations, demands, and conflicts encountered by families, and functions as an advocate for both the family and the team.

Social work intervention begins with assessing (and constantly reassessing) the impact of the syndrome on the entire family unit and supporting all attempts by the family maintain the ability to function and meet the needs of their special child. In other words, from a social work perspective, the *family* with a child with PWS becomes the *client* rather than just the child.

Conceptually, systems theory guides social work intervention. It forms a framework for identifying and understanding family strengths and limitations and can provide guidance in identifying the need for additional support and, where needed, redirection.

Briefly, a systems theory perspective views the family as a small social unit. It asserts that the family is composed of interacting units, each with its own set of functioning parts, each unit a component of a larger whole (Anderson & Carter, 1974). This model addresses all aspects of individual and family functioning with the goal of optimizing growth, development, and adaptation. It recognizes viable family structures beyond the traditional two-parent family such as single parent families, extended family caretakers, and homosexual couples raising children.

A systems approach is also compatible with studies that document the impact of family "process" over family "composition" in determining developmental outcomes (Anderson & Carter, 1974). For the family with a member with PWS, understanding family "process" is key to management. Part of family process includes the fact that membership in the family unit is virtually permanent and remains so even when a member is physically absent. Moreover, process incorporates the concept that family relationships are primarily affectional, that emotional bonds of attachment, loyalty, and positive regard are paramount; both affection and a sense of belonging have a high value. All this information helps the social worker determine how family and community units interact and should be incorporated into interdisciplinary team interventions in clinical, school, and social settings.

Assessment

Teams are effective when an accurate assessment of family process and dynamics, subsystems, finances, community resources, stress levels, coping mechanisms, and the ability to make future plans is available. Figure 12.1 illustrates family and community systems, their respective subsystems, and how they impact each other. As a team member, the social worker is the logical choice to investigate these facts.

With the birth of a child with PWS, the changes in the dynamics and process within the family unit may foreshadow a shift into a less functional system. "The birth of a sick or handicapped child may create a set of dilemmas for a new parent for which there is no preparation" (Traot, 1983). Over time, the resources and capacity of family members may be overtaxed to the point where parents doubt their capacity to fulfill their prescribed roles. Parents capacity to nurture and bond is sometimes adversely affected by food foraging, increasingly difficult behaviors, emotional lability, and the need for constant vigilance; emotional ties become distorted.

It is difficult for outsiders, including professionals, to realize that the drive for food and much of the aberrant behavior is beyond the control of the child. In effect, the presence of the syndrome is like an additional recalcitrant member of the family and tends to substantially diminish the family's ability to cope.

Parents often have conflicts regarding child-rearing and discipline that, if left unresolved, are detrimental to the entire family. Restrictions imposed by the presence of the syndrome cause nonaffected family members to feel trapped and helpless. It is important that the social worker assess, monitor, and, when necessary, intercede in these inter-action patterns to avoid incapacitating the whole family.

Once the assessment process is completed, the team is able to create an appropriate habilitation and management plan. Because the family is responsible for day to day care, this plan should include realistic ap-proaches that enables them to meet the challenge. For example, multiple

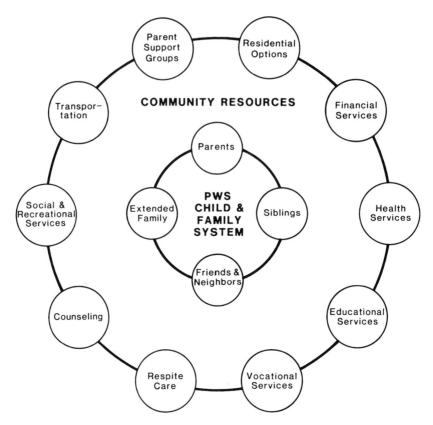

FIGURE 12.1. A social work perspective that illustrates how a PWS family fits within the framework of services from community resources.

therapy appointments may require rearrangement to fit the work schedules of parents or extended family.

Interventions

Interventions begin with the simple question "What is the family asking?" As this question is answered (often over some period of time), knowledge about the family, its strengths, and weaknesses will surface. Facts regarding parenting issues, marital relationships, sibling concerns, the strain on the extended family relationships, and financial and guardianship matters emerge. Inquiry into the physical environment offers insights into the ability of the family unit to comply with team recommendations for management. Entitlement status also can indicate availability of personal and community resources.

The social worker has several roles, the first of which is an advocate or family representative to the interdisciplinary team. A team member, frustrated by lack of compliance with a recommended intervention, needs information about family coping mechanisms that may cause the resistance. Plans may need reassessment and reinterpretation in light of identified family stressors. A second role is as a team member: to review, reinforce, and, where necessary, clarify team recommendations to the family. Yet another function is to establish and maintain an ongoing supportive relationship and a logistical link to the team and community resources. This role begins with the confirmation of diagnosis and continues throughout the child's life. In short, the social worker is the family representative on the team.

Parenting Issues

The ultimate goal of intervention is to enable families to create an environment that optimizes their childs' potential. However, little can be accomplished until the parents have truly "heard" the diagnosis and mourned the loss associated with this news. For some families this grieving process will be immediate and intense as they confront shattered dreams. Unlike the finality of death, their grief is an ongoing, frequently revisited process. Special life cycle events such as birthdays, entry into school, impending adolescence, graduations, and marriage become occasions for renewed sadness or "chronic sorrow" (Olshansky, 1962). Parents often speak of their efforts to acknowledge and adjust, but true acceptance is rare and day to day coping remains a struggle. Indeed, if truly debated, how is such a fate ever accepted?

This grief issue is one that professionals must keep in mind as they intervene with families. It is hard to face a trauma for which there is no explanation and from which there is no escape. Until very recently, parents were in the difficult position of not having had their children identified early in life (Porter, 1988). Despite knowing something was "wrong," sometimes diagnosis was delayed until weight gain was noted (Zellweger, 1981). Often it was communicated that what was "wrong" was the parent. Even though the eventual diagnosis offered some measure of relief, it effectively closed the door to hopes for a normal child and dormant feelings of grief emerged. While diagnostic criteria are now available (see Chapter 1), parents of older children still struggle with their feelings. Where the clinical relationship has been established, the social worker can serve as a sensitive resource and assist the family to stabilize and seek support services.

Early in their interactions with the social worker, some families will request as much information as possible, attempting to reach some understanding about PWS and absorb it. Others simply want to know "what to do next," acknowledging at some subconscious level that true understanding is illusive. Therefore, information must be factual and presented in a realistic and sensitive manner based on the family's capacity to deal with it. However, the trauma of learning about PWS may distort the ability to listen and absorb fact. Therefore, it is recommended that written information be available to be taken home and reviewed.

Financial concerns are usually prevalent until the child reaches age 18. Worries about payment of medical bills and the cost of other services (e.g., respite) can be overwhelming. Once the diagnosis has been determined, families should be encouraged to apply for Supplemental Security Income (SSI) at their local Social Security Office. In some states, eligibility for SSI automatically qualifies the recipient for Medicaid assistance. Thus, the family should also check with their local Department of Human Service (DHS) regarding this possibility. If SSI benefits are denied on the basis of family income, reapplication should occur any time the financial resources of the family change. Families should be encouraged to avail themselves of other entitlement programs. For example, some state medicaid waiver programs offer respite services as well as other in-home services. All states have some form of MR/DD services for which this child and his family are eligible. The parents should be encouraged to use these benefits.

One difference between families who "cope" and those who cannot is the availability of a support system. With a low incidence disorder such as PWS, it is almost certain that no family member will have had experience with this syndrome. Referral should be made to a support group of other parents with children with the same syndrome. If none is nearby, a heterogeneous group of parents with other disabled children may be of help. Information regarding the National Prader–Willi Syndrome Association (USA) should be made available. Parent support does not always ensure family adjustment, thus may also be necessary to recommend family counseling.

Marital Relationships

Marital relationships are very vulnerable to stress. It is certainly not unusual for each parent to be at different stages of adaptation to the presence of PWS *and* unable to respond to the emotional needs of one another. One parent may feel that the child with PWS should be allowed to be "fat the happy" while the other is compelled to restrict food for health reasons (LeConte, 1981). Both may feel angry and trapped. Potential behavior problems limit access to qualified badysitters so there is little or no time for couple interactions. Add to these concerns the fact that spouses have to balance child care, a career, and other children. Sometimes, the depth of frustration and unhappiness does not emerge for some time and expression of feelings, toward their child and each other, remains blunted. If, during the assessment process, it is determined that the marital relationship is strained, couples therapy may be recommended.

Sibling Concerns

The degree to which siblings are able to adjust to a brother or sister with a disability is one of the most neglected aspects of family functioning. When parents are obliged to constantly focus on the needs of their affected child, the rest of the family inevitably suffers. Siblings of a child with Prader–Willi syndrome often have very conflicting and confusing feelings about their brother or sister. They may be embarrassed by the abnormal eating behaviors and resent the need for controlling access to food. They may hesitate to invite friends to their home while, at the same time, such reluctance may generate feelings of guilt. Occasional aggressive behaviors may be feared. Even jealousy may rear its ugly head at the attention given the affected sibling (Trout, 1983). Siblings are sometimes pressured into parenting roles, given additional responsibilities, and forced to "grow up" too quickly.

It is important to give siblings permission to express *all* feelings regarding their brother or sister. In addition to their fears regarding "catching" PWS, older siblings usually voice concern about having a child of their own with PWS. They have questions about what is being done to and for their sibling and are entitled to factual information. Parents may have to be taught to help their "normal" children express their feelings and learn to accept them in a nonjudgmental manner. Parents can model for their children by identifying and talking about their own feelings. Clinic appointments are attended by parents and the affected child while siblings are usually left at home. By inviting siblings to participate in clinic visits, they can see first hand what is happening and can ask questions. Sibling groups have variable success, but should be offered. Investigation of this aspect of family function is important as is locating resources to provide counseling when difficulties arise. On a more positive note, some normal adult siblings feel they have developed a greater understanding and acceptance of differences and a sense of empathy for the disenfranchised (Powell & Ogle, 1985).

The Extended Family

Porter (1988) points out that most families have subsystems of grandparents, aunts, uncles, and cousins, all of whom can be a source of support (child care, finances, or emotional help). But they need time to adjust, understand, and ask questions. Concerns about a recurrence risk in their own families are voiced. Grandparents may be particularly sensitive to having a disabled grandchild and it may take longer for them to adjust. Extended families need to understand the importance of controlling access to food, limiting intake, and establishing consistent behavioral approaches. If the extended family and friends continually challenge the parents, a meeting should be arranged to provide information and facilitate more support.

Major Concerns

The very nature of the relationship with the family allows the social worker to reinforce team recommendations and discuss their impact. Nutritional and behavioral management, community resources, education, and guardianship are topics for social service assessment.

Nutritional Management

Nutritional management is a primary problem and usually is a difficult topic for parents to discuss. When their child has gained weight, they tend to become defensive, fearful that the team will perceive them as "bad" parents. They express guilt because their child cannot have all the "goodies" that children are "supposed" to have and become weary and resentful of the constant focus on food and of having someone else telling them how to feed their child. Birthdays and other special occasions are difficult times and making the decision to lock refrigerators and cupboards may take time as the family sees it as unnatural and embarrassing.

Behavior

Behavior is the other major challenge for families, particularly as children grow older. For those families able to identify their areas of concern, the team can make recommendations for behavioral management. However, the impact of the recommendations on the family life must be taken into consideration. Acting out and tantrumming make families reluctant to go out in public or invite others to their home, encouraging isolation. The social worker is responsible for making the team sensitive to the family's feelings, routines, traditions, and culture. Recommendations must "fit" the family. Failure to take this into account tends to increases noncompliance, frustrates the professional team and the family, and limits success.

Community Resources

The family's need for community services will vary according to the age of the child. Across all ages, it is important for the family to have access to a nutritionist, preferably in their local community, who is knowledgeable about PWS. The nutritionist assists with diet and weight management and serves as a valuable resource for other team members working with the child.

All parents need an occasional break and local respite services are critical to how well families function. Parents of a child with PWS are constantly fatigued and stressed by the 24 hr vigilance. Unfortunately, respite is limited for children with special needs and even more so for those with PWS. Respite can take the form of a few hours, overnight, or even a period of days. Conversely, the child may need a respite from the parents. Participation in recreation and social activities through a local ARC or other special recreation programs such as summer camps is encouraged. A social worker can help identify local resources and, when necessary, obtain funding for these services.

Education

Under PL 99-457, young children are entitled to participate in an early intervention program through the local school district. Parents should be encouraged to enroll their children in such a program as soon as they receive a diagnosis. Physical therapy, speech and language services, and behavior interventions are available through these programs and should be instituted as soon as possible (see Chapter 11). In addition to specific therapies and activities, these programs are a source of support for the parents. School personnel not familiar with PWS may call on the social worker to arrange an inservice to familiarize themselves with the syndrome and answer questions regarding management. A day care for children with special needs may also be needed at this age. Special education services through PL 99-142 serve the child from ages 5 to 21 and IEP goals should anticipate and program for special services (see Chapter 11).

For older adolescents, issues center around the transition from high school to a workshop or supported employment position. Transition planning should begin with prevocational and vocational planing during the first years in a high school setting. Vocational service staff will need considerable education about the very special aspects of PWS.

Discussion regarding alternative living arrangements becomes a high priority at this time. Making the decision to allow the young adult with PWS to move out of the family home to another living arrangement is often a very difficult decision for the family, a decision they frequently need considerable time to make. The social worker should gently bring up the subject regarding future living plans early with the family. The family needs to be encouraged to discuss their feelings and fears around this. Parents need time to absorb that it is "normal" for a young adult to move out of the family home, even a young adult with special needs. Feelings of guilt are not uncommon. This decision may be especially hard for PWS families as group homes specifically for individuals with PWS are few. Families will need assurance that the placement will provide complete control of food, constant supervision, and opportunities for social activities. The social worker will need to assist the family in contacting the local support person for group home placement (see Chapter 15).

Guardianship

Guardianship and long-term financial planning also become issues as the young adult approaches 18. The laws of each state vary but are usually readily available through the local ARC. The social worker can provide parents with basic information about guardianship issues and direct them toward the appropriate legal resource for further action.

Summary

Social workers function as members of a professional team whose purpose is to assist individuals with PWS and their families. Using a social systems model, the unique needs of this population are assessed, after which the social worker advocates and coordinates services.

References

Anderson, R.E., & Carter, I.E., (1974). *Human behavior in the social environment: A social systems approach*. Chicago: Aldine.

LeConte, J.M. (1981). Social work interventions for families with children with Prader-willi Syndrome. In V.A. Holm, S.J. Sulzbacher, & P.L. Pipes (Eds.), *The Prader-Willi syndrome* (pp. 245–257). Baltimore: University Park Press.

Olshansky, S. (1962). Chronic sorrow: A response to having a mentally defective child. *Social Casework*, *43*, 190–193.

Porter, J. (1988). The role of the social worker. In L.R. Greenswag & R.C. Alexander (Eds.), *Management of Prader-Willi syndrome* (pp. 154–161). New York: Springer-Verlag.

Powell, T.H., & Ogle, P.A. (1985). *Brothers and sister: A special part of exceptional families*. Baltimore: Paul. H. Brookes.

Trout, M.D. (1983). Birth of a sick and handicapped infant: Impact on the family. Child Welfare, vol. LXII, no. 4, July August, pp. 337–348.

Zellweger, N. (1981). Diagnosis and therapy in the first phase of Prader-Willi syndrome. In V.A. Holm, S.J. Sudzbacher, & P.L. Pipes (Eds.), *The Prader-Willi syndrome*. Baltimore: University Park Press.

Part IV
Socialization

I think young retarded men and women should be allowed to live together provided they cannot produce children . . . it could be much less expensive than housing two of them separately. They have the same emotional needs as normal people. And with the same supervision provided as individuals, they could make it as couples.

It has been difficult coping with this problem, trying to understand it and have patience. It was difficult for the other children growing up . . . it took so much of my time that I should have devoted to the other children. The worst part was the staring and whispering of people when we were out . . . I would never go through this again – to raise another child with this disorder.

13
Understanding Psychosexuality

Louise R. Greenswag

As the life span of persons with Prader–Willi syndrome (PWS) lengthens, psychosexual growth, development, and education become legitimate concerns for parents and other care providers. Adolescents and adults with the syndrome verbalize their sexual thinking and a desire for sexual expression. Their parents, acutely aware of the social dimensions and implications of this sexual "awakening," often are at a loss as to what to expect and how to manage their offspring. Recently, enlightened attitudes toward sexuality have opened the door to a more frank discussion of this very "human" subject. Such openness is important because, if guiding the sexual growth and behavior in normal children is difficult, helping short, overweight, cognitively impaired, permanently sexually immature children is an even greater challenge. Fortunately, parents and care providers are now more willing to play an active role in channeling the natural tendencies of affected individuals in appropriate directions.

This chapter offers information that may help individuals with PWS and their families adapt to the sexual limitations imposed by the presence of the syndrome. It includes a commentary on human sexuality and sexual expression in the mentally retarded population, guidelines for management based on a developmental perspective, and suggests roles for parents and professionals. It also acknowledges that the topic of human sexuality is a sensitive issue, one that is profoundly influenced by personal value systems. At no point does this discussion endeavor to substitute knowledge or mechanical information for morality.

Conceptualizing Human Sexuality

Sexuality has been described as an enduring part of each person, the sum of one's feelings about being male or female that arise from cultural attitudes and value systems and is related to the assignment of sex roles (Hogan, 1985; Mims & Swenson, 1980). It encompasses many subtleties that coexist in social/sexual relationships where discreet behaviors need not be overtly genital or associated only with physical acts. As a means of expression, it cannot be isolated from other aspects of life.

Sexuality and Mental Retardation

Historically, overt sexual activities by the mentally retarded evoked fear, which in turn fostered laws that segregated "defectives (sic)," encouraged sterilization, and prohibited marriage (Craft & Craft, 1985). Even now, in an "enlightened" era that purports to acknowledge that sexual expression is appropriate for mentally retarded individuals, public attitudes and acceptance lag far behind. Undocumented myths still place the mentally retarded at one of two extremes on the continuum of sexual expression. Mentally retarded people are either oversexed and sexually irresponsible or totally lacking any drive at all. In fact, "the sex drive of the mildly retarded is no different than the nonretarded" (Simons, 1981, p. 173) and most mild to moderately impaired individuals who do not have PWS develop normal reproductive function (Salerno, Park, & Giannini, 1975). And, although mating, marrying, and having children is a normal sociosexual model, when retarded persons express or act out these desires their behavior is likely to be considered inappropriate (Hall, 1975). Despite research that indicates that individuals with lower IQs exhibit delayed sexual maturation and lowered drive, these persons do express sexual awareness (Hall, 1975; Salerno et al., 1975; Watson & Rogers, 1980; Wolfensberger, 1972).

The role parents play in helping their children achieve sexual maturity cannot be underestimated. In a real sense they orchestrate their children's future and should be aware not only of their offspring's developmental processes, but also the extent to which they influence their children's sexual identity. This awareness is fundamental to the promotion of appropriate sociosexual interactions regardless of their children's developmental level. Onset of puberty for normal offspring is a particularly stressful time. Parents tend to become anxious when questions arise about hygiene, menstruation, masturbation, nocturnal emissions, dating, homosexuality, sexual interactions, intercourse, and potential sexual abuse. Craft and Craft (1985) pointed out that "many normal children mature in spite of, rather than because of, parents" (p. 495). Furthermore, although many parents feel they *should* have a good "woman-to-woman" or "man-to-man" talk and discuss sex and reproduction, few actually do (Farrell, 1978).

Psychosexual Evolution and Growth as a Developmental Process

Understanding sexual expression requires an appreciation of inter-relatedness of cognitive, social, and psychosexual development. Social development and sexual behavior generally go hand-in-hand and it usually takes several years even for normal teenagers to be comfortable with pubertal body changes. Evolution of a "sexual self" begins very early in life and progresses through fairly predictable stages of development. For instance, in the normal population, masturbation is a common, self-stimulating activity that begins early in life and continues thereafter in one form or another. The issue is not whether such behavior is appropriate, but rather how and when it is expressed at different points along the developmental continuum. What is socially acceptable in toddlerhood changes as the child grows older. Another example of how sexual development evolves is the way in which children express their curiosity about body functions. Playing "doctor" is a behavior commonly observed in 5–7 year olds and is usually accompanied by giggling about bathroom activities and discussion of breasts and genitalia. By preadolescence, bathroom humor shifts to use of more explicit terms, to jokes with sexual implications, and to budding attraction to the opposite sex.

Developmental tasks associated with normal intellectual, psychological, social, and sexual maturity, which have implications for individuals with PWS, are identified in Table 13.1. It may be a useful guide for assessing/evaluating sexual behavior in individuals with PWS and serve as a guide to appropriate management. [Note that the chronological age range identified in the table ends with early adolescence (13–15 years) because most individuals with PWS rarely reach beyond this developmental stage physically, cognitively, or emotionally.]

Human Sexuality in Prader–Willi Syndrome

For parents and providers, sexual activity in the PWS population may seem almost a contradiction in terms. The first question that comes to mind might be, "Why discuss sexuality in a population where males are impotent and have very small external genitalia, where females rarely menstruate, where neither sex develops more than rudimentary secondary sex characteristics, and none are known to reproduce?" (Zellweger & Schneider, 1968). Such a query indicates a need for further understanding of human sexuality as a multidimensional concept.

While the presence of at least mild mental retardation usually appears to affect the capacity for psychosocial adaptation, most individuals with PWS tend to remain just as impressed by seductive, sexually suggestive media advertising as the normal population. They also watch their normal siblings grow up and participate in family life cycle events where sexual expression of some sort is at least an implied activity. During the school years, children with PWS are frequently mainstreamed into physical education classes where budding sexuality is highly visible. The discrepancies between sexually underdeveloped teenagers with PWS who tend to be somewhat awkward, socially immature, and emotionally labile and normal adolescents are quite evident. Few will develop the cognitive

Table 13.1. Stages and tasks in normal sexual development that are relevant for individuals with Prader-Willi syndrome.[a,b]

Physical	Emotional	Social
Embryo		
Sex determination chronosomes; male, XY; female, XX		
Fetus		
Male: develop testes at 6–7 weeks. Female: ovaries at 12 weeks.		
Birth		
Gender assignment		
Infancy: 0–1 year		
Oral pleasure. Physical response to genital stimulation by self or others. Erective capacity. Touch response, Able to tell self from others.	Self-centered. Self love, sense of feeling of pleasure and displeasure. Trust/mistrust.	Interacts with primary family, 6–12 months = fear of strangers. Likes an audience.
Toddler: 1–3 years		
Total body exploring. Learns muscle control and toilet training. Masturbation to pleasure self. Learns about physical sex differences.	Needs to achieve. Anxious about being accepted. Developing self-control. Senses "goodness or badness" of body. Core gender identity and sex differences evolve.	Uses force to get own way. Likes getting affection. Less fear of strangers. Explores sex differences of others.
4–6 year olds		
Genital manipulation to explore self, to feel pleasure, to relieve mysterious "tension." Sex play and exploration with playmates.	Awareness of genital differences leads to a sense of guilt. Internal controls increase as conscience develops. Attachment to parental figures.	Time for learning basic skills of inter-personal relationships. Development of appropriate social behavior. Identification with parent of same sex. Begins to assert self and reinforce sex identity and gender role.

TABLE 13.1. *Continued*

Intellectual	Cultural	Examples of behavior
Imitates others.	Parental influence is supreme.	Warm physical relationship with nurturing person stimulates sensory perceptions. Likes to cuddle for wearmth and safety. Wants to be held.
Sense of success and failure begins. Reassures self about own genitalia. Learns sex role expectations. Vocabulary related to genital anatomy, elimination, reproduction. Begins to understand right and wrong.	General acceptance of limited nudity in public.	Impulsivity channeled into socially acceptable behavior. Lack of awareness of sexual significance of masturbation; just "does it." Sensual/erotic activities such as hugging, kissing, rhythmic motions reflect desire for pleasuring self.
Vocabulary of "dirty" words increases. Differential thinking leads to understanding how sexes differ. Interactions with opposite sex begin to be overtly structured. The concept of a relationship with the opposite sex is noted (i.e., marriage). Asks questions about "where babies come from." Can learn to use proper terms such as "penis" or "vagina."	Social customs beginning to have impact. But parental influences still paramount. Responsive to sanctions to activities such as masturbation. The idea of "not nice," "nasty," or "don't touch" has impact. Feelings about being male or female culturally integrated.	Giggles and uses "dirty" words. Fascination with bathrooms and bathroom activity. Curious about sex differences and different postures for urinating. Wants to marry parent of opposite sex. Begins to develop childhood romance. Pretends to be "in love" by sitting close and giving gifts. Purposefully explores own body. Play "doctor" games.

(*Continued*)

TABLE 13.1. *Continued*

Physical	Emotional	Social
Early school years: 6–10 years (latency)		
Gradual build-up of hormones triggered by the pituitary gland at about age 8 (adrenarche). Accurate knowledge of genital anatomy. Physical change is not evident until late in this "latency stage."	Begins sexual daydreadming. Repression of sexual expression increases as understanding of significance of sexual activity develops. Freudian concept of "latency" does not mean that "sexual thinking" is not present, but rather that it is low-keyed.	Child learns that sex is not "discussed" in everyday conversation. Social identification with parent of same sex. Sex role rehearsal increases. Sex awareness increases along with increased self-consciousness. Plays with peers of same sex. Ambivalence toward opposite sex. Give-and-take in social interactions; sharing fears and fantasie; with friends of same sex, but rarely with parent. Expects to select a nonfamily member as a partner but not sure why.
Preadolescence: 10–12 years		
Onset of menses. Secondary sex characteristics: pubic and axillary hair. Beginning of seminal emissions, continued self-exploration and stimulation.	Concern over body image increases. Self-concept tied to signs of sexual growth. Guilt over sexual ideation causes confusion. Worries about onset of puberty if lacking information. Lack of positive experience leads to poor self-concept.	Learning about self-control. Testing of behavioral limits incorporates sexual identity. Same-sex relationships are "safe" but ready to shift.

TABLE 13.1. *Continued*

Physical	Emotional	Social
Understands the social significance of sexual behavior. Much curiosity and questions are very specific. Moral attitudes and values are intellectually integrated. Appropriate behavior is understood. Verbal "banter" now has significance.	Parental influence still predominates but peer pressure, media influence, and school begin to have impact. Close observation of non-family members' sexual behvior noted and questioned. Heterosexual interactions still limited. This is a critical time for integrating male/female sexual cultural attitudes. Parents tend to worry about child being "appropriate." Same-sex association to learn "good" role model encouraged. This is the one stage of sexual development when homosexual relationships are encouraged.	As interest in bathroom activities decreases, curiosity about more subtle overt sex differences increases (beards, beasts, pregnancy. etc.). Ages 5–7: play house, doctor, pretend having a baby. Much sex play with same sex but it is more covert. Inspection of genitals of same sex. Ages 8–10: Less role playing but verbal discussion and interest increases. Females curious about menses. Males want details of fertilization and pregnancy. Refuse to be seen nude by parent of opposite sex. Begin to rate self for attractiveness. Sex jokes rather crude, based on primitive knowledge base. Normal voyeurism. Dirty words for shock value. When sexes are mixed, teasing increases and kissing games are common.
Able to make cognitive connection between anatomy and use, but self-conscious about asking about specifics. Will seek a nonparent figure for information.	Parental values strong but peer values being integrated in secret. Cultural norms very influential. Rigid parental values will cause conflict and merely delay development of internal value system. Parental level of sexual comfort has impact on adaptation.	Interest in sex demonstrated through preoccupation with body changes and sex-related jokes. Interested and awed by changes in self and others. Conflicted ideas based on biases against opposite sex along with a defined but limited romantic interest. Tries to copy older role model. Heterosexual activity begins with teasing and rough-housing with the opposite sex as an excuse for physical contact. Boys report homosexual experiences between ages 11–13, girls

(*Continued*)

TABLE 13.1. *Continued*

Physical	Emotional	Social

Early adolescence: 13–15 years

Masturbation common. Capacity for erection. Pubic and axillary hair prominent. Breast development. Broad variation in height and growth. Nocturnal emissions in normal males.	Sexual thoughts and fantasies common. Need for recognition as male or female. Much anxiety over appearance of sexual growth. Fear of being different from peers. Loneliness if not accepted. Feelings of inadequacy if not like others.	Desire for opposite-sex relationships. Puppy love. Awkward heterosexual interactions. Social attempts create worries about acceptance by peers.

[a] From *Comprehensive Psychiatric Nursing* (pp. 176–178) by J. Haber. A. Leach. S. Schudy. and B. Sideleau, 1982, New York: McGraw Hill: and *Sexuality: A Nursing Perspective* (pp. 62–70) by F. Mims and M. Swensen. 1980. New York: McGraw-Gill. Adapted by permission.

[b] These stages and tasks of development are listed only through very early adolescence as research indicates that individuals with PWS rarely develop secondary sex characteristics or reach this era cognitively or emotionally.

capacity required for more mature relationships but their sensitivity to being "different" does not diminish. Wolff (1987) indicates a need for "opposite sex friends even if sexual feelings were minimal" (p. 719). Mental limitations and a healthy self-esteem should not be considered mutually exclusive concepts. Clearly, psychosexual adaptation for the PWS population is a difficult, painful process.

Although there are reports of *lack* of strong sexual drive in individuals with PWS (D. Thompson & M. Wett, personal communication, 1985), these adolescents and adults tend to verbalize identifiable, albeit unrealistic, expectations about relationships with peers of the opposite sex, marriage, and parenting. Parental anecdotes document some dimensions of social/emotional expression that indicate an awareness of sociosexual conventions (Greenswag, 1985). One parent commented:

He is a very affectionate boy and likes girls very much and they like him. He likes to dance and put his arm around them, and even kisses them, but he has never given any indication of anything more.

Another parental comment reveals that males with PWS have been teased about their small genitalia and their obesity, which produces the appearance of having breasts:

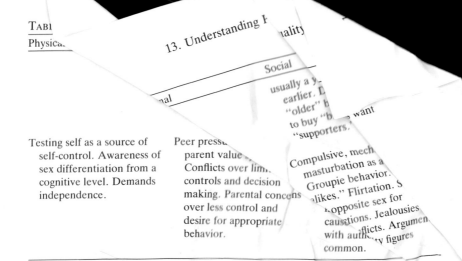

Physical		Social
		usually a y_ earlier. D "older" b to buy "b _ want "supporters.
Testing self as a source of self-control. Awareness of sex differentiation from a cognitive level. Demands independence.	Peer press_ parent value _ Conflicts over lim_ controls and decision making. Parental concerns over less control and desire for appropriate behavior.	Compulsive, mech masturbation as a Groupie behavior. _likes." Flirtation. S _opposite sex for caustions. Jealousies with auth__ty figures conflicts. Argumen_ common.

We haven't discussed the typical differences from other boys except when he was small and was made fun of because of his breast. We just try to comfort him by downplaying the whole thing. We found it was very difficult to explain without confusing him.

A third parent stated:

He knows the basics, he has a girlfriend, but their relationship, because of her condition and his, is an occasional kiss. Talk about marriage is limited because neither realizes or copes with the process of children. Actually, not being able to reproduce is one blessing we see for our Prader–Willi son.

Parents of females with PWS observe that their daughters desire to be like normal girls and fantasize about boyfriends, marriage, and having babies. One parent wrote:

She seems preoccupied with wanting a baby, seems to understand where they come from, but doesn't know how they are made. She accepts the fact than mothers and fathers produce babies with their love. She has always been fond of babies and works as a volunteer one day a week in a daycare center.

Another indicated:

It was difficult for our daughter to understand and accept the fact that she will never have children. This fact was presented to her as gently as possible. She internalized sexual information and occasionally would play out sexual roles, acting out fantasies and romantic ideas. When the doctor told her she would never have any children it was a great psychological shock. She wants to be normal, to marry, and to have children.

It is apparent from these comments that the human dimension of sexuality should not be downplayed or ignored.

Parents

Parents tend to be ... sexuality with their
... offspring, those ... disabled children may
... normal even more diff... task for parents of children
... ent is further compli... ... ion of sexual issues may be dis-
... work of pubertal ... ent on parental individuals with PWS adapt psycho-
... cking and awkward ... a child's needs (Buscala, 1983). Parents should be
... ally depends to ... ... perception of th... own attitudes about sexual expression as well
... couraged to dis... sexuality as a social dimension of PWS. Some will
... need help in d... ... oping realistic responses to the questions put to them
by their chil... en with PWS about getting married and having children.

Perhaps th... current sociological phenomenon of "voluntary childlessness"
may se·ve as an examp... that not everyone need be a parent.

Some parents believ... their children with PWS are asexual; they ignore
evidence of sexual thoughts and attempt to suppress sexual expression.
Others feel that purposeful talk about sex will only stir up "bad ideas"
and discourage provision of information and/or sex education. Some hold
the view that sex should remain a simple, uncomplicated issue associated
with procreation within the sanctity of marriage; since the expectation is
that their children with PWS will neither marry or reproduce, they see no
need to discuss sex at all. In some instances parents unwittingly transmit
mixed messages; they admit their children need healthy social interactions,
but are fearful of encouraging "closeness." Concerned that simple hand-
holding may lead to overt sexual activity, they tend to purposefully
overprotect to eliminate the sexual expression of our children when
about, "who will supervise the sexual expression of our children when
they no longer live at home?"

The question remains: "Can an individual with PWS be whole if the
potential for sexual expression is repressed?" Perhaps the healthiest
response is for parents to acknowledge that their children are entitled
to human relationships and have needs for gratification and emotional
closeness. Since most affected persons are capable of learning to express
their feelings, they should be encouraged to learn to engage in interactions
appropriate to their developmental disabilities so that any sociosexual
relationships may be fulfilling.

The Role of the Professional

Professionals, aware that sexual expression is a relevant aspect of life
for the developmentally disabled, are now giving considerable thought
to managing these issues. Interventions (counseling, teaching, group
facilitating, etc.) require them to be comfortable in their own sexuality, at
ease with the topic, and skilled communicators.

Assisting PWS individuals to adapt pyschosexually has four major dimensions. First, understanding the characteristics of PWS is essential along with acknowledging that the potential for sociosexual activity exists within the constraints of the condition. Second, when parents collaborate with professionals to nurture sexual awareness in PWS children, the process becomes legitimized. They should be included in the counseling/learning process because their attitudes and acceptance play a major role in if, how, when, and where this human sexuality is expressed. The fact that they "know their child best" aids in individualizing approaches and their first-hand knowledge about what the children understand may deescalate anxieties about this sensitive issue. Healthy psycho-sexual adaptation can also be strengthened and enhanced through interdisciplinary collaboration. For example, the social worker's assess-ment of the family unit may offer special insights into family dynamics, living arrangements, and vocational expectations. A marital counselor may have a better view of parental strengths and limitations. Educators may be in the best position to evaluate how PWS individuals relate to peers (of both sexes).

A third dimension concerns the need for honest, uncomplicated sex education programs that incorporate discussion of appropriate sexual topics. Optimally, parents provide sex education during day-to-day interactions. However, where gaps exist in this teaching process, carefully structured, formalized programs are available that can be adapted to the special needs of PWS. The Sex Information and Educational Counsel of the United States (SIECUS) is an excellent resource that recognizes the importance of human sexuality in the developmentally disabled and the need for interactions with the opposite sex. It supports the premise that, with guidance, appropriate behavior can be learned. The curriculum focuses on awareness of self, physical differences between the sexes, and body changes. It emphasizes development of healthy interpersonal relationships that may progress from self-respect to respect for privacy and focuses on the importance of responsibility to society as males and females participating in a variety of life-styles (single, married, etc.) (Spurr, 1976).

Finally, understanding psychosexuality in individuals with PWS would not be complete without addressing the issue of potential sexual abuse of this population. Several accounts of abuse of children, where the children were bribed with candy, have been reported. However, data do not suggest that these children are sexually abused more than comparably handicapped children. Heinemann (1983) identified persons with PWS as being at risk because they are cognitively limited, desire physical attention, and may be easily bribed. Furthermore, they are likely to be in setting where adults are "in control" and are vulnerable to advances by anyone who befriends them.

Prevention of sexual abuse of individuals with PWS is no small task. The difference between "good touch" and "bad touch" should be emphasized to the children and cognitive limitations require that this lesson be periodically reinforced. These children need to be taught that it is "all right" to say "no" to an adult and that physical and emotional limits need to be enforced. Reduction of sex role stereotyping, particularly submissiveness or passivity, is also important. It is essential that children know that any of their concerns or fears will be carefully heeded and that "secret" behavior is to be avoided. The topic of sexual abuse is a challenge and is best addressed within the larger context of body safety. Initiate this discussion of body safety when the children are very young. Be specific. Ask "what if" questions, be nonjudgmental, and believe the child. Recognize that it is not the child's duty (nor always within his or her capability) to recognize and terminate inappropriate sexual advances. The ultimate responsibility of inappropriate behavior is with the perpetrator.

Summary

Understanding human sexuality from a developmental perspective offers parents, providers, and professionals a framework for cultivating realistic attitudes and feelings about sociosexual behavior in persons with PWS. Significant elements of human sexuality that may be associated with this population follow. These elements have been adapted from de la Cruz and La Veck (1973). Gordon (1974), Perski (1981), and Mims and Swenson (1980), Robinault (1978).

1. Individuals with PWS are not asexual; they have drives and interests and, most significantly, will develop strong gender role identification. Individual family, religious, and social values play a major part in how their sexuality is expressed.
2. Psychosexual maturation occurs at a later chronological age as compared to person of normal intelligence. However, sexual interest tends to remain lower where intellectual functioning is lower.
3. Although the average age at which most developmentally disabled individuals reach physical maturity is essentially the same as normal pubescence, sexual maturation in PWS is usually indefinitely delayed.
4. Difficulties in gross motor coordination in PWS often result in less participation in group activities that normally encourage social exposure and may contribute to the delay in acknowledgment of sex roles.
5. The sexual activity of most individuals with PWS is basically exploratory and innocent in nature. Genital manipulation and masturbation are most often fostered by boredom, lack of activities, and a failure to understand what is acceptable public social conduct.
6. Many individuals with PWS have difficulty expressing their feelings appropriately, regardless of the extent of their verbal skills.

7. Affected adolescents have been known to express a desire for companionship and dating and either ask or infer sex-related questions and thinking. They have the same needs for intimacy, privacy, and relationships as anyone else.
8. Ongoing support is essential. When encouraged to deal with the realities of their psychosexual limitations early in life, most can learn to adapt. Parents and providers should:
   a. understand that most "know that they are different" and that this "differentness" increases stress during adolescence.
   b. recognize that many individuals with PWS have the capacity for some measure of sexual expression.
   c. acknowledge that society currently accepts females in nonmaternal roles and some partners remain childress voluntarily.
   d. teach persons with PWS to be responsible for their public and private sexual activities.

While few PWS adolescents and adults are physically prepared to participate in intimate sexual activities, their capacity for sexual expression should be viewed as an important aspect of their psychosocial development and they should be offered guidance about appropriate sexual behaviors. In the final analysis, it should be emphasized that the inability to develop a traditional sex life does not mean that individuals with PWS are less male or less female; their capacity to be sociosexual beings is not diminished.

References

Buscala, L. (1983). *The disabled and their parents*. Toronto: Holt, Rinehart, & Winston.

Craft, A.N., & Craft, M. (1985). Sexuality and mental handicap: A review. *British Journal of Psychiatry*, *139*, 495–505.

de la Cruz, F., & La Veck, C. (Eds.). (1973). *Human sexuality and the mentally retarded*. New York: Brunner-Mazel.

Farrell, C. (1978). *My mother said. . . .* London: Routledge and Kegan Paul.

Gordon, S. (1974). *Sex rights for people who happen to be handicapped* (Monograph Number 6, pp. 351–381). Syracuse, NY: Center on Human Policy, Syracuse University.

Greenswag, L.R. (1985). *Sexuality for people with Prader-Willi syndrome: Is ignorance bliss?* Proceedings of National Conference of Prader-Willi Syndrome Association, Windsor Locks, CT.

Hall, J. (1975). Sexuality and the mentally retarded. In R. Green (Ed.), *Human sexuality: A Health practitioner's text* (pp. 181–195). Baltimore, MD: Williams & Wilkins.

Heinemann, J.T. (1983). *Caution, children at risk; dealing with sexual abuse in developmentally disabled children*. The Missouri View, Prader-Willi Syndrome Association, St. Louis, MO.

Hogan, R. (1985). *Human sexuality, a nursing perspective.* Norwalk, CT: Appleton-Century-Crofts.

Mims, F., & Swenson, M. (1980). *Sexuality: A nursing perspective.* New York: McGraw-Hill.

Perski, R. (1981). *Hope for families.* Nashville: Abington Press.

Robinault, I. (1978). *Sex, society and the disabled: A developmental inquiry into roles, reactions and responsibilities.* New York: Harper & Row.

Salerno, J., Park J., & Giannini, M. (1975). Reproductive capacity of the mentally retarded. *Journal of Reproductive Medicine, 14,* 123–129.

Simons, J. (1981). Sexual behavior in retarded children and adolescents. *Developmental and Behavioral Pediatrics, 1*(4), 173–179.

Spurr, G. (1976). Sex education and the handicapped. *Journal of Sex Education Therapy, 2*(2), 23–26.

Watson, G., & Rogers, R.S. (1980). Sexual instruction for the mildly retarded and normal adolescent: A comparison of educational approaches, parental expectations, and pupil knowledge and attitude. *Health Education Journal, 39,* 88–95.

Wolfensberger, W. (1972). *Normalization: The principal of normalization in human services.* Toronto: National Institute of Mental Retardation.

Wolff, O. (1987). Prader-Willi syndrome—psychiatric aspects. *Journal of the Royal Society of Medicine, 80,* 718–720.

Zellweger, H., & Schneider, H. (1968). Syndrome of hypotonia-hypomentia-hypogonadism-obesity (HHHO) or Prader-Willi syndrome. *American Journal of Diseases of Children, 115,* 558–598.

Part V
Delivery of Services

He has no friends outside school, does not like to do anything physical except dance to records. Watches TV and plays games with his sister. Has taken physical and verbal abuses from children in school but does not complain because he is starved for peer relationships. When visitors come to our house, which is very rare, their kids are always snacking and totally ignore [the] PWS, which is very hard on him.

14
Legal Advocacy for Persons with Prader–Willi Syndrome

Sondra B. Kaska

Early in their child's life, the parents of a child who has Prader–Willi syndrome confront what may become a life-long battle to obtain the supports and services necessary for their son or daughter to recognize his or her potential. As that child matures, the person with PWS may assume some of the responsibilities of advocating for his or her rights. In order for parents, legal guardians, or the individual with PWS to advocate successfully, it is important for them to be aware of some of the legal protections available to persons with PWS or other disabilities and some of the mechanisms in place to assist them in their advocacy or self-advocacy efforts.

Because an exhaustive review of all applicable laws would require volumes rather than a few pages, this chapter highlights three federal statutes that will assist persons with PWS in accessing the system. First, an overview of the Developmental Disabilities Assistance and Bill of Rights Act is provided. Second, the Individuals with Disabilities Education Act is reviewed, due to the importance of education in the life of a child with Prader–Willi syndrome. Finally, one of the most liberating pieces of federal legislation enacted to protect the rights of persons with developmental disabilities, the Americans with Disabilities Act, is discussed. It should be remembered that laws and their interpretations vary from state to state and may change over time.

The DD Act

The Developmental Disabilities Assistance and Bill of Rights Act (the DD Act) was enacted to ensure that all persons with developmental disabilities receive the services, assistance, and opportunities necessary to allow them to achieve their maximum potential through increased independence, productivity, and community integration. The DD Act is also designed to strengthen the role of the family in assisting persons with developmental disabilities to reach their maximum potential; provide interdisciplinary training and technical assistance to persons with disabilities, their families, and professionals and paraprofessionals who work with them; advocate for public policy change and community acceptance of persons with disabilities; and promote community inclusion of all persons with disabilities, regardless of the severity of their disabilities. Additionally, the purposes of the DD Act include promoting the interdependent activity of all persons with disabilities, recognizing the contributions made by persons with disabilities to all aspects of life, and supporting a system designed to promote the human and legal rights of persons with disabilities, such as PWS (Young Lawyers Division, Iowa State Bar Association, December, 1992).

Originally enacted in 1976, the DD Act creates a three part system for the implementation of its purposes: state planning councils, university affiliated programs, and a protection and advocacy system. The State Planning Councils, viable in every state, are charged with advocating for persons with disabilities by carrying out priority area activities and reviewing, monitoring, and evaluating the state plan that each state must have in effect in order to receive the federal financial assistance available through the DD Act. The University Affiliated Programs (UAP), now effective in nearly every state, are operated by private nonprofit entities or public entities and associated with a college or university. The UAPs provide interdisciplinary training for persons involved with individuals who have disabilities, demonstrate exemplary integrated services for persons with disabilities, provide technical assistance, and disseminate research findings regarding the provision of services. The protection and advocacy system in effect under the DD Act must have the authority to pursue administrative and legal as well as other appropriate approaches to ensure that the human and legal rights of persons with developmental disabilities are protected. Each state has a protection and advocacy system. The DD Act defines developmental disability as:

a severe, chronic disability of a person 5 years of age or older [that:]

(A) is attributable to a mental or physical impairment or combination of mental and physical impairments;
(B) is manifested before the person attains age twenty-two;
(C) is likely to continue indefinitely;
(D) results in substantial functional limitations in three or more of the following areas of major life activity: (i) self-care, (ii) receptive and expressive language, (iii) learning, (iv) mobility, (v) self-direction, (vi) capacity for independent living, and (vii) economic self-sufficiency; and
(E) reflects the person's need for a combination and sequence of special, interdisciplinary, or generic care, treatment, or other services which are of lifelong or extended duration and are individually planned and coordinated;

except that such term, when applied to infants and young children, means individuals from birth to age 5, inclusive, who have substantial developmental delay or specific congenital or acquired conditions with a high probability of resulting in developmental disabilities if services are not provided.

In the majority of cases, particularly those in which the person has accompanying mental retardation, persons with Prader–Willi syndrome are considered to have a disability under the DD Act. Thus, persons with PWS are eligible for protection and advocacy services.

The Individuals with Disabilities Education Act

The importance of early intervention for children with Prader–Willi syndrome creates a natural starting point for the examination of laws that provide a mechanism for advocacy. The Individuals with Disabilities Education Act (hereinafter sometimes IDEA) is a federal law that provides protection for children with disabilities from as early as birth through age 21. The IDEA has been in effect since 1975, and is in place in every state. Under their state plans, states may provide more than the federal act requires but may not provide less.

The purpose of the IDEA is:

to assure that all children with disabilities have available to them, . . . a free appropriate public education which emphasizes special education and related services designed to meet their unique needs, to assure that the rights of children with disabilities and their parents or guardians are protected, and to assist States and localities to provide for the education of all children with disabilities, and to assess and assure the effectiveness of efforts to educate children with disabilities.

Under the IDEA, children with disabilities are defined to include those who have "mental retardation, hearing impairments including deafness, speech or language impairments, visual impairments including blindness, serious emotional disturbance, orthopedic impairments, autism, traumatic brain injury, other health impairments, or specific learning disabilities" and who require special education and related services as a result of the disability. Each state, at its discretion, may also include children from ages 3 to 5 who are experiencing developmental delays and need special education and related services as a result of those delays. The mental retardation that frequently accompanies PWS as well as the other health impairments that may be connected with the syndrome generally qualify a child with PWS for services under the IDEA.

Procedural Protections

The IDEA contains procedural and substantive safeguards. The importance of the procedural protections provided under the IDEA cannot be overemphasized. Because each child with a disability is so unique, it is impossible to provide a uniform definition of "appropriate" that meets the needs of each child. Therefore, Congress repeatedly emphasized these procedural safeguards as a way of ensuring that the individualized needs of each child with a disability are met. The U.S. Supreme Court in *Board of Education of Hendrick Hudson Central School District v. Rowley* (1982) found compliance with the procedural protections to be the first of a two-part analysis used to determine whether a school district had met the requirements of the Act. Highlights of the procedural protections follow.

Access to Records

The parents or guardians of a child who has PWS have a right to examine all relevant records with respect to the identification, evaluation, and educational placement of the child, and the provision of a free appropriate public education to that child. This requirement includes parents' rights to inspect and review any education records relating to their children that are collected, maintained, or used by the educational agency. Upon request, the agency must provide parents a list of the types and locations of education records that it collects, maintains, or uses. The agency must also keep a record of any persons other than the parents and authorized employees of the agency who access the child's files. The record must include the date accessed and the reason access was given.

The agency must respond to a parent's request to review records without unnecessary delay and before any meeting regarding an Individualized Education Program (IEP) or a hearing. Parents may also request copies of the documents. Although educational agencies may charge a fee for copying the records, they cannot do so if the charge would infringe on the parent's right to review and inspect the records. The fee is for copying costs, not for searching for or retrieving the requested information.

It should also be noted that parents have the right to request an amendment to the records kept by the educational agency if they believe that the information in the child's file is inaccurate, misleading, or violates the privacy or other rights of the child. The agency must decide whether it will amend the record within a reasonable amount of time following the parents' request. If the agency refuses to amend, it must inform the parents of the right to a hearing to challenge the refusal. Even if the agency determines at the hearing that the information contained within the record is accurate, the parents have the right to put a statement in the child's record setting forth their disagreement. The parent's statement remains a part of the educational records of the child as long as the document in dispute remains a part of the record.

Independent Evaluation

A child with PWS becomes eligible for special education services following an evaluation done by school personnel to determine the child's eligibility and needs. This evaluation can be performed only after proper notification to and consent from the parents of the child. Parents who dispute the evaluations of their child done by school personnel have a right to an independent evaluation at public expense. Although the educational agency has a right to request a hearing to demonstrate the accuracy of its own evaluation, parents are not required to request a hearing to prove that they are entitled to an independent evaluation; it is theirs as a matter of right. The process by which parents request an independent evaluation should not be a cumbersome one, nor is it permissible for them to be required to fill out forms or go through some type of review process to determine whether their request has merit. Additionally, upon request, agencies must provide parents information about where an independent evaluation can be obtained. Advocacy agencies may be able to assist in recommending an entity with expertise in PWS to perform the independent evaluation.

Even if the educational agency prevails at the hearing held to determine whether its evaluation was appropriate, the parents are entitled to an independent evaluation at their own expense. Public expense means that the agency pays for the entire cost of the evaluation or ensures that it is otherwise paid for so that the parents incur no cost of their own.

It is also possible for a hearing officer, on his or her own initiative, to request an independent evaluation, usually because the hearing officer does not believe that he or she has adequate information on which to base a decision. An evaluation ordered by a hearing officer is at public expense.

Notice

Another right afforded parents and guardians of children with disabilities is the right to prior written notice whenever the school either refuses or proposes to initiate or change the "identification, evaluation, or educational placement of the child or the provision of a free appropriate public education to the child." Such notice must include:

1. a complete explanation of all the procedural safeguards afforded the parents;
2. a description of the action that the agency proposes or refuses to take, the rationale for the position taken by the agency, and a description of the other options considered and the rationale for their rejection;
3. information regarding each method of evaluation, test, report, or record that the agency used in determining its position; and
4. an explanation of any other factors relevant to the agency's position.

It is also important to remember that such notice must:

1. be written in generally understandable language;
2. be in the native language of the parents;
3. be translated, if necessary, to a mode of communication that the parents can comprehend; and
4. include written evidence that the parents understand the notice.

Due Process Proceedings

One of the most critical protections afforded under the Act is the right of the local education agency and of the parent of a child with a disability to an impartial due process hearing whenever there is disagreement about the identification, evaluation, or placement of the child or about the provision of a free appropriate public education to that child. The hearing must be conducted by an impartial hearing officer. The educational agency is mandated to provide the parent with information regarding any free or low-cost legal and other relevant services that are available in the area. This would, of course, include protection and advocacy services. It should be noted that, although not a requirement of the system, many states now offer mediation prior to or after the initiation of a due process appeal and are finding it to be a worthwhile alternative to a hearing.

The parties to a due process hearing have the right to be accompanied and advised by counsel and/or by persons with special knowledge or training regarding disabilities. The parties may present evidence and confront, cross-examine, and compel the attendance of witnesses. The parties are entitled to a verbatim record of the hearing, either electronic or written, and to written decisions and findings of fact.

The decision of the hearing officer is the final agency decision, unless the state rule provides for an agency review. Either party may appeal the final agency decision to state or federal court. It is important to remember that, unless the parties otherwise agree, the child remains in his or her then current educational placement pending the final outcome of the action. If the issue involved is the initial placement of a child with a disability in a public school setting, the child shall be placed in the program, if the parents consent, until the completion of all proceedings.

In any action brought under the IDEA, courts are authorized to "grant such relief as the court determines is appropriate." This may include equitable relief, tuition reimbursement, and the costs and attorneys' fees incurred by the parents in pursuing litigation.

Development of the IEP

It is clear that the key operative feature of the procedural requirements of the IDEA is the IEP. It is through the development of the IEP that the program is "tailored to the unique needs of the child with a disability."

Courts have held that parental involvement in the development of a child's IEP is so critical that if parents are not given an adequate and meaningful opportunity to participate in the formulation of their child's IEP, the IEP may be invalidated without reference to its substance, or the burden of proof on the question of appropriateness of the IEP may be shifted to the school.

Typically, IEP meetings are conducted periodically, at least once a year, upon the initiation of the educational agency. Other meetings are appropriate if the child is failing to progress or if there are other problems with the IEP. All reasonable parental requests for IEP meetings must be honored by the agency. Parents must be notified of all IEP meetings far enough in advance to allow them to participate, and such staffings must be scheduled at a mutually agreed upon time and place. The agency must ensure, through the provision of an interpreter or whatever other method is needed, that the parents understand the proceedings of the meeting. If neither parent is able to attend a meeting, the educational agency must ensure their participation through alternate means, such as a telephone conference call. Only if the agency is unable to convince the parents that they should be in attendance may a meeting be conducted without the parents present, and in that case the agency must meticulously document its attempts to involve the parents. The parents should receive a copy of the IEP. The IEP meeting may be tape recorded.

Generally, IEP meetings should be small in order to facilitate open, active parental involvement and in order to be more productive. In addition to one or both of the child's parents, the following persons should participate in the IEP meeting:

1. The child's teacher.

2. A representative of the agency. It is required that this individual be able to ensure that whatever services are set out in the IEP will actually be provided and that the IEP will not be vetoed at a higher administrative level within the agency. Therefore, the selected individual must have the authority to commit agency resources. In other words, in all but the rarest of cases, decisions are to be made at the time of staffing while all members of the team are present.

3. Other individuals at the discretion of the parent as well as of the agency. The agency must inform the parents who will be in attendance and advise the parents that they may bring others.

4. The child, whenever appropriate. This is especially encouraged as the child reaches secondary level education.

"The IEP meeting serves as a communication vehicle between parents and school personnel, and enables them, as *equal participants*, to jointly decide what the child's needs are, what services will be provided to meet those needs, and what the anticipated outcomes may be" (34 C.F.R. Pt. 300 & App. C, 1992). This means that parents are to have an active role in developing, reviewing, and revising the child's IEP. It is permissible for the agency personnel to come to the staffing prepared with evaluation findings, statements of present levels of educational performance, recommendations regarding annual goals and objectives, and suggestions regarding the kind of special education and related services that they believe to be appropriate. However, parents must be clearly informed from the outset that the services suggested are only recommendations and that as such, they are not finalized unless and until they are acceptable to the parents. It is not permissible for the agency to have completed the IEP before the IEP meeting begins.

The following items must be included on each child's IEP:

1. A description of the child's present levels of educational performance. By this is meant an objective statement of how the child's disabilities affect his or her performance in various areas. A label, such as "Prader–Willi syndrome" or "mentally retarded" will not suffice.

2. Annual goals and short-term objectives, designed to meet the unique needs of the individual child.

3. A specific statement of all special education and related services that the child requires, whether provided directly by the educational agency or by contract with another agency. The amount of services must be stated so that all parties will understand the agency's commitment of resources and this amount cannot be changed without calling another IEP meeting.

4. The extent to which the child will be involved in regular educational programs.

5. The anticipated dates for initiation of services and their expected duration.

6. Objective criteria and evaluation procedures and schedules for making at least an annual determination of whether the educational objectives are being met.

The IEP is not a performance contract, which would mean that the agency or teachers would be held accountable if the child did not reach the projected goals. However, each child's IEP must include all services necessary to meet the child's identified special education and related services needs, and all services in the IEP must be provided in order for the agency to be in compliance with the IDEA.

Substantive Requirements

The IDEA contains two substantive provisions of which persons advocating for a child who has PWS should be aware. An eligible child with a disability is entitled to receive a "free appropriate public education," defined as, "special education and related services that have been provided at public expense, under public supervision and direction, and without charge, meet the standards of the State educational agency, include an appropriate preschool, elementary, or secondary school education in the State involved, and are provided in conformity with the individualized education program required."

Under the IDEA, "special education" is defined as "specially designed instruction, at no cost to parents or guardians, to meet the unique needs of a child with a disability, including—instruction conducted in the classroom, in the home, in hospitals and institutions, and in other settings; and instruction in physical education." "Related services" are also specifically defined under the Act as "transportation, and such developmental, corrective, and other supportive services (including speech pathology and audiology, psychological services, physical and occupational therapy, recreation, including therapeutic recreation, social work services, counseling services, including rehabilitation counseling, and medical services, except that such medical services shall be for diagnostic and evaluation purposes only) as may be required to assist a child with a disability to benefit from special education, and includes the early identification and assessment of disabling conditions in children."

In contrast to the precise definitions given much of the IDEA's terminology, the question of what constitutes an "appropriate" education is not provided a functional definition under the Act. The U.S. Supreme Court first attempted to clarify the meaning of appropriate education under the IDEA in the landmark case of *Board of Education of Hendrick Hudson Central School District v. Rowley* (1982). Rather than listing specific criteria that an educational program appropriate for all children with disabilities must include, the Supreme Court set forth a two-part analysis for determining whether the requirements of the Act have been met:

First, has the State complied with the procedures set forth in the Act? And second, is the individualized educational program developed through the Act's procedures reasonably calculated to enable the child to receive educational benefit? If these requirements are met, the State has complied with the obligations imposed by the Congress and the courts can require no more.

Although nonspecific, it is preferable that "appropriate" is not narrowly defined under the IDEA, particularly for a child with PWS, whose needs are so unique. In determining what was required by the substantive mandates of the Act, the Court stated that "[i]mplicit in the congressional purpose of providing access to a 'free appropriate public education is the requirement that the education to which access is provided be sufficient to confer some educational benefit upon the child. . . . [T]he 'basic floor of opportunity' provided by the Act consists of access to specialized instruction and related services *which are individually designed* to provide educational benefit to the child [with a disability]." Under the *Rowley* "educational benefit test," educational agencies are not required to provide the best possible educational program nor is equality of opportunity for children with and without disabilities the basis for determining "appropriateness" under the Act. However, it is clear that Congress's intent was not to allow a school system to fulfill its obligation under the Act by "providing a program that produces some minimal academic advancement, no matter how trivial" (Hall v. Vance, 1985).

The IDEA also requires that the child with PWS or other disability receive the free appropriate public education to which she or he is entitled in the least restrictive environment. To the maximum extent appropriate, children with disabilities are to be educated with children without disabilities. Only when the nature or severity of the child's disability is such that education in regular classes with the use of supplementary aids and services cannot be achieved satisfactorily can the child be removed from the regular educational setting. The placement of choice is the regular educational setting.

Placement must be determined at least annually and based on the completed IEP. Once the IEP has been developed, the team must determine the placement options that would provide appropriate programming for the child. Then, from among the range of appropriate options, it must be determined which is the least restrictive.

After· spending up to 21 years of life in the educational system, the individual with PWS is faced with the transition into an adult system that may or may not be designed to serve the needs of someone who has PWS. Fortunately, Congress has recently recognized the need for the educational system to prepare a child with a disability for postschool participation in society and now requires that transition services be included on the IEP beginning at age 14 or younger. Transition services include community experiences, the development of employment and other postschool adult living objectives, and instruction.

The Americans with Disabilities Act

The passage of the Americans with Disabilities Act of 1990 (ADA) focused national attention on persons with disabilities in a manner that promises to result in long-term positive consequences. Although other statutory and constitutional protections exist for persons with developmental disabilities, for the first time the ban on discrimination against persons with disabilities was extended to the private sector (House Committee on the Judiciary, 1990). The ADA provides an additional avenue of advocacy for persons with Prader–Willi syndrome. Unfortunately, according to a nationwide Harris poll conducted in June 1993, only 29% of persons with disabilities polled were aware of the ADA.

The ADA was based on notable Congressional findings that include (1) our society continues to have a pervasive social problem of discriminating against persons with disabilities by isolating and segregating them; (2)

discrimination against people with disabilities continues in critical areas that include institutionalization, employment, education, housing, health services, and public accommodation; and (3) our country's goals regarding individuals with disabilities are to ensure equality of opportunity, full participation, economic self-sufficiency, and independent living. Thus, the purpose of the Americans with Disabilities Act is to "provide a clear and comprehensive national mandate for the elimination of discrimination against individuals with disabilities," complete with clear, strong, consistent, and enforceable standards that the federal government takes a central role in enforcing.

The Americans with Disabilities Act is a comprehensive statute. Therefore, an exhaustive review of its provisions is beyond the scope of this chapter. However, because it carries a strong federal mandate that promises the 43,000,000 Americans who have disabilities an end to discrimination, a few of the key principles are highlighted herein.

Examining the ADA in relation to Prader–Willi syndrome, the first determination is whether Prader–Willi syndrome falls within the definition of disability (Tucker & Goldstein, 1992). Under the ADA, disability is defined, with respect to an individual, to include (1) a physical or mental impairment that substantially limits one or more of the major life activities of the individual; (2) a record of having such an impairment; or (3) being regarded as having such an impairment. Although it is reasonable to expect that the majority of persons who have Prader–Willi syndrome will fall within the ADA's definition of disability, a individualized determination must be made. Analyzing the definition in relation to a person with Prader–Willi syndrome, the components to be considered are as follows. "Major life activities" include functions such as taking care of oneself, seeing, hearing, speaking, breathing, performing manual tasks, working, and learning. An individual with Prader–Willi syndrome may have accompanying mental retardation, which could impact the person's learning and working. The individual with Prader–Willi syndrome, if his or her diet has not been carefully monitored, may have obesity, which has resulted in breathing difficulties. Other major life activities may be affected by the syndrome.

Whether a major life activity is "substantially impaired" is determined by comparing the ability of the person with PWS to perform the activity to the average person in the population's ability to perform the activity. Also considered is whether there are restrictions on the manner, condition, or duration under which the person with Prader–Willi syndrome can perform the particular activity, as compared to the manner, condition, or duration under which an average individual in the community can perform the activity. In determining whether a person with Prader–Willi syndrome is "substantially limited" in performing a major life activity, the factors taken into account include the nature and severity of the impairment, the duration or expected duration of the impairment, and the expected permanent or long-term impact of the impairment. Generally, the nature and severity of the impairment of a person with Prader–Willi syndrome may be significant and though the disability is permanent in nature, the degree of impact may vary over time. Permanence of duration is not considered determinative in the analysis under all titles of the ADA. It is important to note that these factors are to be considered without regard to the mitigating effect that medication, assistive devices, or other accommodations have on the disability.

Obesity in and of itself is not considered a disability under the ADA. However, due to the fact that the obesity often accompanying PWS has a physiological etiology and may impair breathing and walking, an individual with Prader–Willi syndrome will likely be considered disabled under the ADA. Additionally, a person who has Prader–Willi syndrome with accompanying obesity may be "regarded" as having a disability, thus qualifying for protection under the Act.

Employment

The ADA contains four substantive titles plus one title containing miscellaneous provisions. One of the most controversial provisions is Title I, which prohibits discrimination against persons with disabilities in employment practices (Tucker & Goldstein, 1992). This prohibition prevents a private employer who has more than fifteen (15) employees from discriminating against a person with a disability. State and local government entities are prohibited from discrimination regardless of the number of persons they employ. A covered employer may not discriminate in the areas of job application procedures; the hiring, discharge, or advancement of employees; job training; employee compensation; and other terms, privileges, and conditions of employment.

In order for the protections of the ADA to apply, the employee or potential employee must be a qualified person with a disability. Such an individual must be able, with or without reasonable accommodation, to perform the essential functions of the employment position. An essential function is largely determined by the employer. A written description of the essential functions of the position prepared before advertising or interviewing is considered evidence of the essential functions of the job.

To be required to make an accommodation for a person with a disability, the employer must be aware that the employee with PWS has a disability. The employee seeking reasonable accommodation for his or her disability can be required to provide verification of the disability. The employer must make reasonable accommodations to an otherwise qualified individual with a disability unless the employer can demonstrate that to do so would create an undue hardship on the operation of the business of the covered entity. Reasonable accommodations include such undertakings as making existing facilities readily accessible to and usable by persons with disabilities as well as acquiring or modifying equipment or devices, providing qualified readers or interpreters, allowing part-time or modified work schedules, and job restructuring, and other similar modifications.

It is import to note that the ADA places the burden on the employer to prove that the necessary accommodation will produce an "undue hardship" on the entity. Undue hardship results when an action requires significant difficulty or expense. Factors that may be taken into account in determining undue hardship include the nature and cost of the needed accommodation; overall financial resources of the facility involved in providing the needed accommodation; the overall resources of the covered entity, including the number of employees and number, type, and location of its facilities; and type of operation of the covered entity.

The ADA allows individuals as well as governmental entities to pursue a claim under the employment title of the Act. The Equal Employment Opportunity Commission (EEOC) works in conjunction with the Office of Civil Rights to enforce the employment provisions of the ADA. Before a person files an action in court, however, administrative remedies must be exhausted. (Kent v. Director, 1992).

Equitable relief is available for individuals who prevail in an action against an employer alleging disparate impact. This relief might include injunctive relief, such as a court order requiring the individual with a disability be hired or an award of back pay. In an award for intentional discrimination, an individual may also be entitled to compensatory and punitive damages. Attorney's fees are available to the prevailing party, other than the United States. Such fees may include the cost of expert witness fees. However, fees are not available against a plaintiff unless the lawsuit was frivolous. Any party to an action may request a jury trial.

Public Services

Title II of the Americans with Disabilities Act prohibits public entities from excluding persons with disabilities from enjoying the benefits of the services, programs, or activities of a public entity (Tucker & Goldstein, 1992). Public entities, defined as any local or state government or agency or department thereof, are required to administer services, programs, and activities in the most integrated setting appropriate to the needs of qualified individuals with disabilities. Congress relied on racial desegregation cases as controlling authority for the desegregation mandate of the ADA. Public entities must make reasonable modifications in practices, policies, or procedures in order to avoid discrimination on the basis of disability, unless such modifications would fundamentally alter the nature of the program. Public entities cannot achieve compliance with the ADA by providing auxiliary aides and services only in segregated settings.

Persons with Prader–Willi syndrome all too frequently reside in large congregate facilities for persons with mental retardation. Staff at such facilities may or may not have knowledge about or expertise in dealing with persons with PWS. Because the ADA includes in its findings the focus on ending the stigma and discrimination of institutionalization, this Act may provide a mechanism for the provision of needed supports in community-based settings (Cook, 1991).

A large part of the focus of Title II of the ADA is on providing access to public transportation. The transportation provisions are divided into two subparts: the first addresses public transportation other than by aircraft or certain rail operations; the second refers to public transportation by intercity and commuter rail service. Without access to public transportation, many people with disabilities would not be able to get to and from work or recreational activities.

The transportation provisions benefit a person with Prader–Willi syndrome who falls within the definition of disability previously discussed and who needs some type of seating accommodation or who uses a wheelchair. The public entity must make good-faith efforts when purchasing new bus or rail systems to obtain systems that include ramps or lifts and fold-up seats or other space to safely secure a wheelchair. There are detailed provisions dealing with the purchase or lease of used vehicles and regarding the remanufacture of vehicles to extend their use.

The ADA also requires that paratransit services be provided for persons who are not able, due to their disability, to use the fixed route system. The Act also requires that there be room for one person to accompany the person with a disability and that more than one person be allowed to accompany the individual with a disability if space allows without denying another person with a disability the service. However, the Act does not require unlimited access, but allows exceptions if providing the services would constitute undue financial burden on the public entity. Essentially, the Act strives to provide comparable services to persons with disabilities as provided those without disabilities.

New facilities built for use in providing public transportation or alterations made on existing facilities must be done in a manner that permits access and use by persons with disabilities, including those who use wheelchairs. A public entity that provides a demand responsive system must ensure that the system is accessible to persons with disabilities or that persons with disabilities are provided equivalent services. The ADA does not require modification of vehicles used in conjunction with the National Register of Historic Places if so doing would significantly alter their historical character. It should be noted that airlines do not fall under the purview of the ADA.

The Department of Transportation has responsibility for enforcing the provisions of Title II regarding transportation. Possible remedies include injunctive relief, loss of federal funds for the offending entity, and possible monetary damages. Although there are administrative remedies available through the Department of Transportation, it is not necessary to exhaust these remedies prior to filing an action in court.

Public Accommodations

Title III of the ADA deals with public accommodations and services operated by private entities. Due to their complexity, the provisions of the Act regarding transportation provided by private enterprise are beyond the scope of this chapter. However, it should be noted that considerable controversy was generated regarding the requirements of this section and compromises were made in order to ensure passage of the legislation.

In addition to private entities that provide transportation, a person with a disability is entitled to full and equal enjoyment of the services, privileges, advantages, goods, facilities, or accommodations of any place of public accommodation by any person who owns, operates, or leases a place of public accommodation. Under this title, public accommodation is broadly defined to include all types of entities that impact commerce. Included are motels, restaurants, parks, health spas, educational facilities, museums, day care and senior citizens centers, theaters, auditoriums and lecture halls, bakeries and groceries, bankers, barbers, law offices, and other service establishments. Religious entities are exempt from coverage under this section of the ADA.

This title provides not only for physical access to private entities and thus to the goods and services that they make available, but also prohibits discrimination in any of the testing or courses for professions or trades, thus making the provisions of Title I truly meaningful. Under the ADA, it is considered discriminatory to provide an individual with a disability, on the basis of disability, goods, services, or other accommodations that are different or separate from those provided a person without a disability, unless it is necessary to do so in order to provide the individual with a disability an opportunity for participation equal to that provided persons without disabilities. However, even if separate or different programs exist, a person with a disability cannot be denied the opportunity to participate in the program that is not separate or different. Goods, services, and other accommodations must be provided in the most integrated setting appropriate to the needs of the individual with a disability.

Discrimination under this provision includes the following: (1) applying or imposing eligibility criteria that tend to prevent persons with disabilities from fully and equally enjoying goods or services, unless necessary for the provision of goods or services being offered; (2) failing to make reasonable modifications in policies, practices, or procedures that do not impact the fundamental nature of the goods or services being offered; (3) failing to take necessary steps to ensure that no person with a disability is excluded, denied services, or treated differently, including providing auxiliary aides and services, unless taking such steps would fundamentally alter the nature of the goods or services or constitute an undue burden; (4) failing to remove communication, architectural, and transportation barriers where such removal is readily achievable; and (5) where the entity has demonstrated that the removal of certain barriers is not readily achievable, failure to make such goods and services available through alternative methods that are readily achievable.

Private individuals as well as the United States Attorney General may enforce the provisions of Title III. Injunctive relief may include requiring the offending entity to make facilities accessible, change policies or practices, or provide auxiliary aides or services. Punitive damages are not available. Although private individuals may not obtain monetary damages, if the U.S. Attorney General brings a claim based on a "pattern or practice" or on a situation that affects the public interest, monetary damages may be obtained.

Telecommunications

Title IV of the ADA requires that telephone companies provide a system to allow persons with hearing and speech disabilities to communicate with hearing individuals (Tucker & Goldstein, 1992). The Federal Communications Commission is responsible for regulating this title. Such a system must provide full-time services, be no more costly than telephone services available to the general public, and confidentiality must be maintained. The cost is absorbed by all users.

Although efforts were made to provide closed-captioned television as a requirement of the ADA, those attempts were unsuccessful. However, any public service announcement that is funded or produced by the federal government must provide closed-captioning.

Miscellaneous Provisions

Title V contains various miscellaneous provisions applicable to the entire ADA (Tucker & Goldstein, 1992). These include that an individual with a disability cannot be forced to accept a particular accommodation that she or he chooses not to accept; that retaliation and coercion are prohibited; a provision allowing attorneys' fees to a prevailing party other than the United States; and the abrogation of State immunity under the Eleventh Amendment to the United States Constitution. Clarification is provided that present users of illegal drugs are not covered by the ADA and other conditions, such as pedophilia, homosexuality, and compulsive gambling, are excluded from the ADA definition of disability. The Americans with Disabilities Act recommends, but does not require, alternative dispute resolution regarding claims brought under its provisions.

Summary

Empowerment is the key to effective advocacy, whether the advocacy be on one's own behalf or that of another individual with PWS. The first step toward empowerment is for the person with PWS and their families to become familiar with his or rights in order to effectively assert those rights. It is hoped that the concepts presented herein will assist persons with Prader–Willi syndrome and their families to advocate successfully for the supports and services necessary for persons with PWS to maximize their potential and become active, fully integrated, and participating members of society.

References

Americans with Disabilities Act: Hearing Before the Senate Committee on Labor and Human Resources and the Subcommittee on the Handicapped, 101st Cong., 1st Sess. 66 (1989).

Americans with Disabilities Act of 1990, 42 U.S.C.A. section 12101 *et seq.* (West Supp. 1993) and implementing regulations.

Board of Education of Hendrick Hudson Central School District v. Rowley, 458 U.S. 175 (1982).

Brown v. Board of Education, 347 U.S. 483 (1954).

Cook, T.M. (1991). The Americans with Disabilities Act: The move to integration. *64, Temple Law Review*, 393.

Developmental Disabilities Assistance and Bill of Rights Act, 42 U.S.C.A. Section 6000 *et seq.* (West Supp. 1993).

Hall v. Vance City Board of Education, 774 F.2d 629 (4th Cir. 1985).

House Committee on the Judiciary, H.P. Rep. No. 485, 101st Cong., 2d Sess., pt. 3, reprinted in, *1990 U.S. Code Cong. & Admin. News* 473.

Individuals with Disabilities Education Act, 20 U.S.C.A. section 1400 *et seq.* (West Supp. 1993).

Kent v. Director, Missouri Department of Elementary and Secondary Education and Division of Vocational Rehabilitation, 792 F. Supp. 59 (E.D.Mo. 1992).

Tucker, B.P., & Goldstein, B.A. (1992). *Legal rights of persons with disabilities: An analysis of federal law* (Chs. 20–23). Horsham, PA: LRP Publications.

Young Lawyers Division, Iowa State Bar Association, *A guide to the legal rights of Iowans with disabilities and mental illnesses* (December 1992).

34 C.F.R. Pt. 300 & App. C (1992).

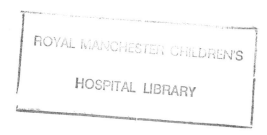

15
Residential Options for Individuals with Prader–Willi Syndrome

Louise R. Greenswag, Sandra L. Singer, Nancy Condon, Harvey H. Bush, Sharon Omrod, Mary M. Mulligan, and Patricia L. Shaw

As a natural outgrowth of earlier diagnosis, case finding, and appropriate nutritional management, individuals with Prader–Willi syndrome (PWS) now live well into adulthood and effective services have been provided to over 400 individuals with the syndrome in a variety of residential options over the past decade. However, additional programs are needed to care for this expanding population and increasing the availability of services requires careful planning to ensure optimum programming.

This chapter proposes that out-of-home placement can be successful in a variety of residential settings when policies, procedures, and programming are based on a core of generic guidelines. These common themes should consist of establishing a safe environment, employing qualified personnel, and instituting creative programs that regulate weight, maintain optimum health, and manage behaviors for persons with PWS. The authors hope that this information will be useful to providers and reassuring to parents.

General Considerations

One of the most critical periods in the life cycle of families occurs when the children leave the family nest. And, if letting go of normal offspring is not easy, how much more difficult it must be for parents of children with developmental disabilities such as Prader–Willi syndrome to relinquish their roles. Have they fulfilled their parental obligations? Are they "putting their child away"? Thoughts about separation and placement intensify feelings of inadequacy, ambivalence, and guilt.

Once children with PWS have completed their schooling, parents and guardians are justifiably apprehensive about their future. A few parents choose to keep their offspring with them idefinitely and have made arrangements for family members (such as siblings) to take responsibility as needed. However, most acknowledge, albeit painfully, that expectations for their children to become socially mature and able to function completely independently are unrealistic. What eventually seems to happen is that, although most parents wish to maintain their children at home, the erratic behaviors associated with PWS tend to intensify over time, even where weight has been controlled. This "unpredictability" coupled with years of stress in a rigid, abnormally structured household eventually makes family life unendurable. Although the decision is difficult, residential placement becomes an attractive option for emotionally exhausted parents who want to enjoy their later years and also acknowledge their own mortality.

For years parents have petitioned for services that will provide a caring, comfortable, safe environment for their children and historically, the earliest residential programs were established primarily through the effors of parents who had few resources beyond their own dedication and persistence. Getting through the maze of bureaucratic roadblocks was a major challenge. The mental retardation guidelines originally used by state funding agencies tended to be so narrowly defined that persons with PWS fell between the cracks in a system where few professionals were knowledgeable about the syndrome. Just the process of seeking federal monies through state agencies was a daunting task. Local help had to be forthcoming from civic minded attorneys, bankers, social workers, psychologists, and physicians who could support the start-up process. Even after one nonprofit corporation was chartered by interested parents (and continues to function independently), it became evident that a "sponsoring agency" with a good track record for providing programming, qualified staff, and community resources had to be located. Despite overwhelming obstacles, some PWS designated residential facilities began to emerge, such as the Oakwood program that opened in 1981 in Minneapolis, MN; it is described later in this chapter.

Parents now know that their children are eligible for Supplemental Security Income (SSI) under section 1614(a)(3)(A) (Mental Health Law Project, 1991), which defines a disability as due to physical and/or mental impairment. Children with PWS are classified under "other related conditions" and as "functionally" retarded. Application for SSI is made through a local Social Security Office. Finding specialized services begins when contact is made with the local Office of the Department of Health and Human Services (DHS) (see Chapter 12). Documentation of eligibility to receive assistance due to the presence of PWS is now clearly referenced in *Index Medicus* (U.S. Department of Health and Human Services, 1983), in the "related conditions" classification of The American Association on Mental Retardation (AAMR) (Grossman, 1973), and as a disability due to a rare birth defect (Goldenson, 1978). Clearly, persons with PWS fit within the service delivery guidelines.

Program Development

Developing residential services raises important questions about how to design programming. What is it about PWS that requires unique services? Are there common or "generic" threads that can be used to establish guidelines? Are there residential options already providing opportunities for weight control, behavioral management, social interactions, work, recreation, and participation in community life? How can other existing programs for persons with developmental disabilities adapt their services to meet the special needs of persons with PWS?

Several important issues associated with most long-term residential programs profoundly affect the extent to which persons with PWS are able to adapt. First, most long-term facilities focus on normalization, i.e., development of social skills, creation of work programs, healthy recreation, and community participation. They are also remarkably similar in that there is usually easy access to food preparation and consumption and only limited supervision. These features require considerable modification to be suitable for persons with PWS. Anecdotal reports of inappropriate placements in nursing homes and in institutions for the mentally ill are a sad commentary on the extent to which lack of knowledge about PWS compromises their lives.

Second, most residential programs build on the premise that clients have a right to live in a "least restrictive environment" that maximizes opportunities for self-fulfillment. At the same time, settings should provide the necessary protective milieu and be defined in terms of client needs rather than the convenience of the providers or a less expensive alternative (Pieper, 1985). This concept requires review when designing services for persons with PWS. Practical experience indicates that, for these individuals, a least restrictive setting translates into PWS designated services or integrated programs that are capable of maintaining a delicate balance of 24 hr supervision, specialized services, and a willingness to go the extra mile to make them effective.

Finally, protection and preservation of the "human rights" of clients is an issue that is often muddled and misused by clients, their families, and caregivers. Any agency that provides services for persons with PWS is responsible for their health and well being. Where "human rights" are perceived to "interfere" with discharge of these responsibilities, they need reassessment.

Simply put, while normalization, a least restrictive environment, and human rights must be addressed, unlimited access to food and only limited supervision puts persons with PWS at great risk. To ignore these issues and disregard the distinction between persons with PWS and their peers with non-PWS disabilities can undermine opportunities for successful adaptation, regardless of the setting.

Guidelines for Services

Life plans and activities simply do not always "go right". Nothing "works" all the time and this certainly holds true for residential programming for persons with PWS. This population has the best chance to adapt where guidelines are clearly defined. Programs/services need to be geared toward long-term placement supervised by competent, sensitive personnel in a structured, safe, physical environment. While it is necessary that persons with PWS do some adjusting and that providers allow some flexibility (depending on individual capabilities), the fact remains that skills may increase and erratic behaviors may decrease. Problems tend to recure wherever and whenever structure changes and external controls are inconsistent. On the other hand, sometimes structure may work too well and fuel the natural tendency of this population to resist changes in procedure and plans, even when it is to their benefit.

Situations have been reported wherein disgruntled, frustrated clients who formerly lived with their families and "had their way" have moved into structured residential programs and found them not to their liking. Their reactions are similar to those they demonstrated when living at home: rages, physical aggression, and destruction of property. Because such behavior successfully destroyed resistance of the family to most demands, it is possible that these individuals assume that continuing such conduct will result in dismissal from the residence. In some cases, inappropriate activities have gone on for extended periods of time and have been described as an endless tantrum. However, *where residential programming is effective, dismissal does not occur, no matter how difficult and controlling the resident might attempt to be.*

Too often parents and providers nurture the idea that a residential facility should be "just like home," where individuals interact as a family unit. While the concept makes sense, experience with this population indicates that a small, intimate, "home-away-from home" is not always a realistic expectation. Yes, there is some sense of unity among persons in specific programs. However, the compromises, negotiations, and mediations that exist in healthy family units are, for persons with PWS, usually limited by the egocentric aspect of their personalities that restrict their ability to cooperate beyond meeting their own needs.

Human Resources and Staff Development Considerations

All personnel, e.g., program administrators, primary staff, and community service providers, must not only be knowledgeable about the syndrome but must also be capable of accepting and appreciating the uniqueness of these individuals who struggle with conflicting physical and emotional drives. Effective staff focus on creative, joint decision-making and follow established programming procedures on a consistent basis. Occasionally, personnel tend to think that serving persons with PWS is no different than serving persons with any other developmental disability. Nothing could be further from the truth. Regardless of their training, new employees will develop a true understanding of PWS only after they have had the opportunity to interact with these individuals. A residential "manual" of information can be an excellent resource for staff. In addition to continuous updating of information about PWS, it should contain "house rules" for all services, e.g., meals, behavior, activities, personal care, transportation, and a summary of individual program plans. Written evidence of guidelines can reduce confusion and the potential for conflict, particularly when new staff are being oriented.

Staffing usually includes a residential director credentialed in nursing, psychology, social work, counseling, or a related field who is experienced in administering programs for persons with developmental disabilities. Essential staff consist of a program and activities coordinator, food manager/cook, nurse, and direct care personnel. Where house managers are employed rather than a three-shift pattern, their duties usually include building maintenance and transportation service as well as staff responsibilities. Where a 24 hr-a-day, three-shift pattern is in place, staff must be able to cover all aspects of programming. The direct care staff ratio is usually 1:3 or 1:4 and in addition to identified weekend staff, full time personnel should rotate. Most often, the major direct care interactions with clients occur during the hours from 3 to 11 PM and a 1:3 ratio is essential.

Competent direct care personnel are able to appreciate the strengths of persons with PWS, demonstrate good listening and communication skills, and can use their position of authority without rancor. They are mature enough to avoid power struggles, recognize and minimize opportunities to be manipulated, not take personal offense when verbally attacked, and have a good sense of humor. They are perceptive to rapid mood changes, sensitive to potential crisis situations, acknowledge the need to be flexible, knowing it is not necessary to win every battle. On-going problem oriented in-service training is essential for staff development and support. Qualified staff who show common sense and genuine caring are the key to the success of any residential program.

The Physical Setting

Although residential options will vary according to provider attitudes and resources, some common guidelines for establishing a physical facility, i.e., location, floor plans, and furnishings have been described in earlier literature (Thompson, Greenswag, and Eleazer, 1988). These descriptions, reviewed in the following passages, should be considered regardless of whether a planned program will be free-standing unit or part of a larger, established facility.

A group residence does not require new construction in an expensive neighborhood. However, the size, cost, staff ratio, and programming will be determined by the number of persons who will reside there. Locale should be in a safe area, accessible for families. Competent staff may be attracted to work in a program if the location is close to public transportation. Parks, community centers, and year-round swimming facilities are an asset, but access to shopping should *not* be within walking distance. An apartment complex can work where a section is devoted to the residential program and, of course, individual services in a single home require an entirely different approach.

Living space requirements include adequate room for food preparation, dining, sleeping, bathing, office area for staff, recreation/exercise, laundry, storage, and all aspects of programming. Where the structure has more than one floor, walking stairs provides good, albeit, involuntary exercise. Several smaller rooms that can accommodate groups for projects, group interactions, and socialization are better than a large, open living area. Smaller rooms provide relatively quiet surroundings, limit distractions, encourage individual interests, and offer privacy for interactions with family or staff. Although most residents are away from the residence for a considerable part of the week-day and evening activities are usually planned, they do spend "home" time. When the quarters are too close, personalities may clash.

The kitchen should be well equipped with room for food preparation and storage. If there is no barrier to the kitchen, cupboards, closets, refrigerators, freezers, and areas where cleaning supplies, equipment, and paper goods are stored must be locked and off limits. The dining room should seat all residents and staff with ample space to move around the table(s). Carpet or acoustical tile helps control noise. This area can also be used for meetings and activities. Keeping the floor clean usually presents no problem since food is rarely spilled.

Single or two-person sleeping quarters work better than a dormitory arrangement. Families can help to furnish the bedroom with pleasant and familiar objects such as a bed, table, chairs, and personal belongings. Single rooms eliminate the need for "time-out" space somewhere else in the home. Bedroom doors should have locks, not just for privacy but to discourage stealing, prevent interpersonal conflicts, and allow for differences in housekeeping. Where separate rooms are not possible, a permanent room divider can help along with large divided closets and dresser drawers that also can be locked. Persons with PWS are notorious collectors and they like space to accumulate items.

Private baths are *not* recommended. Supervision is required since arguments tend to lead to retaliation in the form of clogged sinks and toilets or overflowing tubs. Bathrooms, assigned by sex, should be close to bedrooms with one sink and stool for four persons plus one tub/shower (or shower stall) for six. A private bath should be available for staff and visitors and all baths must be wheelchair accessible.

Lockable storage units should be available. Since hoarding can be a problem, storage space may reduce overcrowded bedrooms and provide space for out-of-season clothing. Laundry facilities that require coins are an issue only in so far as tokens should be used in machines along with packets of soap and softeners because it seems to be difficult for some individuals to measure accurately.

Office space for the director and staff is best located near program areas to ensure adequate supervision. Medical records and medicines must be kept locked since this space may be used for examination, treatment, consultation, and staff respite. Thermostats and fire alarm boxes need specially reinforced covers and the location of the telephone should be carefully considered.

Any residential facility should have exercise, entertainment, and maintenance equipment. A stereo unit, tape recorder, and/or videocassette player can assist in activities such as dancing, relaxation, and aerobics. Unless there is considerable space available, omit pool or ping pong tables since their use is not usually worth their cost. One large television set for one viewing area is sufficient since many residents have their own. On the other hand, a piano/organ is handy for socialization. Exercise equipment encourages regular use that can help with weight loss and maintenance of muscle tone; exercycles are best. In addition, any items needed to maintain a home are valuable, especially light weight sweepers and long handled dusters, since housekeeping tasks are part of the responsibilities of each person.

For safety and soundproofing, carpeted floors are best (except in game/dance areas). Large pieces of wooden furniture are most substantial and long lasting; heavy-duty fabric for upholstery is more durable than vinyl or leather. Comfort is an issue since most persons with PWS remain very short. White or light walls accented with bright colors are pleasant. Tables with stain resistant tops work best for puzzles and games and all picture and wall decorations should be firmly fastened. While living plants in plastic containers brighten an area, basically the decor should be kept inexpensive since some damage is likely during emotional outbursts. Wash and wear tablecloths and/or placemats are best for the dining area, but plan to purchase bargain, open-pattern silverware because it seems to disappear very often.

Programming

It goes without saying that if left unattended, most persons with PWS would literally eat themselves to death. Therefore, weight loss/control is critical to the success of all programming. The insatiable appetite that triggers food seeking behaviors together with metabolic differences that cause weight gain on fewer calories makes individual nutritional guidelines, access to edibles, and the mealtime environment a major concern.

While it is difficult to always find a balance between controlling access to food and the nonfood aspects of group living, it can be accomplished. The multidisciplinary team comprised of direct care staff, nutritionist, and cook play a major role in this aspect of programming. This topic is discussed in depth in Chapter 7. Daily exercise should be linked to scheduled programming, community activities, and recreation. An important "rule of thumb" is that while food is a necessity, beyond mealtimes persons with PWS should be kept occupied with nonfood activities. Dietary supervision and maintenance of health go hand in hand. The potential for medical complications associated with obesity include compromise of the cardiopulmonary and circulatory systems. Issues associated with compulsive skin picking, decreased sensitivity to pain, thermoregulatory problems, and sleep disturbances require constant attention.

Observable egocentric and capricious behaviors can be managed with consistency and structure. This requires establishment of policies and procedures for both rountine and nonroutine activities. Successful programming also reflects individualization since significant discrepancies may exist between cognitive, social, and interpersonal skills. Perhaps one of the most challenging aspects of developing behavioral programming is the dichotomy that exists between high proficiency levels in some cognitive areas such as verbal skills and the capacity to cleverly manipulate the environment. Persons with PWS are remarkably talented at finding "loopholes" in any system. Furthermore, a strong drive to be independent necessitates safeguarding against life threatening dangers that they lack the insight to recognize (Singer, 1994). The approaches to managing behaviors discussed in Chapter 9 vary depending upon the presenting behavior and its purpose (i.e., whether it is for attention, avoidance).

Current Residential Options

The *ideal* out-of-home environment for many or most persons with PWS may be a small group residence designated just for persons with the syndrome. Approximately 40 such programs, geared to long-term placement, serve nearly 200 persons throughout the United States. However, designated programs either may not be feasible or may not be the choice of parents or providers. Many private, not-for-profit agencies currently serving the DD/MR population are philosophically opposed to homogeneous programming but are interested in providing services in integrated group homes, supervised apartments, and/or supported living programs. Another 200 persons live in over 100 such settings. Some programs that serve a younger population offer residential schooling.

Where a PWS designated small group home is the goal, it is suggested that parents/guardians seek out an established not-for-profit agency (local, state, or national) with a respected reputation for serving persons with developmental disabilities that is willing to develop a designated group home. These "umbrella" agencies have considerable experience in the bureaucratic process, particularly funding issues, and understand the requirements for differing levels of service. The agencies are also advantageous because they are usually already linked to community programs, have the resources to find qualified staff, can offer on-going training, and are sensitive to the needs of the parents. When seeking to open an Intermediate Care Facility for The Mentally Retarded (ICF/MR), very strict federal guidelines must be met in order to obtain federal funding for the physical setting, staff development, and daily programming. Some states serve their own developmentally disabled populations and individual state Divisions of Developmental Disabilities contract with private agencies and provide funding. Some states also allow the parents/ guardians to retain the right to remain the payees of SSI money for their children but are then billed by the state for service. Programming costs can vary from $26,000.00 to $50,000.00 annually.

A Designated Group Home (15 Beds)

Oakwood, Residence, Inc., a 15 bed residential facility located in Minneapolis, Minnesota, provides services specifically for individuals with PWS. It is funded through Title XIX monies as an ICF/MR. Oakwood was developed by a group of parents and concerned citizens who saw the need for services for people with the syndrome; it has been in operation since September 1981. This group home provides residential, recreational, health, and social services, through training in independent living and leisure skills. It encourages optimum growth in physical, social, intellectual, and vocational areas.

During the past 12 years, Oakwood has served 20 people with the syndrome, 10 women and 10 men. Two residents died of leukemia, two have moved to smaller facilities, and one was discharged due to atypical behaviors that were not manageable. Entrance age has been set at 15 years or older. The current population is between 26 and 42 years of age, is ambulatory, and capable of managing in emergency situations such as fire or severe weather.

Many of the more common characteristics of PWS are noted in the residents. Most are short in stature, have a typical distribution of body fat, are sexually underdeveloped and immature, exhibit an insatiable drive to eat, display considerable emotional lability, and are cognitively limited.

The Environment

The program provides a safe, predictable environment that is continually monitored and reevaluated. The building is a converted two story structure located in an older, urban, residential area with easy access to community resources. All living areas are comfortably furnished, cheerful, and aesthetically pleasing. Each resident is afforded privacy with a separate bedroom that has, over time, reduced personality conflicts and theft by peers. There are a variety of living spaces that can be used for small group or individual activities, or as quiet areas for relaxation. The kitchen, food storage areas, and staff offices have locks and the exit doors have an alarm system. There is a small apartment located on the first floor for a live-in staff person.

Human Resources and Staff Development

The operations of the program are overseen by the Program Director, who is the Qualified Mental Health Retardation Professional (QMRP). The Program Coordinator, responsible for ensuring the day-to-day welfare of the residents, supervises the direct care staff. A Residential Counselor III is primarily responsible for leisure/recreational activities. This individual also is the chairperson of the facility's Human Rights Committee, coordinates the Resident Council, and provides direct care services. Residential Counselor II(s) carry a caseload of three residents, develop and implement individual program plans, and oversee any personal or financial needs. The remainder of the direct care staff are Residential Counselor I(s) who directly supervise and implement program plans. A registered nurse is employed on a part time basis as the Health Services Coordinator to meet the health needs of the residents and supervise the dietary department. A dietitian, physicians, dentists, psychologists, psychiatrists, and other consultants are also under contract. Oakwood residents are supervised 24 hr a day and there is a full time staff ratio of 1:4 during primary times and one "awake" staff on the overnight shift. A Residential Counselor is *specifically* employed to live in the small apartment and is on call in case of emergencies.

Other support staff include a full time manager of food services, a full time office manager, and a part time maintenance coordinator.

When initially employed, staff receive general orientation in the areas required by ICF/MR regulations. This orientation includes an overview of principles associated with developmental disabilities services, concepts of normalization, the general characteristics of PWS, and Oakwood's environmental and procedural guidelines. After careful review of the general characteristics of PWS, staff are educated regarding each resident's program plan, medical information, and strategies for behavior management. On-going education is provided not only to comply with regulatory requirements but also to keep staff informed of any advances in the fields of developmental disabilities and PWS. Weekly and monthly staff meetings are conducted to maintain communication regarding the needs of individual residents, to orient staff to new program plans, to coordinate all activities, and to assess the effectiveness of general procedures.

General Programming

Programming is constantly reevaluated to ensure the effectiveness of services. Because persons with PWS have difficulty accepting changes even when it is to their benefit, house rules exist to provide guidelines for routine activities. These rules include specification of the times and procedures for serving meals, doing laundry, and taking showers. Protocols are in place regarding smoking and for accessing and spending money. Weigh-ins are completed on a specific day. "Per event" procedures have been instituted to help prepare residents for major changes or initiation of new routines.

Weight Reduction/Maintenance

Weight reduction/maintenance is an integral part of the program. The greatest success with calorie-controlled diets has been based on implementation of the American Diabetic Exchange System; it is easy to understand and meets nutritional requirements. The kitchen, food, and garbage storage areas are kept locked. Weight is usually monitored weekly, although, in special instances, it is checked daily. Times and procedures for meals have been established and issues regarding food are deemphasized by avoiding its use as a reinforcer.

During the earliest years of operation the weight loss regime for the residents was very successful. The original 15 residents lost approximately 1,000 pounds, after which a better balance between controlling weight and enhancing the quality of life became the goal. Unfortunately, the attempt at this balance resulted in some unhealthy weight gain due to the inevitable access to food at work sites and other community settings. Recently staff have developed another approach. In consultation with the dietitian and physician, individual weight ranges and caloric intakes were reevaluated and changed in accordance with current research findings. More structured guidelines for weight control have been developed wherein staff supervise and monitor access to food when residents participate in community activities. On-going communication with day program staff seems to have a positive effect on the extent to which food is available in work settings.

Another important variable in weight reduction and maintenance is exercise. There have been many changes in the manner in which exercise has been approached over the years. In the past, staff have consulted with both physiologists and exercise specialists about appropriate methods of exercise and ways to motivate the residents. The current program, which includes specified times per week during which exercise activity is required, is based on the health and weight of individual residents. Every effort is made to create a variety of on-going activities (this is a regular topic at weekly staffings). Several treadmills and other machines now in use are excellent motivators as well as reliable measures of the intensity of exercise activity.

Health and Medical Care

The behaviors of residents range from demanding to see a physician as an attention seeking device to belief in magical cures, to refusal to report potential problems, and/or failure to accept treatment. It takes considerable skill on the part of staff and providers to balance the tendency to exaggerate or dwell on physical symptoms against the problems associated with the characteristic symptom of decreased sensitivity to pain.

Regardless of behavioral issues, it is necessary to supervise and monitor the health needs of the residents. All full time staff are certified to administer medications. They also have the ability to provide routine treatments, including dealing with the skin picking so that this characteristic behavior does not become a major medical concern. Finding professional service providers who are willing to listen and learn is essential. Oakwood has developed a relationship with specific physicians to ensure appropriate and consistent health services. An information packet that includes a synopsis of PWS and an overview of services is given to new medical and allied health care personnel.

Behavioral Management

Development of strategies to control behaviors is a very important component of the program. Considerable success has been achieved in decreasing the frequency, duration, and intensity of the more obvious and intense behaviors through behavior management, although they still occasionally emerge. The more subtle aspects of the personality traits require that management strategies constantly be reviewed.

Individualized guidelines for interventions are designed to enhance each resident's ability to function as independently as possible and, at the same time, prevent or at least minimize problem behaviors. Personalized program plans consider specific behaviors and efforts are made to teach alternative skills, self-control, and responsibility for individual actions. Anticipation of potential problems associated with "changes" usually requires specific guidelines. In some instances the program plan may need to be altered rather than attempting to "change" a resident's perceptions. Standard prompts such as "calm down and we can talk" or a directive such as "you need to be calm in order to leave the house" are examples of the inventory of verbal responses the staff uses on a consistent basis. "Planned ignoring" and redirection are other interventions. When necessary, use of physical intervention procedures are implemented to control more dangerous behaviors.

Individualized Programming

One of the most diffcult issues to deal with is resistance to programming and/or the lack of motivation to participate. While every attempt is made to develop interventions to meet individual needs and abilities, it is acknowledged that the hunger drive is not amenable to behavioral training and the lack of ability to generalize information also reduces the effectiveness of some behavioral strategies. Programming is based on a Provider Implementation Plan developed by the interdisciplinary team that consists of the resident, Oakwood staff, day program staff, county case managers, parents, or other family members. A variety of techniques are implemented to assist residents to maintain previously learned skills and to attain and retain new ones by teaching, supervision, and prompting task completion.

Day Programming and Vocational Opportunities

Oakwood residents have attended several different programs in the past and, for the most part, the current programs seem to be reasonably successful. The less successful day program services have usually been those unwilling to make adjustments associated with accessibility to food. However, since choices for day programs are limited, it is necessary to work with what is available. From Oakwood's experience, access to food is inevitable, therefore good communication with day programs is essential and every effort is made to teach and train day staff about PWS. It appears that paid work increases the self-esteem as well as the "buying power" for residents. Therefore, where health is *not* an issue, it is important to balance access to food in the workplace with these "other" benefits of paid work.

Several residents with severe behaviors and little control of food seeking activities attend a licensed Day Habilitation and Training Center. This facility offers environmental controls required for management. Other residents work in supported employment at community work sites, sort mail, or do lawn care and seasonal work in horticulture. Those, who have some control over their food-seeking behaviors, work full or part time in a sheltered workshop. There is access to food in cafeterias but in most instances, successful workshops have staff who are willing to do some monitoring and network with residential personnel on a regular basis. Most of the Oakwood residents have worked in supported employment in the community on a full, part time, or temporary basis.

Access to Community Activities

Every effort is made to offer age-appropriate activities that fit the interests and abilities of residents. Because access to food and money can limit independent community participation, careful planning is necessary. Appropriate supervision is required so that community experiences are successful and rewarding. All potential activities are discussed at weekly staffings and a schedule is created. Individualized community experiences may also be developed based on a resident's special needs.

Summary

Structure and consistency in services as well as collaboration between the team are the keys to overall success. Family members, residential staff, day program, vocational personnel, and health professionals, etc. need to support all efforts to create a consistent approach to services.

A Designated 8 Bed Off-Campus Group Home

The Training School at Vineland, New Jersey is a subsidiary of Elwyn, Incorporated, a non-profit agency which contracts with the State of New Jersey, Division of Developmental Disabilities to provide services both on campus and in the community. In 1985 the Training School established a seven bed designated unit for individuals with PWS known as The Dorothy Group Home away from the main campus. Many of the policies and procedures in the home reflect fulfillment of mandates for licensing by the state.

This home is located approximately 15 miles from the main residential campus in a rural residential area and seven clients, 5 males and 2 females, current age range 30 to 51 years, live there. Four of the seven clients have been in the home since 1985, while each of three others has resided there for 4 years, 1 year, and 6 months, respectively. Vacancies in this home were created when the one non-Prader–Willi client initially placed there was moved to a home more appropriate for his needs and two clients with PWS were transferred to a Supervised Apartment project after 6 years in the home.

Prior to opening the home, these clients with PWS lived in another group home that was mismanaged and that the state wished to close. In spite of the fact that the provider agency (The Training School at Vineland) had no prior experience with persons with PWS or in operating a group home for them, it was willing to undertake this project. Considerable effort went into planning. Prior to having the clients move into the house staff were provided with background information, classroom lectures, menu planning based on the American Diabetic Plan, a 3 day course on behavior management and crisis techniques, and materials from the National Prader–Willi Syndrome Association (USA). Parents were encouraged to provide input.

The Environment

This group home is located in an area where the individuals can take walks and form friendships with neighbors and has outdoor space for a small garden or outdoor games. The interior utilizes very sturdy furniture that cannot be easily picked up or damaged. Even the lamps are hung rather than placed on tables and decorative items are inexpensive in case there is a need to locate replacements. Each client has a separate bedroom that permits privacy, lessens incidence of stealing, provides a place for keeping possessions (usually hoarded), and gives staff the opportunity to teach clients to take responsibility for their personal possessions and the area. Two or three rooms are set aside as common space. This allows for relaxation, listening to music, watching TV, conversation, participation in exercise activities, and pursuit of hobbies. All areas and appliances that contain food are off limits and staff are reminded constantly to keep areas locked.

Human Resources and Staff Development

All staff function as a team and include the direct care personnel, a behavior specialist, parents/guardians, and consulting professionals. Training is a continuous process that requires review of the most recent information about PWS, management of time, diet issues, and implementation of appropriate interpersonal and social skills. Staff turnover can present problems since persons with PWS do best where the staff remains stable and guidelines for interventions are consistent. Refresher training is conducted three to four times a year and first aid and CPR techniques are regularly reviewed. Monthly direct care staff meetings provide opportunities for ongoing discussions, suggestions, and development of new approaches to solving current problems related to either the home or a specific individual. Staff at the home are also trained in all aspects of food management and caloric intake so they are not manipulated into giving seconds or additional food to the clients. They make sure that no food is brought into the home from outside sources and that meals and snacks are not consumed while staff are supervising other activities. A solid relationship between day program staff and group home caregivers is essential in order to provide consistent management of all activities. For example, an evening meal or snack may be adjusted to accommodate any extra food procured without permission at the day program.

Programming

General guidelines, rules, and "per event" procedures are the result of collaboration between the clients and staff. Set routines are established and clients fully participate in the decision-making process. Weekly meetings include discussion of menu planning and preferences, home chore assignments, and plans for community activities. Daily meetings are held directly after clients return from work not only to discuss the day's events but also to plan the rest of the afternoon and evening.

Money belonging to the clients is placed in individual bank accounts; only a limited amount is kept at the home (and locked). Withdrawals may be made for specific purposes and must be co-signed by the client and a staff person. Checkbooks are kept secure and staff know which local sources (for eating and purchase of food) accept checks. Ongoing training helps clients learn to budget their income to buy necessary items and save for larger purchases.

Weight Control/Nutritional Considerations

As previously mentioned, when the program was first established, one of the clients did not have PWS. This made a difference in initial planning. When activities involved food, those with PWS were frustrated, envious, and generally stressed because they were "different" and could not eat whatever they desired. Of course, this also caused the client without PWS tension and he now lives elsewhere.

Caloric intake is determined on an individual basis by a nutritionist and a physician with some input from the client. Weekly weigh-ins are conducted and any caloric changes require written orders from the doctor. House staff work together with each client to prepare a balanced menu and correct serving sizes. The written menu is reviewed if questions arise. If an item is not specifically written into the diet plan, it is not made available to the client. If a client is caught taking unauthorized food, the staff must take responsibility for lack of supervision.

Weekly program plans include having clients perform cooking assignments in the kitchen. This may seem an unusual approach, given the food-related concerns associated with PWS. However, clients are provided with supervision, learn to plan menus, and measure ingredients accurately. This procedure seems to encourage self-esteem and pride in their capacity to prepare a meal for themselves and their peers.

It is expected that individual diet plans will be followed. When this does not occur, adjustments are made and the rationale pointed out to the clients. This is particularly important since clients attend day programming with a mixed population and have less supervision. Clients with PWS quickly learn that while food intake is restricted in the home, there are opportunities to obtain food from others or steal saleable items for food and/or drink during the day program. Prior to eating in a restaurant or attending any activity, every effort is made to find out what is being served. This gives clients a chance to choose their meal based on their caloric allowances. Overall, experience has led to planning menus with 50 to 100 calories less per day to adjust for manipulation or stealing of food items.

Health/Medical Issues

Finding a physician familiar with PWS is critical since upper respiratory infections and skin picking are constant problems. Several clients who smoke appear to have more frequent chest congestion. Some are capable of taking their own drugs with limited supervision from staff. They take pride in being in control of their medications, accept responsibility for making doctors appointments, and know their medications and when to take them. They even question the physician regarding either elimination or reduction of drugs. Of note is the fact that many clients enjoy seeing a doctor, tend to become somewhat hypochondriacal, and, on occasion, illnesses are faked in order to see the physician. Now and then, items have been swallowed necessitating a hospital admission. This happens because there may be a chance to consume extra food until hospital staff become aware of the ruse.

Behavioral/Emotional/Social Issues

Many plans have been established to manage emotional outbursts associated with food, changes in routines, or interpersonal conflicts. Most require frequent readjustments and staff have become accustomed to changing programming and rewards often. Aberrant behaviors can be avoided when staff recognize antecedent behaviors. However, in some instances, no "preceding event" is identified. One positive reinforcement that seems to work consistently is the individual attention from a staff person. Problems seem to occur less frequently when staff understand the importance of consistency among each another and use the same intervention strategies.

Emotional outbursts also arise from either lack of family interest, or too much family input. Clients lacking family contact tend to be jealous of peers who do and lash out. In some instances, clients play family against staff. When this happens, it usually takes considerable time and continuing communication between the caregiver and parent to build (or rebuild) a trusting relationship.

Social problems arise because persons with PWS have difficulty forming friendships with non Prader–Willi individuals. Friendships that have developed between the persons with PWS and other MR/DD individuals appear to be rather one-sided with persons with MR/DD able to take advantage of situations, always requesting "things" in order to remain a "friend." The person with PWS, wanting to be liked and accepted, often succumbs to these social pressures. Also, relationships with caregivers tend to be transient, particularly if the relationship cannot be manipulated. However, friendships with others with PWS seem to be somewhat more harmonious.

Individualized Programming

Individualized programs emerge from each client's Individualized Habilitation Plan that are reviewed on an annual basis. The client together with the team discuss progress and problem areas and devise plans that encourage more independence. These plans are carried out throughout the year, with the direct care staff assisting through verbal prompts, reminders, praise, and encouragement. It is not always possible to individualize an activity or skill in the group home, but every effort is made to do so whenever possible or on a rotating basis.

Integration into Community Services and Activities

Day services and community activities are an important part of overall programming. Participation is usually supervised by staff who provide transportation, manage ventures that involve money, and escort clients who wish to attend church. Lack of public transportation in this location requires that clients make arrangements in advance to fit with other schedules. At this point in time no close relationships exist between the clients and their neighbors. This may be due to lack of sharing information about persons with PWS to those living nearby.

Summary

It appears that individuals have more success when the home has a stable staff, the day program is appropriate, staff understand the individual needs, and there are no unknowns concerning the environment or routine. The program is most successful when clients have an opportunity to plan, organize, and implement their routines and are included in the decision-making process.

A Program in a State Facility

There are state facilites for the mentally handicapped that serve persons with PWS and, as this population base seems to be increasing, more administrators of these facilites are prepared to establish both designated and integrated residential units. In many instances, programs already in place are either an outgrowth of a previous but inappropriate placement or for clients no longer able to live at home. However, a state school placement may be more difficult for parents to accept because of the "institutional" ambiance and the stigma associated with mental retardation.

Denton State School (DSS) Denton, Texas provides campus and community-based services to persons of all ages with developmental disabilities. This facility is located on 200 acres 30 miles north of the Dallas/Fort Worth Metroplex in Denton, Texas. The campus consists of residential units, work areas, recreation sites, a pond, swimming pool, parks, and a snack bar. The campus is served by the local trolley-shuttle system and is 1 mile south of a major shopping district. Denton is also home to the University of North Texas and Texas Woman's University.

DSS seeks to identify and serve all individuals with developmental disabilities in its catchment area who are in need of residential services and habilitation. Priority for admission to the campus-based services is given to those individuals with the most severely disabling conditions and/or needs, which, of course, includes persons with Prader–Willi syndrome (PWS). Programming for all individuals is determined by an interdisciplinary team (IDT).

DSS receives funding from the state of Texas, which in turn receives Title XIX monies as an Intermediate Care Facility for the Mentally Retarded (ICF/MR). It is also accredited by the Accreditation Council on Services for Persons with Disabilities. While this secondary accreditation does not provide any direct source of additional funds it does acknowledge the quality of services provided. Providing services to clients with PWS presents a major challenge that is being met through the creation of an integrated eight bed apartment unit located on the campus. This home houses two men with PWS and six other mentally retarded males with nutritional problems such as uncontrolled diabetes.

Initially, DSS experienced extreme difficulties meeting the needs of the clients with PWS on campus. Their living and programming arrangements needed considerable attention and improvement. A decision was made to adapt a remodeled residential apartment to address the specific needs of these individuals and integrate them with a group of non-PWS persons, all of whom either had uncontrolled diabetes or demonstrated some type of nutritional problem that required constant supervision. All of the individuals had previously lived in other residential units on campus.

The Environment

A large one-story campus building was extensively remodeled into four 2,700 square foot apartments. Each apartment contains a living, dining, and laundry room, kitchen, four bedrooms, and office space for the unit manager, a Qualified Mental Retardation Professional (QMRP). All the apartments, under one roof, share a patio, garden area, and a common lobby. The bedrooms have very large closets and are designed for semiprivate living. Each apartment has separate locks and a private front door connecting the shared lobby with the living rooms of each unit.

To create a safe, structured, monitored environment for this special group of clients, the keys to this apartment and to the kitchen area are secured by staff. The dining room is large enough to seat all residents and staff at mealtimes and is also used for leisure activities. It is adjacent to the living room as well as to the locked kitchen. While the phone is located inside the kitchen area, a portable one is available for convenience and privacy. The thermostat is protected by being hidden in a vent and the back door is equipped with an alarm that can be turned on as needed. The bedrooms can be locked with keys maintained by those occupying them; an extra one is maintained for staff use. One bedroom has been modified to provide for individual closets while all other closets are shared. Two bathrooms were modified to include a more sturdy shower/ tub combination.

The decor includes sturdy, attractive furniture, plants, pictures, an entertainment center with a television, VCR, and stereo. The dining area includes two separate tables and chairs. Placemats and centerpieces are used. Each bedroom is decorated by the men who live there and their families. While the common lobby includes furnishings and pictures, no additional flammable items have been added, since one client has been known to set fires.

The environment also reflects specific restrictions/guidelines for the residents. These individual guidelines are determined by the IDT with approval of a Human Rights Committee (HRC). A built-in provision in all individual programming requires that any client may have any restriction removed when the client indicates the on-going capacity to act responsibly. However, to date guidelines such as limits on purchases made at the snack bar and access to earnings remain in place for individuals with PWS and food storage areas are totally off limits to unsupervised access. Guidelines are in place regarding search and seizure (for both food and nonfood stealing), methods for personal restraint, and use of psychotropic medications to manage behaviors as needed.

Issues associated with human rights can be problematic. The key to successful address of rights issues at DSS is education of direct contact staff serving persons with PWS, their families, and the members of the human rights committee who oversee delivery of services. Direct communication with these providers about the syndrome, its associated risks, and the need to consider the safety of these clients has proven helpful. Documentation about these "rights" issues from an outside expert in PWSA has served to clear away many misconceptions.

Human Resources and Staff Development

It is very important for staff to receive educational information about all aspects of PWS including health, nutritional, and behavioral management issues. Staff/providers must understand that PWS is a very complex, multifaceted condition that requires very specific program design. Even personnel who have previously worked with non-PWS clients with developmental disabilities require training. Staff need to cultivate a sense of humor and the ability to compromise and to be patient, characteristics that are rarely observed in persons with PWS. A consultant with expertise in PWS can be an excellent resource for on-going training.

As previously indentified, this particular residence on the campus of the DSS is one of four units in the same building. The unit being described is supervised by a QMRP, who in turn oversees a residence supervisor on each work shift. This person has an assistant and several primary-contact staff (or trainers) under his or her direction. There is a minimum of four staff on duty between two of the four apartments from 6 AM to 10 PM and an awake staff on duty in each unit at night. Most of these staff are concentrated in the apartment with persons with PWS so that frequently there are three staff on duty in that apartment. The unit is also provided with a psychologist, behavioral therapist, social worker, nurses, and clerical and additional administrative services on an as needed basis. In addition to dietary guidance, other supports include medical and psychiatric services, occupational, recreational, and chaplaincy services.

Recognizing the role of food in the lives of person with PWS is essential. At DSS, a central campus service plans and prepares all food every day of the week and delivers all meals to the unit. This precludes the need to do any meal preparation in the kitchen of the apartment. Only snacks such as popcorn and diet sodas are usually kept at the unit. It should be noted that while most of the clients with PWS do possess the skills to learn more about food preparation, food seeking behaviors and the potential for uncontrollable consumption are deterrents to including this activity in program planning.

Programming

Program activities (both work and social) are a challenge. The general rule of thumb is "three meals a day plus appropriate snacks and keep them busy." How well an integrated residence functions depends on how individual case plans are developed and followed and the ability of the staff to collaborate with one another.

Each person with PWS has program goals related to "living" and "leisure/relationships." The goals and objectives focus on personal hygiene and domestic skills (chores in the unit, keeping bedrooms clean, and doing laundry). All clients are encouraged to cultivate hobbies and activities that do not involve food. For example, one individual possesses considerable artistic ability, which is used as a frequent activity. Board games stimulate improvement of social skills. Exercise is encouraged through walking and, where possible, biking. It is the responsibility of staff to provide choices among a variety of structured non-food-related activities, particularly during evenings and weekends.

Management of maladaptive behaviors is based on understanding the developmental levels of the clients, application of strategies that reflect external management, and prevention rather than modification of behaviors. Controlling the behavioral idiosyncrasies of these clients requires considerable creativity and imagination by the IDT. While potentially maladaptive behaviors are discussed elsewhere in this text, one particular characteristic of this population that seems to have the most severe impact is their capacity to manipulate staff, other residents, and family members. For example, a client who has lost close to 30 pounds and has been more productive at work continues to have incidents of maladaptive behaviors. This client, aware of deteriorating relationships among the members of his family, has been more successful in manipulating and preserving the adversarial status between staff and family and programming continues to be a challenge. However, due to the successful collaboration between the IDT and the family members, another client has lost 92 pounds since moving to this unit and incidents of aggression and destruction of property have diminished. This particular individualized program is fully described in Appendix E.1.

The telephone is an example of a tool that can be used to manipulate family and staff alike and all program plans include specific guidelines for use of the phone on the unit. When a family member receives multiple calls from a client complaining of staff wrongdoing, it is difficult for the family to question the veracity of the situation. Family and staff need to collaborate in order to discourage misinterpretations of verbal interactions between the client and family. Staff must acknowledge that when a family member makes inquiries based on a complaint made by phone, this exchange of information is not an attack on staff. Instead, the conversation represents a need to clarify facts and for family members to ensure themselves that their son is all right, albeit angry at some necessary restrictions that have been put in place. Staff *also* needs to be supported when they are unfairly attacked. All too often persons with PWS realize that they can effectively pit family against staff.

On a more specific note, questions may arise as to how well the persons with PWS get along with their non-PWS peers in this setting. The answer to that inquiry is "quite well." Most persons with PWS are only mildly retarded and like being the "boss." This residential unit where non-PWS peers are lower functing gives the residents with PWS many opportunities to be in control. However, staff must be ever vigilant so that residents with less cognitive ability are not manipulated.

Work Opportunities

Another campus department is responsible for job placement and administering the sheltered workshop programming. However, direct-contact staff usually accompany some of the clients to their work settings. Programming for the clients with PWS consists of all day work in either a sheltered workshop or supported employment/job placement. In the past, problems tended to arise when the person with PWS chose not to work on a regular basis. Eliminating their ability to seek food when not going to work and increasing activity requirements in the residential unit during work hours have changed these patterns. While there continues to be occasional outbursts and obstinacy, these clients do well at work and are justifiably proud of their successes most of the time.

Sample Daily Schedule

6:00 AM	Wake up, get dressed and personal hygiene
7:15 AM	Breakfast
8:00 AM	Catch bus to work
8:30 AM	Work
10:00 AM	Diet soda break
10:15 AM	Work
12:00 PM	Lunch
1:00 PM	Work
3:00 PM	Diet soda break
4:30 PM	Catch bus home
5:15 PM	Supper
6:00 PM	Chores
7:00 PM	Recreational activities
9:00 PM	Shower, grooming
10:00 PM	To bed (may stay up later)

Pros and Cons of This On-Campus Integrated Program

It was necessary to create this integrated residential unit to serve the individuals with PWS living at DSS because there were too few clients to warrant establishment of a homogeneous apartment. Two persons with the syndrome have lived at DSS for over 20 years. Until this special unit was established, they lived in less supervised housing where, due to lack of information about PWS, inconsistent supervision and programming resulted in morbid obesity. It is fortunate that the administrators of DSS recognized that a carefully structured program could "mix" clients with PWS with non-PWS, overweight, cognitively impaired diabetic individuals and offer a less institutionalized, more homelike environment in a supervised apartment unit.

The major problem associated with establishment of this unit is the fact that staff need considerably more on-going education and training. Food and food-related activities will always be a higher source of concern in this setting. In retrospect, it might have been just as easy to design a whole new treatment plan when the residential change was made rather than attempting to adapt the initial program to the new setting since any change in structure is going to result in some behavioral reaction.

Summary

Any program, integrated or not, must be individually designed. An integrated system can be effective where the special needs of this unusual disability are understood and addressed. DSS administration recognized the need to provide such specialized services for clients with PWS. To this end, an on campus apartment unit was established that also integrated six residents without PWS who also require dietary management. This program seems to work because the unit population is quite small and closely supervised. The fact that all of the residents require dietary controls tends to eliminate a major problem associated with PWS and close supervision by direct contact providers, in most instances, tends to reduce the potential for behavioral disturbances. This approach to providing services is a valid strategy where the population is too small to warrant establishment of a PWS-specific residential unit. The program at DSS has resulted in positive changes in the health and well-being of residents living there.

An Integrated Residential Program

While parents/guardians recognize that the family member with PWS should live away from the family home, many cannot accept the fact that the few designated programs not only may not have space, but are located too far away. In some cases their predicament has been resolved by locating a placement in an integrated residential program that is nearby. Granted, a mixed client population (Prader–Willi and non-Prader–Willi) presents challenges and dilemmas such as the need to protect the rights of non-PWS clients, difficulties with erratic behavior, and food restrictions in the home or apartment. However, with careful planning, on-going staff training, and much effort, integrated programs can be effective.

The Humboldt Workshop, Inc., is a private, nonprofit agency located in a small community of 5,000 persons in Iowa. This agency, a Residential Care Facility for The Mentally Retarded (RCF/MR) facility, provides habilitation, rehabilitation, and related services for adults who are not able to live independently because of a physical or mental handicap or other developmental disabilities. It maintains residential groups homes scattered throughout the town. These homes are one component of services that also provide sheltered workshop programs and opportunities for community participation for its clients. The goal of the program is to assist residents to achieve or maintain optimum self care and self reliance. For some residents, this integrated group home serves as a transitional setting prior to advancing to a supervised apartment or independent living. The residential unit, one of the "homes," is The Humboldt Group Home (HGH), an integrated residence for two persons with PWS and 12 non-PWS residents. A third client with PWS is with the residents at the workshop program during the day but continues to live with his family.

The Environment

HGH is located in a residential area convenient to grocery stores, restaurants, churches, library, swimming pool, theater, and several schools, and is within walking distance of the downtown area. The physical unit is a brick building on a large lot that allows for plenty of space for gardening and outdoor games. The home, licensed for 15 residents, has a central kitchen (locked when staff are not present), a large dining room, and large living room. There are three double bedrooms and two single rooms on each side of the building each with three bathrooms and a laundry room.

Human Resources and Staff Development

In addition to established policies of the agency for staff employment, the direct care personnel who work with PWS require considerable background information about the syndrome. Particular attention is paid to the need for consistency, structure, and constant supervision. Care providers need to be mature, resilient, have a sense of humor, be sensitive (but not thin skinned), and able to establish realistic expectations based on experience and common sense. The Humboldt Workshop, Inc. provides on-going training through in-services.

Programming

Program plans for persons with PWS are developed in the same way as for other residents. Each has an individualized program plan (IPP) based on need. HGH advocates integration of all residents. Once admitted, the first 30 days are spent observing and evaluating the resident, after which staff create an IPP. Program coordination and scheduling are designed to ensure that each resident receive integrated services that meet established goals and objectives. The plan is reviewed every 6 months. Behavior strategies are especially important because all the residents are involved in vocational day programs where management of behaviors is essential and staff need consistent guidelines.

   The IPPs for the residents with PWS include basic living skills training with planned instruction in personal health care, exercise, and improving interpersonal skills. This training varies with each person and encourages learning to manage laundry, housekeeping, management of time, shopping, use of public services, and, where possible, menu planning and food preparation with supervision. Leisure time and recreation training include planning, guidance, and participation in hobbies, games, gardening, sports, and community events. Where special services are required to deal with physical or mental health problems, individuals are provided medical and psychological assistance.

Behavioral Interventions

Behavioral strategies are based on use of a token economy and positive reinforcement. This management approach acknowledges that external controls are essential. Where necessary, professional consultants work with staff in care conferences to design individualized strategies. Guidance for programming consists of coaching, advising, modeling, encouraging, and informal instruction by direct care staff to reinforce or change behaviors/performance.

This program serves three persons with PWS. Two live at the group home and attend the day program from 9:00 AM to 3:00 PM. The third person lives with his parents and attends the day program. While the residential providers have no control over the individual who does not reside in the group home, the other two residents receive calorie-controlled diets and their weight is monitored. One has been very successful because it seems relatively easy for her to understand the parameters. The other resident, with less cognitive ability, has more difficulty loosing weight. Even though the kitchen is locked, there are numerous opportunities for foraging and stealing food. A variety of exercises are planned but few are enjoyed. However, all residents walk five blocks to and from work.

Summary

This program is able to serve two persons with PWS while preserving the agency's philosophical integrity of integrating a variety of individuals with developmental disabilities into a common program. The key to success lies in the willingness of agency administrators to offer staff on-going teaching, support, and professional resources as needed.

A Small Nonprofit Multiservice Agency Offering Both Integrated and Nonintegrated Services

Laura Baker School Association (LBSA) is a nonprofit multi service agency in Northfield, Minnesota, a small college community of 15,000 located 35 minutes south of the Minneapolis, St. Paul metropolitan area. It opened in 1897 and currently serves over 100 persons from eight states, who have developmental disabilities and other related conditions and are over four years of age. The mission of LBSA is to serve and enhance the lives of functionally disabled individuals by reducing the social and environmental barriers and by offering them choices and opportunities for increased independence. Although LBSA does have some private pay residents, placement of most clients is through states and counties and local or state human service moneys underwrite the costs. LBSA does not receive medicaid funds for residents who live on campus.

Laura Baker School (LBS) currently serves 42 individuals on a campus in a residential section of Northfield. The remainder of its clients receive supervision and services in a variety of living arrangements off campus in the community. Education is provided for school age residents on campus. In addition to academics, the school offers speech, music, occupational, and physical therapy. Programming for *all* residents is tailored to meet individual needs and focuses on the development of semi-independent living skills, vocational training, and community integration.

The campus consists of five separate buildings, three of which house the residents; a fourth is a dining, kitchen, and educational complex. The fifth building contains administrative and health services, together with a library and activity rooms. All of the residential buildings are coeducational; two are one-story, 16-bed units that are wheel chair accessible and contain living rooms, kitchens, and laundry areas. The third, a two-story building, contains a 15-bed unit on the first floor and a 14-bed unit on the second floor. Both of these units contain living and laundry facilities, but the second floor unit also has a kitchen.

LBSA began offering services to individuals with Prader–Willi syndrome (PWS) in 1985, when one person with the syndrome came to live on campus. Currently 13 adults and children are being served, the youngest of whom is 14 years old. Eight residents with PWS live in integrated units with persons who have a variety of developmental disabilities. The other five live in a unit on the second floor of the two-story building that was opened early in 1994 specifically for persons with PWS. This unit was created because LBSA administrators became aware that other agencies across the country were being encouraged to develop homogeneous small group homes as the "ideal" setting. The decision was made to create such a unit on campus to determine if persons with PWS were managed more effectively when living in this type of homogeneous setting. The most recent independent evaluation indicates that residents with PWS function well in both the integrated and designated units due to the consistency of management by staff in both settings.

The Environment

The campus of LBS is in a lovely, tree-shaded section of Northfield conducive to walking and hiking. The living units have a homelike atmosphere and are tastefully decorated with sturdy furniture. Residents are encouraged to personalize their bedrooms and living room. In the designated unit, residents have the ability to lock their bedroom door with a key lock. This has proven effective in minimizing stealing. Staff, of course, have a master key for each bedroom.

Human Resources and Staff Development

All staff receive approximately 65 hours of orientation when they are initially employed. This orientation includes education and instruction about LBS's philosophy of care, the needs of individual residents, and the unique characteristics of PWS. Additional training is offered throughout the year in a variety of areas such as CPR, first aid, physical interventions, epilepsy, dietary management, administration of medications, and crisis prevention and intervention (CPI).

Staff meet on a regular basis to share techniques for successful interventions and discuss any issues that arise. Each living unit has a communication book where all unit correspondence is placed. This allows for on-going networking among staff and keeps information about each resident current. Each unit has a resource manual about PWS. It includes material on a variety of topics associated with the syndrome such general characteristics, diet, medical concerns, behavior, and recent research. Staff also have access to *The Gathered View*, the newsletter of the Prader–Willi Syndrome Association (USA). Each year some staff attend this national organization's national conference and share information at in-service training sessions.

Programming

General programming is designed to provide an environment where the health and behaviors of *individuals* with PWS are carefully managed and monitored. Teams consisting of the clients, the parents/guardians, a social worker, direct care, health administrative staff, a behavior analyst, day program personnel, and other professionals collaborate to create individualized program plans (IPP). These IPPs assess and address each client's needs, identify realistic goals, and develop strategies to maximize the capacity for adaptation.

Weight Reduction/Maintenance

Each client has a physical examination by a physician where an ideal weight is determined along with the caloric guidelines required to reach or maintain it. The food service supervisor, a trained dietician, is responsible for ensuring that the proper caloric intake for clients is reflected in their daily diets. A weekly menu is posted that allows some choices. The dietary supervisor must approve any variation in the type or amount of food and is consulted when activities involves food. When off-campus activities include trips to a restaurant or a place where snacks will be served, adjustments are made in meals served on campus. Also, all decisions about foods to be allowed when off campus are determined ahead of time. Each resident is weighed weekly and medical consultation is sought regarding weight loss or gain as needed.

All residents eat the majority of their meals in the central dining room. The kitchen area is kept locked and inaccessible to all residents when staff are not present. Throughout the campus, all cabinets containing food and all refrigerators are locked. Staff are taught to discard food scraps directly into a main garbage area that can be observed rather than disposing them in the trash cans located around the campus.

Some residents with PWS are working to develop and improve their cooking skills. All seem to enjoy this task and seem to be most successful performing them only when the amount of food required for preparation of their individual meal is provided.

Health/Medical Issues

The health staff at LBS work closely with physicians in Northfield and Minneapolis St. Paul. The agency also has access to The Mayo Clinic in Rochester, Minnesota, The University of Minnesota Clinic and Hospital, and other health care facilities that offer any specific medical services that the residents may require.

Behavioral Management

Two behavioral analysts are on staff. Their role is to work with the team to create individual behavioral strategies. These include teaching alternative communication skills and techniques to address inappropriate behaviors and implementing positive reinforcement tools. Staff have found that their CPI training in verbal deescalation techniques has been very helpful. A consulting psychologist is available to any clients who need counseling.

Several proactive strategies have been effective. For example, concrete house rules are carefully defined and discussed with residents until there is identification that these guidelines are clearly understood. Any mistake caused by staff is acknowledged, explained to the resident(s) and an apology is made for the error. It has been noted that this process seems to enhance feelings of trust between residents and staff. Staff are encouraged to use very consistent responses based on established program protocols for any given situation. This is particularly important when outbursts occur.

Integration Into Community Services and Activities

LBS staff encourage residents to become involved in off-campus community activities. Day program options include EPIC, a vocational program for adults, and a supported employment program. Use of public transportation, local banks, the post office is possible for those residents who are working on improving their life skills. Shopping trips are possible and staff support is provided as needed.

Northfield offers a variety of opportunities for cultural and sporting events. It has a bowling alley and a multiscreen movie complex. Special Olympics is another option. The community's Educational and Recreation Department has a excellent program for individuals with special needs that offer arts and crafts clases and many specialneeds that offer arts and crafts classes and many special events. Residents at LBS can select activities in which they choose to participate and can register through the Community Education Program. Staff provide assistance for those residents who wish to attend church and religious workshops.

Summary

Laura Baker School offers an integrated and a designated program for individuals with PWS. Both settings have been effective in meeting the individual needs of these residents. By providing an environment where weight and food intake is monitored, exercise encouraged, and staff interactions are consistent and team strategies for interventions are followed, success for individuals with PWS is not only possible, it is the norm.

Supported Living Programs (SLAS)

Another alternative to the previous options is that of a Supported Living Arrangements (SLA) model, a broad category of highly flexible, individualized services designed to provide the necessary assistance so that persons with developmental disabilities can live as independently as possible. SLA is an option that exists somewhere between traditional group homes and independent living. It is *not* a fixed model. The key to the success of this option creation is of individualized environmental and technical supports that promote as much independence as possible. The intensity and extent of support depends on the individual needs and abilities. One arrangement is to have an individual live alone. Another is to share a home with a peer roommate or a nondisabled roommate, paid or unpaid, who may or may not provide support. For persons with PWS this concept may more aptly be described as semindependent living. The key point is that what is effective for one person with PWS may not be best for another. Two variations of SLA models are described.

The first variation is a supervised apartment program created in 1991 by Elevyn, Incorp, the same agency that also administers the previously described seven bed PWS designated home in a residential neighborhood off campus.

This SLA option is located in a complex with approximately 50 apartments where The Training School at Vineland (TSU) rents five units, two of which are designated for four clients with PWS, two males and two females, age range 24 to 35 years.

The apartment complex is near public transportation that can be used to expand the potential for participating in community activities. Each unit contains a telephone system that allows residents to contact staff with problems or for help. Residents also have keys to their own apartments and medication box. However, it should be pointed out that the basic factors that set persons with PWS apart from other MR/DD populations that live in an SLA are food related. Even in the apartments, access to food and appliances that contain food is restricted.

Two of the individuals who lived in the seven bed designated home expressed a desire to move to an apartment with fewer restrictions. A team decision led to offering these two clients such an opportunity. After approximately 6 months, two other persons with PWS were included, one who had lived at home with his family and one who had came from a private facility but was unsuccessful living with mixed clientele.

The resident who lived at home prior to coming to the SLA is more aware of community options, is able to use the telephone, has a checking account, and is involved in local activities. However, the resident who moved into the SLA from an integrated program continues to have difficulty adjusting to routines and expectations. Her family has been manipulated and induced to meet all her needs so that, at this point, she has little incentive to attend day programming, participate in community activities, or socialize with peers.

Many of the routines established in TSU's Dorothy Group Home continue in the apartment setting, but there is less emphasis on strict structure. As the clients have become more familiar with their new setting, they are able to make choices and plan their daily and weekly routines. Depending on individual capabilities, they can remain unsupervised for periods of 2 to 6 hrs and this time can be expanded with compliance. Staff are encouraged to allow individuals to perform as many tasks as possible with the least amount of supervision.

Control of weight is regulated in the same manner as in the group home, except that residents in the SLAs are responsible for planning and shopping on a weekly basis with supervision. A charge account system has been established with the local supermarket where food is purchased. A future goal is to have residents shop for food without supervision.

Three of the four individuals currently in this SLA program medicate themselves with limited direction from staff. They seem to enjoy being in control and accept responsibility for making doctors appointments and can express their medical concerns to their physician. They have discussed reduction and/or elimination of their medications and even requested prescription for a nicotine patch in order to quit smoking.

Behavioral/emotional/social issues to be considered in a SLA are similar to those identified in the group home setting. Unfortunately, the process of forming friendships with individuals who do not have Prader–Willi syndrome that was discussed in the programming at the off-campus designated group home has not substantially improved in this setting.

Summary

Living in these apartments seems to encourage more independence and control in the daily life and routines. Initial integration into the community for services and activities was initiated by staff. However, the four individuals in this program recently have become more assertive in arranging their own appointments and transportation and choosing their activities.

The second SLA option describes an independent undertaking by parents on behalf of their son who had lived out-of-home for over 20 years, first in a large residential facility, then in a PWS designated home. At age 32, because he wished to leave the group home, his parents decided to offer him the opportunity to have more independent, integrated, and productive experiences. They acquired a house with the long range goal of including additional housemates. He currently lives in this home by himself, renting it from his parents. His sources of income are Social Security Assistance as a dependent and Supplemental Security Income. His parents are his conservators.

With the help of several local agencies who assist persons with developmental disabilities living in the community, this individual has been provided a comfortable, safe supervised living environment where his food intake can be controlled and monitored. It is a three bedroom, four bath ranch house with ample living and dining space. The size of the house was based on future plans to have more housemates. A fully equipped kitchen is large enough for more than one person to prepare meals at the same time. Adjacent to the kitchen is a large locked pantry with a second refrigerator and an accessible laundry area. Since the need for privacy and a sense of security for personal belongings are identified in persons with PWS, each bedroom has its own bathroom, ample storage, and sitting space for watching individually owned TVs when desired. The fourth bathroom is available for use by visitors.

An interdisciplinary team (IDT) of providers is involved in planning and coordinating all support services. His parents continue to make sure that the team receives on-going education about PWS and about their son's abilities and needs. Paid support services include a resource counselor who spends three afternoons a week with him. During these times weekly shopping is done (including groceries), he participates in recreational activities, and practices self-help skills and other daily living tasks such as personal care and household and money management. There is on-going training to acquire, retain, and improve community adaptation by attendance at adult education classes in life skills such as eventually learning to take public transportation. Participation in social and recreational activities is encouraged. In addition to sleeping alone in his home and managing his early day activities, he goes to work until one o'clock each weekday afternoon, exercises, watches TV, and has a social relationship with a girlfriend. Twenty-four hour emergency services are also available as needed.

A standard, low-calorie, low-fat weekly menu has been developed by a dietitian. This young man gets himself up each morning, prepares his own breakfast, and makes his lunch. Using a preprinted list of approved foods and quantities, he shops for groceries once a week. Initially he was supervised in the store by a staff person from the support agency, but currently shops alone once he reaches the store. The person accompanying him to the store makes a quick check of the grocery bags as they are placed in the trunk of the car. Once home, the receipts are checked off to see if any unauthorized purchases have been made. All foods for the 7-day period are placed in the unlocked refrigerator in the kitchen. Using the weekly menus, he has learned to prepare his own meals without supervision and to use a rice cooker and crock pot. Foods are chosen from what is made available to him, but the same basic menu plan is followed. Many low-calorie, low-fat foods are sold in mini packages, just right for single meal servings. Other foods purchased in larger quantities are placed in smaller, individualized serving size packages or containers. Low-calorie or specially prepared frozen dinners are used for evening meals. In addition to managing weight by diet, exercise activities such as swimming and use of an exercise bicycle are encouraged and monitored each day. Walking with family, friends, and provider staff is built into daily activities including the task of walking a neighbor's dog. Weight is checked and recorded weekly.

With supervision, this individual volunteers at a local convalescent hospital, which offers the opportunity to learn job skills and work habits that may lead to paid employment. Transportation to and from this work program is furnished by a special transit service and is paid for by a voucher system as a regional center service.

Summary

This SLA option allows for much flexibility depending on parental decisions. At the present time, they are considering seeking the services of a paid roommate, which will be funded by a regional center and provided by the local agency that oversees supported living programming.

Summary

As the life span of individuals with PWS lengthens, long-term residential services become a paramount concern. Affected individuals should be evaluated as developmentally disabled using appropriate criteria. IQ scores do not indicate the degree to which individuals with PWS are functionally retarded and with few exceptions are unable to live completely independently. Since 1980, considerable strides have been made in creation of a variety of successful out-of-home residential services.

References

Goldenson, R.M. (Ed.). (1978). *Disability and rehabilitation handbook* (pp. 618–619). New York: McGraw-Hill.

Grossman, H.J. (1973). *Manual of terminology and classification in mental retardation*. American Association on Mental Deficiency, Special Publication Series N.2, 11.

Mental Health Law Project (1991). SSI-New Opportunities for Children with Disabilities: Washington, DC.

Pieper, B. (1985) Residential issues for people with disabilties. Chicago: Spina Bifida Association of America.

Singer, S. (1994). *Oakwood Residence, Inc. Summary of residential program for people with Prader-Willi syndrome*. Unpublished manuscript.

Thompson, D., Greenswag, L., & Eleazer, R. (1988). Residential programs for individuals with Prader-Willi syndrome. In L.R. Greenswag & R.C. Alexander (Eds.), *Management of Prader-Willi syndrome* (pp. 214–222). New York: Springer-Verlag.

U.S. Department of Health and Human Services. (1983). *Cumulated Index Medicus*. 24 p 12,878. Bethesda, MD: National Library of Medicine.

16
Vocational Concepts in Prader–Willi Syndrome[1]

ANNA MARIE SAPORITO

Individuals with Prader–Willi syndrome (PWS) whose lives now extend into adulthood require preparation for entrance into the world of work. Once formal education is complete, vocational counseling, evaluation of abilities, vocational education/training, and integration into the vocational service system should begin. This chapter describes legislation that mandates delivery of vocational services to all individuals with developmental disabilities including those services that directly affect persons with PWS. A framework implemented by vocational specialists can identify rehabilitation processes that may maximize the extent to which affected persons can benefit from vocational experiences.

Rehabilitation means implementing realistic methods of coping while understanding that the presence of one or more problems in the same person usually compounds the task of adjustment. If rehabilitation is to be realistic, the concept "cannot be separated from the environmental factors associated with the needs of these adults past, present, or future" (Andrew, 1981, p. 225). The rehabilitation process focuses on the disabled population in general and, for purposes of this discussion, persons with PWS. It is designed to assist in adaptation to life while taking into consideration the physical and psychosocial limitations associated with this syndrome.

If rehabilitation broadly addresses the effect of a disability on the total person, vocational rehabilitation speaks specifically to "the relationship between the world of work and individuals with physical or mental handicaps" (Daniels, 1981, p. 169). The goals of vocational rehabilitation include counseling, evaluating, assisting in planning services, coordinating

---

[1] *Editor's note*: The information in this chapter is an adaptation by the contributor from the contents in the first edition by permission of the Prader-Willi Syndrome Association (USA).

resources, acting as a liaison between persons with disabilities and their communities, and working closely with their families.

Historically, The Vocational Rehabilitation Act of 1943 (PL 78-113) recognized that mentally disabled persons were entitled to funds and services. The next 10 years saw the expansion of humanistic, sociocultural aspect of care. By 1966, the act had been amended (PL 89-333) to enlarge the target populations and at the same time eliminated economic need as a criterion for receiving federal monies. Two terms used in the legislation are particularly important: eligibility and feasibility. *Eligibility* for services requires that (1) the presence of a physical or mental disability that can be documented by a physician, (2) the disability must represent a substantial handicap to employment, and (3) there must be reasonable expectation that services will render the client employable. *Feasibility* refers to the fact that employment should be available in the area for which the person has been vocatioally prepared (R. Roberts, lecture and class discussion, 1982) and that the individual is able and willing to cooperate with an established program. The Rehabilitation Act of 1973 (PL 93-112) mandated the use of individualized written rehabilitation plans (IWRPs) to set realistic, contractual goals and encourage the accountability of service providers.

Unfortunately, there is still a discrepancy between what has been legislated and the conscientious delivery of services within individual states and local communities. Enactment of laws is not an end in itself. Too often individuals and their families are entitled to care but remain uninformed and underserved.

Vocational rehabilitation services vary and depend on the degree to which an individual can function independently. A hierarchy of program options based on this potential for independence includes work activity (prevocational programming), sheltered work (high-extended and low-extended), enclaves, transitional employment, and competitive employment (encompassing supportd work).

Vocational Services for Persons with PWS

The physical, cognitive, and psychological features of PWS discussed in Chapters 1, 5, 9, and 11 clearly indicate the neurobehavioral complexities of the syndrome, including the presence of at least mild mental retardation. It is under the rubric of delivery of vocational services to the mentally retarded population that individuals with PWS benefit from the aforementioned legislation.

As a disability, PWS fits well within the eligibility/feasibility guidelines mandated by law. However, providing appropriate services to individuals with this syndrome is a challenge because the physical, cognitive and behavior problems affect their capacity to function and adapt. Few programs take into account the unique aspects of the syndrome. Affected individuals often are funneled into existing services despite hard evidence that such programs often are simply not suitable.

In vocational settings, adjustment and adaptation are measured by productivity, compliance, and the ability to function in a competitive work environment and most mildly mentally retarded persons are clearly capable of consistent performance at very high levels in typical workshops. It is, however, unrealistic to expect that these same criteria for success will work for individuals with PWS because of their uncontrollable craving for food, as well as these cognitive limitations and emotional lability. Although the majority of persons with PWS function in this mild meutally retarded category, they tend to remain only sporadically capable and productive.

Questions arise: What vocational services are available? How successful are these programs and what can enhance existing services and ensure the effectiveness of new ones?

Finding answers is not easy because PWS is a relatively low-incidence condition. Many vocational providers will never see a case during their entire professional career. The Prader–Willi Syndrome Association (USA) (PWSA, USA) estimates that approximately 81% of adults with Prader–Willi syndrome (PWS) over the age of 18 are currently being served. A survey of 173 families of persons with PWS reported in the association's newsletter, *The Gathered View* (September/October 1991), indicated that 68% worked in sheltered workshops, 9% participated in some form of community work such as supported employment, 16% were in day activity programs, and 4.5% received occupational training. Activities of the remaining 2.5% were unspecified. Only 24% of the placements were viewed as appropriate by the respondents. Few programs exist for individuals who still live at home, and in most instances these services have been instituted only when parents have exerted considerable pressure on a local agency (M. Wett, personal communication, July 1985).

Enhancing existing programs and ensuring the effectiveness of future ones require sensitive counseling, vocational assessment, education of staff, and provision of challenging work *without* the pressure of strict demands for productivity in settings where availability of food is restricted. Vocational services should focus on the natural talents and learned abilities of persons with PWS. These may include very good fine motor skills, vocal aptitudes, the ability to relate to young children, a somewhat sedentary nature, the desire to relate to non-PWS persons, a desire for some measure of control, a need for structure, and perseverance on task.

The Goodwill Industries of Southeastern Pennsylvania Prader–Willi Residential Day Program Project is an existing program that provides progressive and structured vocational services to persons with PWS (Swallwell, 1992). It is designed for collaboration between the vocational services staff and the staff of the group home where these clients live. Its goal is to make accommodations that ensure that clients receive appropriate individualized training, supervision, and monitoring. Programming that was originally designed for persons who have special social, emotional, and vocational needs has been tailored to the specific and varied needs of the population with PWS. To this end, the group home direct care staff accompany the residents to the workshop and participate in supervising their activities. This method relieves workshop staff of *total* responsibility for overseeing these individuals, provides consistency between residential and vocational services, and allows vocational staff to observe how best to provide behavioral management.

The PWS Day Program Project consists of six progressive components that may maximize client choice, reinforce appropriate behaviors, and provide predictable scheduling that may reduce the frequency of outbursts. Initially, a Vocational Conditioning Center (VCC) provides a workshop area for clients who need much supervision. This first VCC step deals with short-term issues. Success is measured by the length of time between outbursts and their intensity. Then, as the need for intense supervision decreases, clients proceed through other components of work programming, the first of which is a specifically designed "enclave." This is a section of the workshop floor devoted to a specific job, where groups of clients work side by side with supervision. This component is a step up for clients with PWS. In the third component, a advancement integration from the enclave level, clients with PWS function alongside others on a variety of jobs, also with supervision. The Work II component follows and allows even more integration into the broader workshop environment with access to an extensive assortment of jobs. The next phase is participation in mobile work crews (MWC), where short-term offsite work experiences are provided and clients are accompanied by staff. This "supported employment" emphasizes development of work behaviors and skills at an actual job outside the main workshop facility and utilizes job coaching. The degree of involvement is individualized to the needs of each client. This setting offers long-term training for competitive employment. The final level is placement through job acquisition and maintenance.

The progression though this hierarchy of programming depends on the ability of clients to adapt and maintain consistency at each level. Realistically, a client may function best at one level and technically not be capable of progressing beyond that point. Careful evaluation and support is necessary in order to provide an appropriate and challenging work. Success is measured by the extent of participation in the program, and for those clients in more advanced phases, maintenance of productive employment in the community.

Although this program can be effective, vocational staff may become frustrated when behaviors become unmanageable and agency alternatives are limited to in-or out-of-house suspension, leaves of absence, or termination; all such choices have a negative impact on both vocational and residential staff and on involved family members. The importance of cooperation and collaboration among professional providers and families cannot be underestimated.

Vocational Counseling

Thoughtful intervention by a vocational counselor is essential to successful programming, because persons with PWS and their families continually struggle to accept the presence of the syndrome and its effect on goal planning and attainment. Furthermore, clients with PWS often have been sheltered by their families and their unique cognitive and behavioral characteristics strongly influence the effectiveness of the counseling process. Therefore vocational counseling should offer interventions as situations and issues arise. Because reflection and inferential thinking are not strong attributes in this population strategies and techniques that focus on behavioral management should be utilized (see Chapter 9).

Vocational Evaluation

Vocational rehabilitation professionals recommend that young adults with disabling conditions and their families open a case with their state vocational agency 2 years prior to high school graduation so that potential needs can be evaluated and available resources explored. Too often students leave school and wait for extended periods of time to receive vocational services. Families need to be made aware of available services and the mechanisms for accessing them. They can initiate the process by contacting their local vocational agency. Alberto (1994) indicates that in order to help assure that the transition from school to postschool settings is successful and made by informed decisions, the process of educating students for transition must begin prior to their final year in school. The Individuals with Disabilities Education Act (IDEA) (1990) requires that school districts include an Individual Transition Plan (ITP) in the Individualized Education Plan (IEP). This ITP must contain "a statement of the needed transition services for students beginning no later that age 16 and annually thereafter and, when determined appropriate, the age may be lowered to 14 or younger." This ITP process, through joint consultations and planning among family members, the student, educators, and adult service providers serves two functions. First, it makes educational and postschool decisions concerning instruction, community experiences, employment, and other adult-living objectives and, when appropriate, acquisition of daily living skills and functional vocational evaluation. Second, it serves as a mechanism for coordinating information from and for family members about all options necessary for postschool life.

Determining work capabilities is a challenge and the initial step is the evaluation process usually conducted by a vocational evaluator, rehabilitation counselor, or work adjustment specialist. This process determines which hierarchical vocational options are best and identifies critical work-related skills. There is a clear correlation between vocational evaluation and practical prescriptions for programming.

The key issue to evaluating persons with PWS is recognition of their limited cognition since their mental abilities tend to level off somewhere between the second and fifth grade with math skills lower and reading abilities higher (see Chapter 11). This means that while affected individuals can take personal care of themselves and may be somewhat self-directed, their verbal skills and ability to manipulate their surroundings belie their true functional capacity and mask their ability to adapt. Were it not for their insatiable appetite and emotional lability, most would be capable of considerable independence.

Evaluation begins with the gathering of information on educational/technical background, previous work experience (including volunteer work), and interest areas (work and leisure). It then calls for analysis of adaptive, functional, and work skills (Mund, 1978). These adaptive skills include self-management, impulse control, taking directions, responding appropriately to authority, adjusting to change, staying on task, conforming, and learning new things. Professionals familiar with individuals with PWS will immediately recognize that their potential for developing adaptive skills is a major concern, because of difficulties related to adjusting to new situations and controlling their impulses.

Functional skills evolve from natural aptitudes such as mechanical ability, artistic talent, use of tools, and sociability. As a population, the skills and limitations of individuals with PWS are similar but individual differences can present extreme variation. Persons with PWS are likely to be stronger in one sphere than in another with noted strengths in fine motor skills but weaknesses in social situations.

Definitive assessment of motor skills should begin at an early age during physical and occupational therapy activities. This is critical since the natural capacity for fine motor talent is a firm basis for *all* hands on vocational training. Prevocational assessment and training are discussed within the context of physical/occupational activities (see Chapter 8). Work skills accumulate via actual training experience and need to be job-specific. This is important for persons with PWS who, if given both verbal and hands-on visual instruction, may function well with supervision.

The evaluation should continue with administration of a series of standardized tests and work samples. Information is then reviewed and synthesized and a profile of the individual as a worker emerges. It is important for evaluators to keep in mind that although persons with PWS have similar characteristics, each has very unique aptitudes and skills, strengths and weaknesses, motivations, and interests.

Evaluations may differ from agency to agency. Some provide formal assessments, situational assessments, or a combination. Most formal tests are pencil and paper type, and are generally timed to maintain standardization. A recommended resource to evaluate perceptual motor performance is The Developmental Test of Visual-Motor Integration (Beery, 1967), which assesses how well motor behavior and visual perception meld and indicates the potential for performing a variety of motor performance tasks. As previously mentioned, because vocational services must take into account the capacity to adapt, behavioral evaluation is very important. The aptitudes of persons with PWS can be assessed by the following tools.

1. The Vocational Behavioral Checklist (Walls, Zane, & Werner, 1978), while not designed for a specific disability, is of value in identifying prevocational skills, assessing areas of sensory development, determining the ability to attend and respond to simple discriminations, and utilize visual, auditory, and tactile modalities.

2. The Adaptive Behavior Scale (ABS) (Nihira, Foster, Shellhaas, et al., 1974) is designed to provide an objective description of the ability of emotionally maladjusted, developmentally delayed, and retarded persons to cope with normal environmental demands. It measures independence in daily living and social competencies when used in conjunction with information about individuals from other sources of information as well. The ABS is relevant for persons with PWS because assessment of physical development, self-direction, social skills, math and time concepts, and identification of maladaptive behaviors affect vocational programming.

Other formalized testing instruments include standardized work samples, that utilize specific work-related tasks from selected occupational areas to determine skills, aptitudes, and level of interest for a variety of work settings.

Selection of evaluation instruments should take into account all of the characteristics of PWS. For example, many persons with PWS exhibit difficulty in concentrating while sitting for long periods of time. Distractibility and, at times, sleepiness may have a negative effect on test results. Therefore, tests that are not lengthy may provide more valid and reliable results. It is also important to limit distractions in the work area for the same reasons. Standing for short periods of time while being tested should be allowed and encouraged to prevent sleepiness from having a major effect on the test-taking experience. Evaluators are cautioned that significantly obese individuals may have edema or infections in their lower extremities that may require elevation of the affected limb(s).

Individuals with PWS frequently present unique expressive and receptive language skills that also will have an inherent effect on the testing situation and its outcomes. See Chapter 10 for more detailed information on speech–language skills. These individuals may acknowledge comprehension of instruction, but, in actuality, may miss relevant details or misinterpret instructions. This can often lead to argumentativeness or excessive question-asking behavior. To minimize potential problems during evaluation, the amount of information presented at one time should be limited and clients should be asked to repeat instructions. Request for clarification of any discrepancies should be made before continuing. It is important to maintain a supportive, positive interactive style.

Vocational Rehabilitation Options

Considering the range of intellectual, cognitive, behavioral, and physical functioning of persons with PWS, it is important to take a critical look at vocational options for this population of adults and where they are currently being served.

Vocational Training Programs

Secondary school years are very difficult for many mentally retarded idividuals, primarily because by adolescence, abstract skills have a high priority (Robinson & Robinson, 1976). This is particularly true for persons with PWS as they progress through special educational programs because less appropriate behaviors seem to increase with age. It makes sense that high school vocational/technical programs be made available where reasonable coping and work related skills may be acquired.

The term "training" in vocational literature usually refers either to merely exposing the client to the work programs rather than training or to placing clients in job situations where it is hoped that training may occur (Gold, 1972). Persons with PWS require cohesive, supportive vocational/educational training that focuses on the relation strengths of individuals with PWS. For students with PWS, an instructional delivery model can assist in the vocational transition process previously identified. This model uses community sites as an extension of the classroom. During high school years students can be rotated through various community businesses for assessment of vocational aptitudes, likes, and dislikes. It can identify necessary environmental adaptations and required instruction in general work, social, and communication skills. This information results in a accumulation of a data base upon which postschool vocational selection can be made (Alberto, 1994).

Chausow (1986) suggests that because persons with PWS have relatively good fine motor skills, are patient, and tend to be sedentary, repetition office (clerical) tasks, simple laboratory assignments, and piece work at a sewing machine are viable training options. Basic office skills include sorting, filing, stuffing envelopes, and use of copiers, adding machines, and simple calculators. Individuals with good finger dexterity are able to learn some data entry computer skills. Library work (recording book titles and cataloging) and laboratory tasks such exact titration are possible because, by nature, persons with PWS are frequently precise and persistent. Trouble relating to authority figures and strong parenting instincts are two characteristics of PWS that, under ordinary circumstances, are rarely congruent. However, training as a child care aide can be an effective work option because persons with PWS not only desire to nurture but also enjoy being in a position of authority without fear of rejection. Naturally, fine motor talents also make training in basic carpentry skills a possibility, including operating simple power machinery and simple finishing work.

Offices, laboratories, and child care centers are not the only options. Still another vocational training alternative is in the area of horticulture. Greenhouses and landscape businesses deal with plants, ground maintenance, floral goods, services, and customers (Richmond, 1983). This environment offers a rare combination of physical and cognitive activities on a continuum from simple to complex tasks that have the potential to improve problem solving, communication, and making decisions. Although not normally "outdoor" people, outside work provides persons with PWS the opportunity for physical exercise. Greenhouse tasks such as potting, floral arranging, and, in some cases, sales offer opportunities to be creative. Working in a horticulture setting provides occasions to increase self-esteem via "show and tell" experiences through participation in seasonal community events that highlight on-the-job projects. In offers what Lewis and Gallison (1976) call "people-to-plant value." People need to feel needed and a living plant is almost totally dependent on person care. This type of work can diminish dependency, engender competence, and encourage personal growth (Copus, 1980).

Sheltered Workshops

Sheltered workshops (SW) are a very positive vocational options and exist to provide remunerative employment, training, and, appropriate job placement for individuals unable to function independently in a competitive setting. Individual interests, abilities, social, and behavioral patterns, and potential are continually evaluated and challenged.

SW training emphasizes personal and social adjustment. (Chinn, Drew, & Logan, 1979). While persons with PWS usually have higher cognitive and functional skills than many nonaffected workshop clients, their limited adaptive abilities make sheltered workshop settings a realistic option. Sometimes, however, their extensive vocabulary and verbal skills tend to delude caregivers into thinking that this population is simply "too bright" for a sheltered workshop environment and families wish to avoid the stigma of such a setting. Unfortunately, few persons with PWS adjust beyond this work milieu without dangerous weight gain and diffculties with authority figures. Moreover, their lack of ability to adjust to "new" situations can be a major barrier. Successful workshop programs are those where staff is willing to "go the extra mile" while teaching and supervising persons with PWS. Where the functional, adaptive, and work potential of persons with PWS are consistently evaluated and revised, vocational adaptation can increase. Realistic work expectations and consistent behavorial management can maximize the potential of this population.

Three sample workshop evaluation forms that address individual goals and objectives appear as Figures 16.1 through 16.3. They outline a sample set of expectations for improving the adaptive behaviors of a person with PWS and a daily workshop check-in sheet that accompanies the adaptive behavior plan. Figure 16.3 describes a take-home note that indicated hour-by-hour and day-by-day progress. Other workshop checklists for task completion for carpentry work, use of power machinery, and horticulture appear in Appendix G.

Supported Employment

Supported work consists of real work performed by clients in a competitive employment situation, where they perform the same tasks as persons without disabilities with the same expectation for production and quality. Once placed, instruction facilitated by a job coach occurs at the job site. Previous training is not usually a prerequisite. Wages received are usually commensurate with wages earned by any person performing the same or similar work. Employment should be in a setting that is physically and socially integrated and where there is access to co-workers and supervisors who can serve as work-role models. Early involvement of employers and job coaches in the design and development of services and their commitment to supported employment is essential. Long-term support services (i.e., job coaching) must be provided for whatever time necessary to ensure continued success. The type and intensity of support usually will vary over time.

As paradoxical as it may seem, there are reports of persons with PWS working in food service settings—washing dishes and performing kitchen tasks, at fast food restaurants. Successful employment may be due to the fact that in these situations literally *all* items are counted, right down to the buns, meat patties, and potatoes. Some tasks in food service are anecdotally reported to be limited to making salads. Long-term assess-

---

Client: <u>Jane Doe</u>   Case Manager <u>G.W.</u>
Date of IWRP: _____   Staff: <u>trainer-laundry/shop area</u>
Starting Date _____   Target Date _____   Completion date _____

  I. Long Term Goal: <u>J. will increase production rate from 55% to 70% of</u>
    <u>community standards in laundry and shop area.</u>

 II. Objective:
    A. Condition behavior/skill: <u>given clear instructions on task: encouragement</u>
       <u>and no more that on warning* each a.m. and p.m. and check-in slip.</u>
    B. Desired behavior/skill: <u>J. will keep hands and feet moving on task.</u>
    C. Desired level of performance: <u>at rate which is acceptable** to supervi-</u>
       <u>sion 90% for 18 days out of 20.</u>

III. Method (include what will by done, where, by done, where, by whom, and any
    special techniques of materials to be used:
    A. <u>Information about acceptable work rates (yes/no) will be on check-in slips.</u>
    B. <u>At the end of each a.m. and p.m. work supervisor will circle yes/no</u>
       <u>reacceptable**.</u>
    C. <u>If "yes", J. may sit in dining room from 3:30–4:00 p.m.</u>
    D. <u>If "no", J. must stay in free time area from 3:30–4:00 p.m.</u>

IV. Collection/monitoring procedures: <u>performance will be monitored through daily</u>
    <u>check-in slips.</u>

 V. Attached data collection graphs, charts, logs: _____Yes _____No
    Signature: _____ Title _____ Date _____

* Warning = staff will simply say, "J., you have had your first warning."

** Acceptable = no more than one warning per a.m. or p.m. for the following
behaviors:

1. Standing or sitting for more than one minute without working.
2. Not sticking to her won program or bossing others.
3. Raising voice to nonconversational tone to staff or other clients.

FIGURE 16.1. Sample objective plan for workshop program for persons with PWS.
(Reprinted by permission of Hope Haven, Inc., Rock Valley, IA.)

ment of this type of job placement is not yet available, but it is suggested
that the best (and very concrete) measure of success in this type of setting
is maintenance of reasonable weight. As pointed out in Chapter 1, some
affected individuals seem to be less emotionally labile when food is
available only at specific times. Therefore, consideration should be
given to the emotional well-being of individuals with PWS who work in
settings where food is always on view, since such sites may be a constant
source of frustration, even for those who are able to maintain a reasonable weight.

```
Name  Jane Doe   Date _____
Punctuality   Acceptable Work*

1. Work on time @ 8:3 _____  a.m. _____Yes _____No
2. Lite Club @ 9:30 _____  p.m. _____Yes _____No
3. Work/free time @ 10:15 _____
4. Work at 12:00 _____
5. Finish Task by 12:45 _____
6. Work @ 2:45 _____
7. Other _____
8. Other _____

* Acceptable means no more than one warning per a.m. or p.m. for the following
behaviors:

1. Standing or sitting for more than one minute not working**
2. Bossing others
3. Raising voice to nonconversational tone toward staff or others.

** Note: These times are to the minute. If J. is one or more minutes late, she is late.
If on time, initial the blank. If late, do not initial the blank. Instead, put "late" on the
blank and in parenthesis indicate the number of minutes late.
```

FIGURE 16.2. Sample daily performance card. (Reprinted by permission of Hope Haven, Inc., Rock Valley, IA.)

Vocational Adjustment Concerns

Under ordinary circumstances, vocational training and adjustment would be considered complete when the trainee is able to work independently and be self-sufficient. This is not usually the case for individuals with PWS. Indeed, their vocational adjustment is a rather elusive, continuing process of encouraging appropriate behaviors, social propriety, and cultivation of healthy interpersonal relationships. Difficulties arise in evaluation and training when affected individuals and/or their families are not ready to acknowledge the limitations associated with the syndrome, particularly the presence of functional retardation.

Discussion of vocational services would not be complete without including a word of caution about some training programs that, on the surface,may seem reasonable. Particular reference is made to training for housekeeping in motels or janitorial work. Two physical characteristics of persons with PWS may interfere with training for this type of work. First, their decreased sensitivity to pain and delicate skin increase the danger of being burned by water that is too hot and/or chemical cleaning agents. Second, the penchant for scavenging for food and money requires that a job coach maintain constant supervision. Where these concerns are appropriately addressed, these work areas may be feasible options.

Name Jane Doe Date _____			
	8:45–10:45 a.m.	10:30–12:00 a.m.	12:45–2:45 p.m.
Back to work on time	X	No	No
Follows directions promptly	X	X	No
Pays attention to task	X	X	X
Uses appropriate voice tone	X	No	X
Does not take items without asking	X	X	X
Follows all work shop rules	X	X	X

Daily Comments:

_____

_____

_____

_____

_____

Supervisory Staff

FIGURE 16.3. Sample take-home slip for reporting daily workshop adjustment for persons with PWS. (From Goldstein, A., & Carr, L. (1985). *Daily Progress Note.* Evanston, IL. Shore Training Center, Shore Community Services for Retarded Citizens. Reprinted with permission.)

Consideration should also be given to if or when to teach money management, since few persons with PWS learn enough math skills to administer their own funds. However, for some unknown reason, they are able to understand the value of money as a bribe or for buying food. Money skills should be addressed on an individual basis.

Vocational adjustment entails reaching beyond "pay for work done." Training goals should include increasing self-worth and dignity gained from being a contributing member of a community. Participation in productive work and social interactions go hand in hand and social responsibility, supposedly a product of the maturation process, will always be a long-range objective of vocational services.

Keys to Successful Adjustment

Employer/Staff Education

It is imperative for all personnel who work with persons with PWS to be knowledgeable about the syndrome in order to maintain consistency in the work area. A special commitment by employers and supervisors is important to make work a worthwhile experience. Information should include a description of the syndrome, dietary information, past behavioral challenges that may potentially reoccur in the work place, management strategies, and specific rules/regulations for the work area.

Family and/or Group Home Participation

Success in the world of work begins *before* the worker arrives on the job. Consistency and structure are key elements for long-term job placement. All care providers (family and staff) must contribute to effective vocational programming. Care providers and the workplace staff need to network approaches to management and delineation of responsibilities.

Vocational Planning

Because individuals with PWS have few opportunities for controlling decisions about their lives, they should be encouraged to participate in planning their programs. Interactions should be structured by providing an appropriate selection of choices and addressing concerns and requests. Inclusion of the individual in the planning of programming may facilitate compliance and participation. Structuring and limiting reasonable choices will aid in cultivating decision-making skills.

Development of Consistent Approaches to Management

1. Access to food should be restricted at all times and supervision at the work site, in lunch and break areas, and the rest room is essential. Caution is suggested when assigning tasks such as running errands and/or making deliveries. Lunches and snacks should be prepacked prior to coming to the work setting to prevent inclusion of items not permitted.

2. Be generous with verbal praise for good work and appropriate behavior. Build opportunities for success within the worker's range of abilities. Pride in one's work is an inherent motivator. Identify incentives such as assisting a staff membr, spending break time with a special co-worker, participating in a special activity, earning an additional low calorie snack, or receiving points/tokens to be redeemed for a reward previously selected by the worker. Discourage bringing money to work unless previously negotiated. This limits bartering.

3. Off-limit areas should be identified to reduce the frequency of "unauthorized acquistions." When such occurrences take place, noncon-

frontational cues should be used (see Chapter 9) to redirect the individual back to the appropriate work area and the worker's direct supervisor should be notified.

4. Specify one supervisor or key person to whom the person with PWS may address work-related concerns or problems. Identify the procedure for addressing these problems before the work begins the job.

5. Because changes in routines can result in frustration and difficult behavior, it is recommended that a written work schedule be established. Provide support (emotional and, at times, physical) and allow additional time for information to be processed when changes in routines must be made. When possible, plan for changes ahead of time.

6. Avoid arguing and verbal debates by placing limits on question-asking. Establishing time limits or number of allowable questions will aid in reducing perseverative questioning (see Chapter 9). Also, provide verbal praise for appropriate attempts to ask reasonable questions and to avoid arguing.

7. A designated place outside the main work area should be provided to vent frustration and regain composure. This avoids distracting outbursts in work areas.

Cognitive Strategies and Interventions

In the proper environment, persons with PWS are capable of learning multistep tasks and simple procedures, but may have difficulty under-standing lengthy, more complex concepts. Therefore, provide a few instructions at a time, in clear, understandable terms, and allow additional time to learn new tasks or procedures. Visual models, demonstration, and hands-on practice facilitate learning. Close monitoring during the learning phase is strongly recommended to ensure that instructions are followed correctly.

Use of Cognitive Strategies in the Workplace

Cognitive strategies such as simple written drections, note taking, verification, clarification, check lists, check sheets, and schedules can facilitating new learning, organization, problem-solving, and self-monitoring. Accommodations may need to be made for slow processing of information, limited ability to understand abstract verbal concepts, academic deficits, and distractibility. Many workers with PWS are not truly aware of their inability to adequately monitor themselves. How-ever, supportive feedback and a nonaccusatory approach will decrease argumentativeness and perseveration. The establishment of concrete standards and expectations discussed prior to beginning work tasks is useful as both a cognitive strategy and a behavioral management technique. It is essential to monitor completed work for quality and accuracy at regular intervals.

Strategic arrangement of the work area and placement of materials can decrease stealing or hoarding of materials, reduces the effect of environmental distractions, and minimizes inappropriate social interactions. For some individuals, it may be necessary to limit the amount of work materials available at the workstation at a given time.

Summary

Vocational programs should be an integral part of the life of individuals with PWS. Services for this population are mandated by law and opportunities for vocational options are expanding. Sensitive counseling, careful assessment, and realistic training initiated prior to completing their schooling are essential. All training must take the natural functional talent, personality traits, food-seeking drive, and the need for structure into consideration. Sheltered workshops provide a good option because the extent to which most persons with PWS can function in a competitive setting with only limited supervision has yet to be determined. In addition to determining a person's present vocational level, recommendations are generally made to ensure success in the workplace such as the need for special work accommodations, use of strategies or interventions to compensate for deficits, behavioral management techniques, and adaptive equipment. Where professionals are ill prepared, written plans poorly conceived, and supervision lacking, failure follows. Reassessment of program goals should be on-going and education of all staff and potential employers is required to ensure that all service providers are sensitive to the needs and individual capabilities of this population. Community liaison is the key to success.

References

Alberto, P.A. (1994). *Education, Work, and Transition*. Paper presented at the meeting of the National Prader–Willi Syndrome Association, Atlanta, GA.

Andrew, J.W. (1981). Evaluation of rehabilitation potential. In R. Parker & C. Hansen (Eds.), *Rehabilitation counselling* (pp. 205–225). Boston: Allyn & Bacon.

Beery, K. (1967). *Developmental Test of Visual-Motor Integration: Administration and scoring manual*. Chicago: Follett.

Chausow, R. (1986). *Position paper on vocational and recreational skills for Prader-Willi syndrome clients*. Unpublished manuscript.

Chinn, P.C., Drew, C.J., & Logan, D.R. (1979). *Mental retardation, a life cycle approach*. St. Louis: C.V. Mosby.

Copus, E. (1980). *The Melwood Manual*. The University of Wlisconson-Stout, Materials Development Center. Menomonie, WI.

Daniels, J. (1981). The world of work and disabling conditions. In R. Parker & C. Hansen (Eds.), *Rehabilitation counselling* (pp. 169–197). Boston: Allyn & Bacon.

Gold, M.W. (1972). Stimulus factors in skill training of the retarded in complex assembly tasks: Acquisition, transfer, and retention. *American Journal of Mental Deficieny*, 76, 517–526.

Individuals with Disabilities Education Act of 1990, Public Law 101–476, (1990). Title 20, U.S.C. 1400–1485: U.S. Statutes at large, 104, 1103–1151. October.

Lewis, C., & Gallison, S. (1976). *Plants for people*. Paper presented at a conference of the National Council for Therapy & Rehabilitation through Horticulture, Gaithersburg, MD.

Mund, S. (1978). Vocational rehabilitation: Employment; self employment; a vocational rehabilitation process. In R. Goldenson (Ed.), *Disability and rehabilitation handbook* (pp. 76–87). New York: McGraw-Hill.

Nihira, K., Foster, R., Shellhaas, M., & Leland, H. (1974). *Adaptive Behavior Scale*. Washington, DC: American Association on Mental Deficiency.

Prader-Willi Syndrome Association (1991). PWSA Surveys Workforce. *The Gathered View*. September–October.

Richmond, C. (1983). *Horticulture: Hiring the disabled*. American Rehabilitation, vol. 9, 1. Washington, D.C.: U.S. Dept. of Education, Office of Special Education and Rehabilitation Services.

Robinson, N., & Robinson, H. (1976). *The mentally retarded child*. New York: McGraw-Hill. Swallwell, T. (1992). Goodwill Industries of Southwestern Pennsylvania Residential Day Program Project. Vocational Services for Prader-Willi Syndrome charts. Lancaster, PA.

U.S. Department of Labor, Employment Standards Administration, Wage and Hour Division. (1982). Regulations, Part 25, Employment of Handicapped Clients in Sheltered Workshops. U.S. Department of Labor. September.

Walls, R., Zane, T., & Werner, T. (1978). *Vocational Behavioral Checklist*. Dunbar, VW: West Virginia Rehabilitation Research and Training Center.

17
A Crisis Intervention Model for Persons with Prader–Willi Syndrome[1]

Jeanne M. Hanchett and Beate Maier

Most persons with Prader–Willi syndrome (PWS) are easy to manage during their preschool and early school age years. They are often charming, cherubic, and healthy members of the family. However, in many cases, these pleasant children become extremely difficult-to-manage adolescents or young adults with increasing episodes of food foraging, stealing, and running away behaviors. Some rapidly accumulate excess weight and develop associated medical problems. Others demonstrate severe behavior problems that are often more difficult to manage than the voracious appetite. When families find themselves unable to cope with problems of medical illness secondary to morbid obesity and severe behavioral disturbances, crisis intervention is required.

There are few medical facilities familiar with PWS; anecdotal reports of caregivers of patients with acute medical/behavioral episodes reveal that most cases are admitted on an emergency basis to a general hospital ICU or acute psychiatric unit. Staff in these settings usually lack knowledge about PWS and are unable to offer services or provide the necessary time to develop new strategies that can carry over into long-term programming. This chapter discusses a crisis intervention program at The Rehabilitation Institute (TRI) in Pittsburgh that has served more than 250 patients with PWS over the past 14 years.

TRI is a private rehabilitation hospital that devotes a 20 bed unit to the care of persons with PWS and related disorders. It is licensed as a unique

---

[1] *Editor's note:* Despite advances in early diagnosis and management, some individuals with PWS have episodes of morbid obesity and/or behavioral problems that require crisis intervention. Unfortunately, there is a dearth of such services. Therefore, we are pleased to provide our readers with a model designed to meet the challenges associated with acute care. It is our hope that this discussion will encourage creation of similar programs.

mental health/psychiatric unit by the state of Pennsylvania and patients come from most of the 50 states and Canada; they are referred by physicians, families, case workers, and group home staff and an increasing number of admissions in recent years have come from residential programs and hospitals. While the primary reasons for admission are equally divided between medical complications and disturbed behaviors, many patients have a combination of both. Staff include a physician, program manager, psychiatrist, psychologist, nurses, dietitian, social worker, speech–language therapist, exercise physiologist, occupational therapist, special education teacher, and a team leader who supervises the direct care personnel on the unit. All have extensive training and experience working with persons with PWS. The unit is not locked and patients are admitted voluntarily.

Medical Issues That Require Intervention

Morbid Obesity

When PWS is diagnosed early in life, families are usually able to set appropriate limits on their child's food intake and therefore avoid morbid obesity at least during childhood. However, over time, persons with PWS become more clever at obtaining food and more free to move independently in the community and weight increases rapidly; it is not unusual to see gains of 50 pounds or more in one year. The term "morbid obesity" is applied when there is a greater than 100% increase over ideal body weight. At this point, there is a high probability of the occurrence of hypoventilation, heart failure, diabetes mellitus, hypertension, ulcerations of the skin, cellulitis, and a decrease in the ability to ambulate.

Marked pulmonary hypoventilation and sleep apnea occur in obese adults (Kopelman, Apps, Cope, et al., 1986) and morbidly obese children and adolescents (Mallory, Fiser, & Jackson, 1989). This has been observed in persons with PWS persons as well (Hanchett, 1993; Kaplan, Fredrickson, & Richasdson, 1991). The most common cause of premature death in PWS is cardiopulmonary failure related to hypoventilation. Several cases of severe hypoventilation have been referred to TRI following an episode of cyanosis and apnea at home presaged by increasingly loud snoring, difficulty walking, inability to sleep lying flat, and marked shortness of breath. After intensive intervention in a hospital (where intubation and assisted ventilation is frequently necessary) stabilized patients are transferred to TRI. (If consulted during the initial time in an ICU prior to admission to TRI, we strongly recommend that a tracheostomy not be performed.)

A complete physical assessment is done at the time of admission. It includes monitoring of saturation levels during sleep to determine the necessity of supplemental oxygen, which is prescribed only if sustained oxygen desaturation occurs. Some severely obese patients are cyanotic and have compensatory elevation of hemoglobin levels. Extreme shortness of breath in all activities including speaking is not unusual. Most patients with this degree of pulmonary compromise also are using bronchodilators, diuretics, and cardiac medications at admission. Rapid accumulation of ankle and leg edema has heralded cor pulmonale (right sided heart failure) and is accompanied by marked pulmonary compromise, usually with cyanosis, orthopnea, and grunting respirations. Heart failure is also indicated by shortness of breath and may be difficult to differentiate from pulmonary compromise. Both are dire emergencies.

Patients are placed on a 600-calorie diet and a multivitamin and mineral supplement and a gradual physical conditioning program is instituted. Because many of the morbidly obese patients have spent virtually all waking time either in bed or in sedentary activities such as TV watching for many weeks or months prior to admission, they are immediately encouraged to walk and given much verbal reinforcement. They often lose weight rapidly on this regimen of diet and exercise, sometimes as much as 15 pounds or more the first week. Thereafter, weight loss is usually 2–4 pounds weekly. Blood pressure and heart rate are monitored during exercise. This procedure assists the exercise physiologist in determining just how rapidly to increase the program, which includes walking, swimming, and eventually stationary bike riding and running. This dual program of diet and exercise results in marked improvement in cardiovascular fitness as well as weight loss. Most patients are discharged on fewer medications and, for some, all medication can be discontinued before discharge.

Diabetes Mellitus and Hypertension

Approximately 30% of morbidly obese patients over the age of 20 have non-insulin-dependent diabetes mellitus (Type II diabetes). On admission most diabetic patients have extremely elevated blood sugars and markedly elevated glycohemoglobin levels (as high as 19%), indicating long-standing poor diabetes control. In a few instances diabetic patients have developed complications including retinopathy, neuropathy, and amputations after only a few years. Following institution of a diet and exercise program, control of diabetes improves, blood sugar levels fall to normal within a few days or a few weeks, and doses of oral hypoglycemic agents and insulin are markedly decreased. In many cases normoglycemia is maintained when all hypoglycemic agents and insulin are discontinued while the patient remains on a low calorie diet. This process of reversing clinical diabetes is an extremely important goal, since the complications of diabetes mellitus result in loss of function, costly medical care, and premature death. In several patients where diabetes has been identified in its earliest stage (prediabetic state), rapid weight loss has resulted in avoidance of the disease entirely. Observations of hypertension are similar to those with diabetes; weight loss and exercise cause an improvement in blood pressure and medications can be discontinued.

Skin Problems

Skin problems are difficult to avoid with massive obesity. Pendulous abdominal fat folds make hygiene difficult; meticulous cleansing and drying of fat folds and daily irrigations with a dilute vinegar solution can control skin irritations. Monilial infections are treated with clotrimazole as needed. Topical medications containing cortisone should be avoided except for short periods of time because of the likelihood of damage to skin with prolonged use. Skin picking behaviors are found in about 80% of persons with PWS and present a challenge in management. While no specific medical treatment has been identified as beneficial, limiting attention to this behavior is helpful. We do not tell patients to "stop picking"; this draws attention and may increase the picking. If there is blood on fingers, hand washing is suggested before further activities. Infections are seen only on rare occasions, despite the presence of numerous open areas and the chronicity of many of the lesions. However, cellulitis of the lower legs in association with obesity and stasis is common and tends to be chronic and recurrent unless there is marked weight loss. Antibiotics are used only when there is evidence of acute infection.

Behavioral Problems That Require Intervention

TRI's approach to behavior management is grounded in a model of human learning and behavior. Behavioral diagnosis is based on identification of various internal and external conditions that foster problems, hypothesize the purpose served by such behaviors, and identify specific personality characteristics that contribute to the difficulties. This multi-component view of behavior embodies the traditional explanation of behaviors and focuses on establishing coping skills necessary to manage anxiety and develop socialization skills. Social attachments between caregiver and patients are allowed to evolve so that the caregiver can become a teacher and a source of rewards. The overall interactions on the unit are guided by the characteristics of the team leader and the staff. This gentle teaching paradigm works well in this treatment milieu because of the warmth, tolerance, and affection that develop between patients and staff. Not all behaviors are addressed at the same time.

Soon after admission, the staff psychiatrist assesses the patient and assists the psychologist and unit staff in developing a behavioral program. If psychoactive medications have been previously prescribed, they are usually continued during the initial period of assessment. An individual treatment plan is developed and problem behaviors are identified. This treatment plan consists of a system of reinforcement for positive behaviors. For example: "staying calm 70% of the time" might be a goal for a person who has tantrums several times daily. "Points" are then earned for achieving a goal. This token economy system results in patients "earning money" to use for nonfood items on shopping trips. When maladaptive behaviors are displayed, staff members employ gentle teaching strategies of ignoring and redirecting described by McGee (1986). Behavior that may endanger the client or others is dealt with by seclusion and "time-out" procedures. This is explained to the patient as an opportunity to regain self-control.

It is important to recognize the concept of dual diagnosis in many cases and acknowledge the presence of both mental retardation and mental illness or emotional disturbance. The most difficult and maladaptive behavior is addressed initially and as the patient improves and accomplishes goals, a new program for behavioral improvement is developed, with the patient's involvement. This usually results in progressive behavioral changes during the length of hospitalization. Grouping patients with PWS together is a powerful therapeutic tool that helps patients identify and adapt to this diagnosis. It also appears to be helpful for patients to assess their own coping skills and behavior in relationship to their peers.

Pharmacologic intervention is an integral part of treatment, particularly when psychiatric evaluation reveals evidence of depression, intense anxiety, or psychotic thought processes as well as assaultive or disruptive behaviors. While medications alone do not resolve maladaptive behaviors, their use in conjunction with behavioral programming allows the patient to benefit from the TRI crisis intervention milieu and learn new coping skills. At the present time the group of medications known as selective serotonin re-uptake inhibitors (fluoxetine, sertraline, and paroxetine) appears to be the most helpful. Thioridazine, haloperidol, and buspirone have been prescribed when there is evidence of disordered thought processes and assaultive and/or disruptive behavior. The progress of each patient is measured by recording the frequency of target behaviors as well as anecdotal observations by the interdisciplinary team members. Chapter 9 discusses drug intervention in depth.

The TRI Rehabilitation Team

The team approach discussed in Chapter 4 serves as the cornerstone for treatment of patients with PWS. Plans for intervention actually begin prior to admission when the entire team is presented with background information on the patient, highlighting specific medical and behavioral problems. This information is based on an extensive process of accumulation of records from hospitals, physicians, vocational settings, counseling centers, and schools. On the day of admission family members, case workers, or group home staff members are interviewed by the attending physician, dietitian, social worker, psychologist, team leader, and program manager. The psychiatrist also obtains information from family members of patients who have particularly severe psychiatric problems. A physical examination is performed and a program is instituted. A staffing conference is held a few days after admission to develop treatment strategies based on observations. All the members of the interdisciplinary team are present as well as the speech–language therapist, occupational therapist, exercise physiologist, and other resource persons. Each is encouraged to participate in the development of programming and subsequently monitors overall effectiveness. This ensures a consistent approach to behavioral strategies and broad-based observations of the patient's behavior as well as physical status. Staffing conferences are then held every 1 to 2 weeks throughout the patient's admission (Figure 17.1).

The TRI Program

The therapeutic milieu is highly structured. Activities are scheduled throughout the day with an effort to alternate physically active therapies and more sedentary cognitive activities. Recreation is selected to promote both physical activity and social skills. Free time and television watching are limited to 1-1/2 hours a day. Each therapist has at least two goals for the patient at all times; the primary one is in the area of expertise of each therapist, such as speech–language, fine motor skills, or physical condition. Equally important is the goal of facilitating overall behavioral strategies within specific therapy settings.

The program psychologist works closely with the staff in developing individualized behavior programs based on interviews with parents, observations on the unit, and information reported at staff conferences. Patients are seen for individual counseling when it is indicated, such as those who have great difficulty adjusting to unit routines.

The dietitian provides nutrition educational services to the patients, individually and in groups. A low calorie, simplified "stop light diet" that uses a red–yellow–green system of grouping foods as described by Epstein, Masek, and Marshall (1978) has proven helpful and effective. Most patients learn this simple system and use it after discharge (Akers & Mandella, 1984). Appropriate behavior is expected during dietary sessions and is rewarded with nonfood items or "points" in the token economy system.

Communication therapy is provided by speech–language specialists and emphasizes participation in the group process, group activities such as

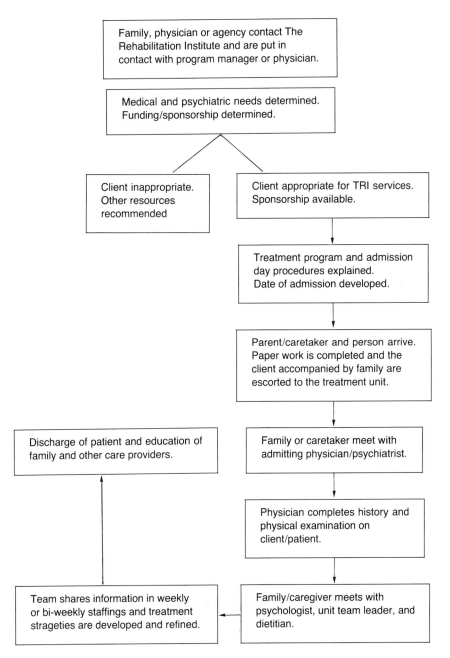

Family, physician or agency contact The Rehabilitation Institute and are put in contact with program manager or physician.

Medical and psychiatric needs determined. Funding/sponsorship determined.

Client inappropriate. Other resources recommended

Client appropriate for TRI services. Sponsorship available.

Treatment program and admission day procedures explained. Date of admission developed.

Parent/caretaker and person arrive. Paper work is completed and the client accompanied by family are escorted to the treatment unit.

Discharge of patient and education of family and other care providers.

Family or caretaker meet with admitting physician/psychiatrist.

Physician completes history and physical examination on client/patient.

Team shares information in weekly or bi-weekly staffings and treatment strageties are developed and refined.

Family/caregiver meets with psychologist, unit team leader, and dietitian.

FIGURE 17.1. Admission flow chart.

role playing, and increasing verbal social skills. Individualized physical fitness programs are developed and supervised by an exercise physiologist. Those with significant cardiopulmonary compromise are monitored. The strength of this program lies in the individual PWS patient establishing a goal to increase stamina and endurance; participants are reinforced even for small gains, and self-esteem improves significantly as fitness improves.

The occupational therapist focuses on improving fine motor skills, organizational, and problem-solving abilities as well as independent living skills. Functional activities such as gardening, sewing, home safety practices, and community awareness address these goals in a manner that facilitates behavioral goals. Craft activities and water exercise encourage the ability of participants to follow directions and to work in a group. Patients with PWS are frequently adept at learning computer skills and problem solving is enhanced by a computer literacy program that teaches basic computer operations and improves attention. The TRI library also uses an innovative program designed to teach seeking out and utilizing information. School-age patients attend a special education program that follows individualized educational prescriptions and applies the same behavioral guidelines within the educational setting. Tolerance for work is assessed by the Vocational and Career Services Division where appropriate interactions between the person with PWS and staff members as well as peers are encouraged. A primary goal in this area is to increase tolerance for on-task activities and to develop the interpersonal skills necessary for vocational success.

Learning about PWS and appropriate developmental tasks within the context of lifetime restrictions of the syndrome are the goals of group sessions facilitated by the social worker on the team, the psychologist and the staff psychiatrist, who sees patients individually and jointly with the social worker or psychologist.

Nurses play a key role in day-to-day management and are adept at sorting through requests and demands for attention and assistance. Many persons with PWS have excessive minor complaints; some are attention getting and others are used in hopes of obtaining sweet liquid medication. A delicate balance between addressing the behavioral needs and at the same time assessing the physical needs of these persons can be achieved by experienced nurses; it requires frequent communication between unit staff nurses and physician.

The Discharge/Follow-up Process

Achievement of crisis intervention goals is essential. However, long-term success is based on good discharge planning. This requires education of family members, residential/group home providers, case workers, teachers, and all other professionals, because upon discharge, patients return to their home, school, or workshop and usual source of medical and psychiatric care. Most team members meet with the family and other care providers at the time of discharge. Use of the prescribed diet is encouraged, along with methods for adapting behavioral strategies to the home or wherever residential services are to be provided. Every effort is made to pass appropriate information to those persons who will be managing the patient; discharge summaries are sent to parents and professionals.

Follow-up is conducted through a system of newsletters and postcards from the dietitian that encourage patients to report their weights on a monthly basis. Families are encouraged to call the dietitian with questions and observations. Many staff members serve as a resource to persons in the home environment and community for long periods of time after discharge. This comprehensive program of discharge planning and intervention has resulted in prolonged benefit.

Acknowledgments. The authors thank Judith Brice, M.D., Judy Bridges, M.S.W., Jennifer Deau, M.S., Joanne Heckel, R.N., Kim Henry, W. Lindsay Jacob, M.D., Byron Jordan, M.Ed., Gwen Moore, Linda Myers, C.O.T.A., Ken Smith, Nancy Spears, Lori Stambaugh, CCC/SLP, and Jessica Valley, R.D., for sharing their expertise and experiences.

References

Akers, M., & Mandella, P. (1984). Red, yellow, green system of weight control. Pittsburgh, PA: The Rehabilitation Institute of Pittsburgh.

Epstein, L., Masek, B.J., & Marshall, W.R. (1978). A nutritionally based school program for control of eating in obese children. *Behavior Therapy, 9*, 766–778.

Hanchett, J.M. (1993). Hypoventilation, oxygen saturation levels and Prader-Willi syndrome. *Proceedings of National Prader-Willi Syndrome Association Scientific Day.*

Kaplan, J., Fredrickson, P.A., & Richardson, J.W. (1991). Sleep and breathing in patients with Prader-Willi syndrome. *Mayo Clinic Proceedings, 66*, 1124–1126.

Kopelman, P.G., Apps, M.C.P., Cope, T., Ingram, D.A., Empeg, D.W., & Evans, S.J. (1986). Nocturnal hypoxia and sleep apnea in asymptomatic obese men. *International Journal of Obesity, 10*, 211–217.

Mallory, G.B., Fiser, D.H., & Jackson, R. (1989). Sleep-association breathing disorders in morbidly obese children and adolescents. *Journal of Pediatrics, 115*, 892–897.

McGee, J.J. (1986). Issues related to applied behavioral analysis. In J. Stark, F.J. Menolaseino, & V. Gray (Eds.), *Mental retardation and mental health.* New York: Springer Verlag.

Mullins, J., & Maier, B. (1987). Weight management of youth with Prader-Willi syndrome. *International Journal of Eating Disorders, 6*(3), 419–427.

Part VI
A Network of Caring

Getting help is so hard . . . it seems like no one believes us, especially R's teacher. Even our social worker said she never heard of PWS and because of her thinking we did not get help for a long time.

Most of the problems are because of our ages and being retired and on a fixed income and being worried about her future. A lot of places tell you right out they will not accept [persons with] PWS.

I am in the "end domino" in his life. His sister has her own life. I would like to see him in a group home that is more like a home than an institution.

Being a parent of a PWS person is a very lonely position at times, as I'm positive that being a PWS person must be extremely lonely and upsetting. It is nice to feel that at last some help and support is around [the National Association].

18
A Chronology of Hope:
A Case Study[1]

Jack Sherman

As with most developmental disabilities, the presence of Prader–Willi syndrome (PWS) has a profound impact on the family system. It would be a disservice to both affected individuals and their families to ignore parental feelings. For this reason, the case presentation that follows integrates the medical, psychological, educational, and social history of a Caucasian female. Her parents assisted the case historian by sharing their recollections and frustrations as the parents of a disabled child whose diagnosis was delayed for over 26 years. Their comments afford the reader a very personal perspective and a sensitive counterpoint to this clinical case review.

The Case Study

Miss M. was born in 1957, just a year after the publication of the article by Prader, Labhart, and Willi (1956) that definitively described what has come to be known as PWS. Both the timing of her birth and the lack of physician awareness about this syndrome played a large part in the delay of accurate diagnosis. From the beginning, very early in her stormy neonatal period, M. was evaluated by pediatricians, internists, endocrinologists, neurologists, and psychiatrists. All these specialists reported symptomatology now acknowledged to be some physical or emotional manifestation of PWS. Unfortunately, it was not until M. was 26 years of age and living in a home for the emotionally disturbed that a psychologist involved with her programming suspected the presence of PWS. At his

---

[1] *Editor's Note:* The initial description of this individual appeared in the first edition of our book. We are pleased that Dr. Sherman has maintained his concern and interest in this case and appreciate his willingness to contribute additional historical information.

recommendation, M.'s parents sought a genetics center familiar with this disorder where a thorough assessment confirmed the diagnosis.

M. was the fourth child born to a 38-year-old father and a 40-year-old mother who had three normal offspring, one miscarriage, and no stillbirths. There was no history of consanguinity nor exposure to teratogens prior to or during the pregnancy. History was also negative for birth defects or mental retardation. Her mother reported no discernible difference in M.'s fetal activity and that of her three previous pregnancies. The older siblings, ages 11, 9, and 6 at the time of the proband's birth, were all normal and healthy. M. was delivered vaginally 2 weeks posterm after an uneventful pregnancy and labor. She weighed 3.3 kg (7 lbs. 4 oz) and was 48.25 cm (19 in) in length. Apgar scores were not reported. Her neonatal course was marked by hypotonia and inability to take oral feedings because of poor suck. At 3 days of age she was transferred from the hospital where she was born to a university-based tertiary care center. She remained there 5 days and was discharged with a diagnosis of cerebral palsy of unknown origin. After her release to home care, M. continued to require dropper feedings. Other than the prolonged feeding times, she was a quiet, placid infant who required little attention.

Our story began when the doctor who delivered our daughter knew something was not normal and suggested immediate hospitalization for more tests at a children's hospital. After one week of tests, their findings were that our daughter had some form of cerebral palsy. One of the most devastating medical contacts we had was when a consultant met with us at 4:30 on Christmas Eve, 1957. We appreciated his seeing us prior to the holidays. Then he said, "Your daughter would probably not survive six months because she could not overcome a simple cold." We were in tears. The timing and lack of finesse were devastating. Of course, every day of those first six months was worrisome.

M.'s father, who traveled extensively for business, stayed in constant phone communication with his wife and said that the entire family prayed for a miracle. He spoke gratefully that they all survived the first 6 months and felt that the experience allowed him to be more willing to accept his daughter's problems because he had expected her to die in infancy.

Yet every day that she survived was a boost to our morale. Somehow (after the 6 months had elapsed) whenever our daughter behaved abnormally, we would go back to that December day . . . that always allowed me [her father] to be more understanding of her.

By 6 months of age her ability to take oral feedings and her appetite improved considerably, and from that time she demonstrated the voracious appetite consistent with PWS. No major illnesses were identified during her infancy and toddlerhood. M.'s developmental milestones were delayed. She sat at 8 months, rolled over and stood with assistance at 10 months; she pulled herself up at 11 months but did not walk until 3 years of age. Speech began at age 2. Although she was reported to have been toilet trained at 3 years, nocturnal enuresis and occasional daytime "accidents" continued until age 8 (Figure 18.1–18.7).

From a behavioral perspective, M.'s parents were disturbed at her weight gain in childhood despite their efforts to limit her food intake at meals. Initially, they thought the weight gain was due to her sedentary habits. They finally realized that she was stealing food. Her memory capacity was considered quite remarkable by her parents since she could remember people whom she had rarely seen and was able to identify the times and circumstances when she saw them 2 or 3 years later.

Entering the educational system was difficult. M. was teased, suffered from name-calling, and lacked friends. Her mother reported that she was pushed around frequently and sustained a fractured wrist when knocked down by another student. Her teachers repeatedly called on her parents to exercise more control over M. because she continued to steal the lunches of other students and took leftover food from the garbage cans at school. M.'s psychometric testing revealed that she had a verbal IQ of 102, a performance IQ of 95, and a full scale of 99. She was in the 47th percentile for reading and 42nd for spelling, but only the 18th for arithmetic. Her IQ scores were considerably higher than those of most individuals known to have PWS. However, her math skills were typical for affected individuals; she maintained below-average scholastic performance throughout her childhood. Her parents report that she was under extreme pressure to keep up with the other students when she entered high school. Furthermore, it was at this time of her life that she

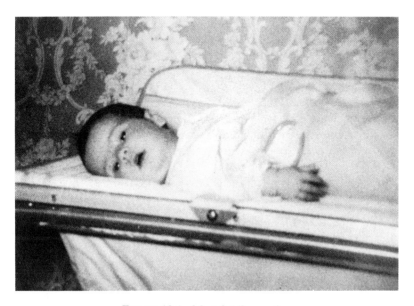

FIGURE 18.1. M at 2 1/2 months.

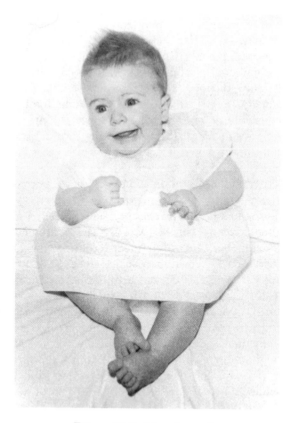

FIGURE 18.2. M at 6 months.

began to steal money, beginning with a few coins here and there but soon progressing to taking considerable sums from her parents and their house guests. She made no effort to hide the money she took.

At 17 years of age, while a sophomore in high school, M.'s emotional outbursts necessitated admittance to a psychiatric unit. After 10 days, the attending physician recommended that she be transferred to a psychiatric hospital for an extended stay. During the time M. remained in this mental facility, her behavior deteriorated further. According to her parents, "she became very angry at us and learned a lot of bad habits".

Four months later, M. was transferred to a private school for troubled children. Interestingly enough, another student at the same private school had been diagnosed as having PWS. However, despite the marked similarities in their behavior and clinical appearance, M.'s parents were assured by the school's doctor and psychologist that she did not have PWS because her IQ was normal, was a "good student," and had no speech impairment. During the time M. lived in the private school, she was evaluated by an endocrinologist, who noted her hypogonadism, mild

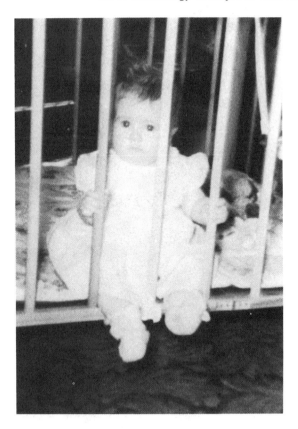

FIGURE 18.3. M at 9 months.

scoliosis, short stature, small hands and feet, obesity, amblyopia, and myopia. He initially entertained diagnoses of Froehlich syndrome, pseudohypoparathyroidism, pseudopseudohypoparathyroidism, and Turner syndrome, but PWS was not mentioned in the differential diagnosis. After nearly 3–1/2 years, M. left the private school and returned home to live with her parents.

Our daughter received an equivalent to a high school diploma at this private school. She had far fewer tantrums and they were not as severe. Food was still a problem, although at school she put on very little weight. She enjoyed the setting and the personnel and we felt she had progressed to the point where vocational training should be pursued.

Once home, M. was placed under the care of a psychologist who diagnosed her obesity as "primarily psychiatric in nature." He further characterized her behavior as typical for a 7 or 8 year old child (at this time, she was 22 years of age). He was impressed with her ability to crochet, hook rugs, and assemble jigsaw puzzles. He

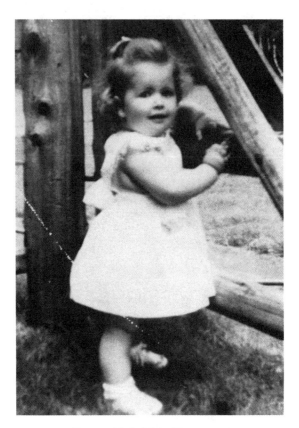

FIGURE 18.4. M at 22 months.

also commented on her "explosive emotional behavior" and her "habit of eating until she fell asleep." The psychologist suggested M. start in a vocational program. She was referred to the state Division of Vocational Rehabilitation, which in turn referred her to Goodwill Industries for job training and placement. Unfortunately, and unbelievably, M.'s vocational training started in a sheltered workshop as a cashier in the cafeteria. At the same time, she entered an independent living program at the sheltered workshop site. In this environment (unstructured and with food available), she gained weight rapidly. It reached an astronomical 131 kg (288 lbs); she could hardly walk and was unable to manage her personal hygiene. Very soon, she was denied employment "because of the severity of her psychophysiological problem."

M. returned home, but her conflicts with her parents became intolerable. Her food-related tantrums continued to the point where her parents begged a psychiatric hospital to admit her. Her physical health was in jeopardy, her mental state fragile, and her parents exhausted. They knew she needed a well-structured facility where she could be cared for appropriately. In March 1980, M. required admission to a small com-

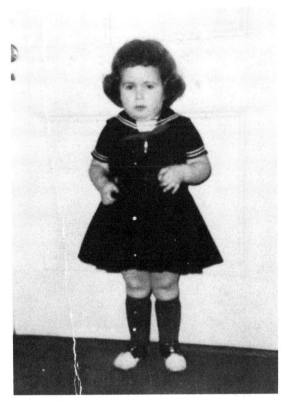

FIGURE 18.5. M at 5 years.

munity hospital because of breathing difficulties. Her "final" diagnosis during this hospitalization was Pickwickian syndrome.

Two years later (1982), M. was admitted to a home for the emotionally disturbed. She weighed 94.4 kg (207 lbs) and was 133 cm (52.5 in) in height. During the third year of her stay in this facility, a psychologist noted her skin-picking behavior. He recalled that a patient known to have PWS whom he had seen at another hospital had the same habit and recommended a genetics evaluation at a center experienced with PWS. M.'s diagnosis was confirmed on the basis of her history, previously mentioned physical findings, her highly arched palate, narrow forehead, almond-shaped eyes, and hands and feet that were below the third percentile in size. Cytogenetic analysis revealed a deletion on the 15th chromosome. Confirmation of the diagnosis of PWS was an emotionally charged event. Her parents cried, thankful that after nearly 26 years they "were not to blame" (Figure 18.8).

Following this definitive diagnosis of PWS, M.'s parents quoted their daughter as saying "I am glad to know what I have. I will be glad to

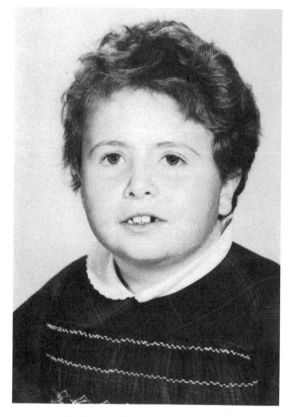

FIGURE 18.6. M at 8 years.

volunteer to go through any tests. I don't want another child to go through what I had to." Later in a newspaper story about the plight of individuals with PWS, she told a reporter that she wanted everyone to know about the condition.

In 1986, M. achieved a long-awaited goal. At the age of 29, she was transferred to a group home established exclusively for PWS adults that came into being due to the unrelenting effort and persistence by members of the state chapter of the national parent support group, the Prader–Willi Syndrome Association. Her medical health has remained generally good but her psychological and social behavior has led to several regressions in her overall life style and level of achievement.

Soon after her admission to the PWS group home, she had conflicts with her roommate and with other peers at the residence. Her assaultive behavior necessitated "in-house" confinement. She did regain her former freedom after a 2-week period of "grounding" and restrictions, but her high cognitive function and ingenuity led to continued inappropriate activities such as ordering numerous magazines and catalog items despite

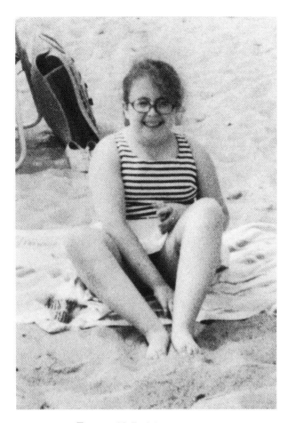

FIGURE 18.7. M at 12 years.

her inability to pay for them. She required a great deal of counseling to gain control of this impulsive behavior. In fact, M. has had several acute-care psychiatric hospitalizations to seek control of severe depression. Although she has been maintained on several medications for her emotional lability, such as haloperidol (Haldol), lithium, and, more recently, carbamazepine (Tegretol), she received no benefit from a trial of fluoxetine (Prozac) prescribed in 1989.

We are encouraged by her present emotional stability. M. has made much progress in the past six months. She is more alert and it appears that adjusting her medication has a great deal to do with her alertness. M.'s social life is outstanding. She attends plays, concerts, shows, shopping, museums, camping at two weeks per year, picnics in parks, boat trips, dances and has gone camping two weeks during each year.

M. keeps a busy schedule at her PWS residence and at her day-care workshop where she has the tasks of soldering and assembling electronic equipment. She is taking educational classes and recently completed

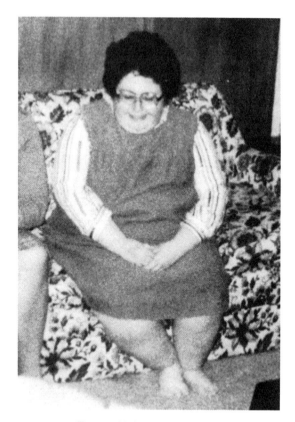

FIGURE 18.8. M at 24 years.

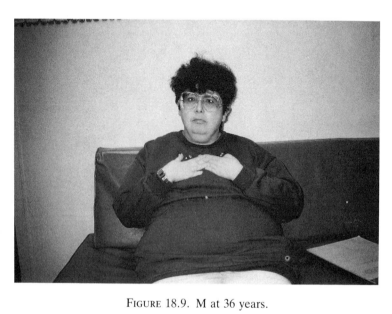

FIGURE 18.9. M at 36 years.

courses in computer science, mathematics, and grammar. She is able to apply these skills as an editor of her day-care center's monthly newspaper and to perform other computer tasks in the center's office. She is considerably more socially active. M. has also attained levels of independence that has enabled her to fly alone from her PWS group residence to her parents' home in another state, although once she lost her airplane ticket and on a very early trip, bought and ate approximately 25 large chocolate candy bars (since that trip, she travels without money) (Figure 18.9).

M. has had significant weight fluctuations since 1986, when she weighed 115 lbs. Her highest weight since then was 145 lbs. in early 1993. Considering her weight of 288 lbs. at the age of 23, a loss of 143 lbs. over 13 years is most encouraging. In December 1993, when she weighed 137 lbs., we felt very optimistic. We have noticed a great difference on her home visits, in regard to food. Prior to the last 7 or 8 months, M. would take an inventory of what food we had in the refrigerator, freezer, and cabinets. Presently, this is not her concern. Perhaps this is because we keep only a minimum amount of food in the house but have a good supply of low-calorie fruit and vegetables available. After her visit during Thanksgiving, she returned to the group home weighing the same as when she left and, in fact, no weight gain has been noted after the last few home visits. It seems that her obsession over food is somewhat diminished and her control of her weight is more of an issue. Essentially, she has neither gained nor lost much weight since mid 1993. She has been on a 900 calorie diet since she moved into her current PWS residence.

Four years later, 130 pounds less and over $600,000 in medical costs, our daughter entered a PWS group home. It seems that over the years we were misguided and misinformed, which led to much confusion as to how to approach her eating habits and cope with her temper tantrums. We had many family problems, many debates, and heated discussions and the situation created more disorganization in the family. Our other three children, all older than M, would get upset because we could not control her. The fact that our family is very close and religious no doubt pulled us through some difficult periods. Because she had not been diagnosed for so many years, our financial cost has been nearly $1 million, most of which, fortunately, was covered by personal medical insurance. But, as parents we also shouldered a large share. Our health suffered. In addition to high blood pressure, we were depressed, nervous, upset, confused, disappointed, and just plain angry. All three of us struggled . . . but all three of us never gave up. Now although some problems remain, the past few years have been pretty good. May it continue.

Summary

It is clear from this case history that delay in diagnosis caused many years of physical and emotional suffering for both M. and her family. Despite having many of the clinical characteristics of PWS, one major issue that significantly delayed and complicated her diagnosis was her level of cognition as indicated by her high IQ score. Her verbal score was 102 and full scale IQ was 99.

The medical community and allied health professionals can benefit by becoming familiar with the characteristics of PWS when confronted with the signs and symptoms suggestive of this disorder. Certainly, earlier identification is now a realistic expectation; it can lead to longer and more healthy lives for affected individuals and more stable family life for all concerned. This is a chronology of hope and M. is doing her best to persevere.

Reference

Prader, A., Labhart, A., & Willi, H. (1956). Ein Syndrom von Adipositas, Kleinwuchs, Kryptorchismus and Oligophrenie nach Mytonicartigem Zustand in Neugeborenalter. *Schweizerische Medizinische Wochenschrift*, *86*, 1260–1261.

19
Two Families' Points of View[1]

JANALEE TOMASESKI-HEINEMANN, AL HEINEMANN,
and LINDA THORNTON

Growing up with Matt: Janalee Tomaseski-Heinemann and Al Heinemann

Janalee

"Prader-Willi syndrome—what's that?" I asked, as most people do, when I met my husband-to-be, Al. At that time he was raising his 6-year-old daughter Sarah and 7-year-old son Matt, who has the syndrome. As a social worker who raised three children of my own, I thought I knew a lot about child rearing. However, as my relationship with Al grew, I decided to research PWS before making a commitment to marriage. Although I read some articles dealing with the syndrome's diagnosis and physical aspects, I discovered that the realities and impact of Prader–Willi syndrome could not be comprehended until I actually lived with it.

Al

"I am slowly losing the fight to PWS" I thought, when I first told Janalee about my son Matt. But I couldn't admit it out loud. Raising my children alone, each day that I struggled to get Matt to and from day care typically there was a tantrum to deal with. Then, in the evening, I would have to deal with a verbal barrage as I weighed out his strict food portions from his Weight Watcher diet. Then later, when I was exhausted and would fall asleep, Matt would make his night raids on the kitchen."

---

[1] *Editor's note:* The first edition of this book included a personalized chapter, written by a parent, that was well received. This chapter is an update by both parents of this same young man, followed by a touching essay by a young mother of a lovely little girl who lives in New Zealand.

Janalee and Al

We have been married over 11 years now and have survived as individuals and as a family, despite the frustrations and tears associated with Matt's diet restrictions and behavior problems. In fact, we have done more than survive . . . we have loved and laughed and grown a lot. Matt is now over 20 years old and lives in a supported living home with two other young men with the syndrome. How have we endured? Well, our solutions will not guarantee complete success nor do they follow the book on discipline, but they represent our point of view about living with a child with PWS. And, if some of our commentary seems disjointed, it's probably because, from time to time, so are our lives.

Matt was diagnosed at 3 months of age, only because our pediatrician knew Dr. Hans Zellweger, one of the few experts familiar with the syndrome. A diagnosis was provided, but no information about how to deal with it. In that first year, the biggest concern was getting Matt to eat. There was no way to possibly comprehend what a major struggle we would have in a few short years to get him to stop eating!

At 8 years of age (Figure 19.1), Matt weighed 108 pounds and had daily temper tantrums. Our goal was to get him down to a "husky" size. It was beyond our wildest dreams to think that by age 20 he would be a

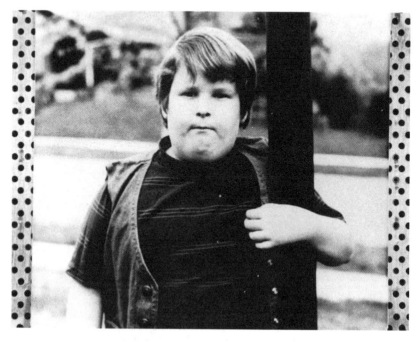

FIGURE 19.1. Matt at age 7, before his weight loss.

slim 145 pounds thanks to locks on the kitchen, family vigilance, and learning about the syndrome. What we did not know early on was that due to the administration of growth hormone, Matt would grow to 5′10″ tall and be able to eat a more normal diet. Also, older psychotropic medications were not considered (Figure 19.2) effective, but now Matt is on new medication that makes him less likely to become upset or perserverate.

When we attended our first national conference, it appeared that every child, teen, and adult was short, obese, and had behavioral problems. At that time we could not see beyond our fears, but over the years, by trial

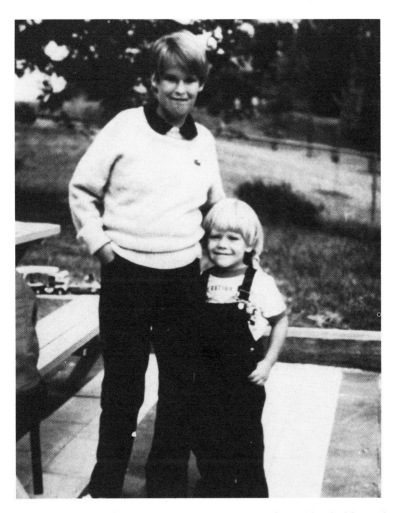

FIGURE 19.2. Matt at age 12, after his weight loss (with him is his nephew, Mikey).

and error, we created some guidelines for food and behaviors that seem to work for us even as he has grown older.

PWS Diet Secrets (for Adults Only)

Al

When I was raising the kids alone, I attempted many diets for Matt with no success. There was always an angry struggle because Matt had to eat differently from Sarah and me and he could never have his favorite foods. "Giving in," plus the fine art of sneaking food, made all his lettuce salads a futile effort to control his weight.

Janalee and Al

Heading a long list of concerns that parents of children with PWS must confront are the issues of food and eating. As parents we recognize that Matt constantly lives in an unfair situation, so we do what we can to make him feel that he is being treated more fairly. Anyone who has lived with a child with PWS knows that when it comes to food, this battle cannot always be won. The good news is that Matt did lose 32 pounds in one year and his weight has remained under control. Although we don't disagree with the dietary guidelines from nutritionists and physicians, it is another issue to live with their recommended restrictions. Our secret is to try to be a little smarter, more alert, and occasionally more devious than he is. Here is our very personal and a bit off beat advice that reduced some grief and aggravation associated with food when Matt was still living at home.

Lock away Temptation

It would have been hard to convince us before, but the pain of putting locks on the refrigerator and cupboards was our heartache, not Matt's. He not only seemed to understand, but also seemed relieved that the responsibility for not sneaking food had been taken from him since he had no control. As he said to us, "I try not to sneak but my hand reaches in the refrigerator and I can't stop it."

The Fine Art of Sneaking

Even if children with PWS have to live in an unfair world, why rub their noses in this inequity? We were appalled to read about behavior management of adolescents with PWS who were allowed to eat only half the food on their plate, had to leave the other half in front of them, and were punished if they touched it. (Perhaps we should also try electric cattle prods on the refrigerator!) Since we are fortunate enough to be able to eat more than Matt, we figure the least we can do is to be discreet.

Sneaky is another work for it! When Matt still lived at home, Sarah was allowed snacks and extra treats, but only if she asked for them out of sight and sound of her brother. This allowed her the same liberty as her peers and Matt was no worse off for what he didn't know. Perhaps when Sarah gets married, her husband will have a difficult time understanding why she prefers to eat behind the bedroom door. As for the two of us, when Matt was still living at home, we had a "stash drawer" and locked ourselves in the bedroom—for more than sex.

The Hand Is Quicker Than the Eye

Matt was not allowed to fix his own food, dish out his own plate, or hover in the kitchen while meals were being prepared. At first he was unhappy at not being able to "help out" in the kitchen (after all, he says, his goal in life is to be a cook, chef, or baker), but he finally learned to accept this rule. Thus he wasn't as aware of when we skimped on his food and we didn't have to worry about whether his hand was quicker that our eyes.

Dinner Time Drama

Serving food can be a fine art. We quit kidding ourselves long ago about emulating the ideal American family at the dinner table. Matt and Sarah were allowed to eat in front of the TV and their food was set up on trays, which solved several problems. Matt was less aware of who got what portion, watching TV reduced his obsession with keeping his eye on the food, and food was served out of pans directly onto plates, reducing dirty dishes (an extra bonus). Best of all, we had a chance to sit down to a peaceful meal and conversation and didn't have to guard the dinner table.

Garnishing the Garnish

Food preparation requires visual skills along with the usual nutritional advice. Matt ate the same food we did but his portions were smaller. A smaller plate and cup were used and the food was spread out on the dish. Extra nonfattening food items such as carrots, dill pickles, or diet jello were added to make the amount on the plate look larger. Since he would get only one-half a banana or apple, it was cut up into slices and served in a bowl to make it less obvious that it was only half a serving. Less visible foods were skipped (i.e., butter or mayonnaise on sandwiches, and potatoes). As a finishing touch Matt began with a bit smaller portion so that he could come back for one more spoonful.

Surviving the Cafeteria

Packing a diet lunch for school is an unrewarding chore we learned to avoid. Matt was allowed to buy the hot lunch and skip one fattening item on the menu (e.g., the french fries or the dessert). The item skipped was his choice, providing it was not the salad. He received great praise from his teacher, who monitored his choice. Of course, this meant nothing if he sneaked leftovers or snacks from the other students. The teacher explained to Matt's classmates that it was important for his health not to give him any of their food. We kept in close touch with the school, his teacher, and the cooks, to see that he was supervised in the lunchroom. We constantly reminded all school personnel that although he appeared to have control over his diet, his hand was no doubt quicker than all of their eyes.

The Payoff—Self-Pride

Children with PWS vary as to how much they can eat and not gain weight. Also, it is very hard to regulate every calorie consumed. Our solution was to have a chart on the refrigerator to record a daily weigh-in. Initially, when he was quite young and would lose 2 pounds, he was rewarded with a small toy. Later we were able to eliminate the reward because Matt seemed to get enough self-satisfaction from his weight loss to want to continue. With a total lack of modesty, and beaming with pride, he would say, "I think I world's champion weight loser!"

Love Means Saying "No"

All of the hard work of weight control will be to no avail if relatives, friends, or babysitters are feeding your child behind your back. People who really care about you and your child will not sabotage your efforts. Parents do not have to apologize when requesting that no treats be given. In fairness to others, however, education is necessary. This may mean swallowing one's pride and explaining PWS in detail, with all its "do's and don'ts." At first it was hard for me (Al) to admit the extent of Matt's problems. Also, it's confusing for the child with PWS to have Grandma (or heaven forbid, Daddy) slip him a treat while Mommy always says, "No!" When the child is treated with consistency, there is no "good guy" or "bad guy." We try to help Matt understand that we are truly sorry that he is always hungry and frustrated, and it seems that he is learning that "no" can still be a loving word.

Behaviors: What Seems to Work for Us

Janalee and Al

When it comes to dealing with behaviors, rule number one is "don't wait for experts to help, you may be it." There is no magic person out there with all the answers. In other words, when you think your boat is sinking, don't wait for professionals to tell you how to handle everything, just grab a bucket and bail. Learn about PWS. Don't close your ears to these experts, just sift through and weigh what they say and see how it fits your needs. (That goes for all this advice as well.) And, by the way . . . if you are beginning to feel like a drill sergeant in the Marines, try to remember that caring and loving need to remain a part of all this. Otherwise guidelines for managing behavior won't mean a thing.

Set the Rules, Explain the Options, and Rehearse

Your child needs to know exactly what the limitations are and what will happen when he does well or if he "blows it." Spell out guidelines for eating and behavior before going anywhere. It used to be impossible to go to a restaurant with Matt without having him push for extra food and having a tantrum when he didn't get it. Now, before we go he is told exactly what he can order and is cautioned that he'll get no more. Though no longer necessary, there was a time when he had to be reminded that if he got upset or pressured us, one of would immediately get up and leave with him, that he'd get no bedtime treat, and would not be allowed to go the next time. This system not only spelled out the rules but also helped us avoid being trapped in an emotional situation. Eventually, Matt was even able to handle a Thanksgiving visit with all the relatives with no upsets or pushing for extra food, a feat we thought beyond our dreams.

Consistency (That Evil Word) and Vigilance

Time and time again the importance of being consistent is emphasized. The bad news is . . . it works! This is because PWS is similar to other organic brain conditions where affected individuals lack the capacity to "reason out" consequences for behaviors. They thrive on routines and guidelines and lack the flexibility to manage exceptions to established patterns. One day of extra food privileges creates days of grief before Matt is back on track. The real challenge is getting *both* parents to be consistent, because behavior management is not a part-time, once learned task.

Rewards: There Are Good Days

There is conflicting advice on whether to use food as a reinforcement. One concern is that the use of food as a reward may encourage even more of an obsession. Tell us . . . how can a child with PWS become even more obsessed about food than he already is? Matt thinks, talks, and dreams food 24 hours a day. We can be driving on a long trip and talking continuously with Matt sound asleep in the back seat. Mention the word "pizza" and he will immediately sit straight up with his eyes wide open and say, "Pizza? Who say that?" The fact is that for us, using food as a reward has worked. Of course, the food reward is minimal. When younger, if Matt was good all day, he would get a small piece of candy as a bedtime treat, but supper would have fewer calories to compensate. On the other hand, a nonfood reward system was used to deal with Matt's "crying behavior" at school. We arranged for his teacher to send us daily "good day" or "bad day" reports. When he collected five "good days" in a row, or 10 cumulatively, he could buy a small toy. Gradually, as he gained more control, the reward was reduced and then eliminated.

Punishment (Time Out for Both Sides)

Because we are heavily into talking problems out with the kids, it took a while for us to learn to keep our mouths shut. Talking things out with a child with PWS *does not work*! This makes more sense to us as we have learned more about problems associated with brain dysfunction. We mentioned earlier that children with PWS don't think abstractly and have trouble experiencing one situation and generalizing it to others. They also have trouble separating important details from less important ones. To them, all issues are critical; they "get stuck" on one concern and cannot go on to the next. Add to this impaired thinking a desperate hunger and emotional "ups and downs" and the stage is set for a large blow-up! We cannot express strongly enough the importance of defusing a situation early and not wasting energy on confrontations, logic, or threats. When still living at home, the minute Matt got upset, he was immediately sent to his room. We tried to stay low-keyed and firm. He was allowed to come out as soon as he was "feeling better." Even now, if he can talk calmly, the problem is discussed. We refrain from harping. Mind you, this approach didn't come about easily. At first, when Matt was sent to his room, he would kick, scream, and tear it apart. The consequences of this behavior were that anything he wrecked was removed permanently from the room and not repaired. If the situation became too intense, one of us would go in and calmly say, "You have five minutes to settle down Matt, and if you haven't done so by then, you will only get a small sandwich for supper." As his room became barren, even of his furniture, he improved and lost a few extra pounds in the process. This tactic was effective at the time. Although totally eliminating a meal is not recommended, delaying and/or cutting back on a quantity is a strong motivator. The good news is that we discovered Matt had more control over these tantrums than we thought he could have.

Don't Set Yourself up

We are painfully aware of the difficulties involved with the suggestions for behavioral change just described. But keep in mind that other alternatives may be even more painful. While you and your child are in the initial stage of deciding who's boss, try to reduce the number of awkward situations in which you unwittingly find yourself. For example, attending a buffet dinner is looking for trouble and going to the supermarket isn't much better. Situations always come up that other people simply will never understand. Once, when Matt was alone in the mixed candy aisle at the grocery store, I (Janalee) must have given him "the eye" because he immediately exclaimed, "I didn't take any Mom, see!"—and pulled his pockets inside out as proof. Some customers looked with pity at Matt and glared at me. I slunk away.

Use Positive Reinforcement

Although there is plenty to criticize, look hard for opportunities to make positive comments. Matt usually thrives on compliments. This same young man who can feel so bad about himself at times, can also be bursting with self-pride. If we can't say anything good, we don't say anything. Fortunately, his teachers also used this approach. For a long time Matt's behavior and weight seemed to us and to him to be totally out of hand. But then he learned to have some control. One day, he came home all excited from school and said, "You know what? I almost have a bad day. Tears started to come out of my eyes, but I say, stop it! stop it!, and the tears stopped!" Later he said, "I'm so proud of me!" That's a whole lot more important than us being proud of him.

Set Rules Out of Love

Being tough on a child already struggling in life is painful. We have often said that when a child can have so few pleasures in life, it's hard to take away what makes him most happy, even if it's not in his interest. I (Al) in particular struggle with these food and behavior issues, but can see how much happier Matt is when his weight and behavior are under control. The fact that Matt's self-concept improved has been our most important reinforcement. No matter how hard it may be to achieve, our ultimate goal is that he will be able to socialize and "fit in" as much as possible, in spite of his special needs. As Matt has said, "When you're fat and mad, you feel sad." An obese, angry, lonely child cannot grow up to be a happy adult. Being tough is difficult but the consequences of not being so are even tougher.

Listen Beyond the Tantrum

When a child with PWS is screaming, crying, swearing, swinging his arms, and telling you he hates you, it is hard to listen and to feel anything but anger. Understanding the speech of a PWS child is often difficult and when the child is out of control, the tendency is to repeat the same words and thoughts over and over. It is as if Matt's foot is stuck on the accelerator of his rage at 100 miles an hour and he cannot let up until he crashes. At that point, who wants to listen to what he is saying? I (Al) have said that during the first moments of a tantrum, it would save a lot of grief if we had a special kind of spray to squirt in his face that would make him fall asleep instantly. During one tantrum, Matt said he hated us for "studying about Prader–Willi." He swore, tore the heads off flowers in the yard, cried, and hollered in his bedroom for 2 hours, then fell asleep. When he woke up, he was contrite and quiet, played patiently for hours with our grandson, and thoroughly enjoyed swimming in the pool with his older brother, Tad. The Prader–Willi "demon" had passed and hopefully would stay out of Matt's soul for awhile. An apologetic note that Matt wrote after a major tantrum (we rate them major, minor, and crying spells) is illustrated (Figure 19.3).

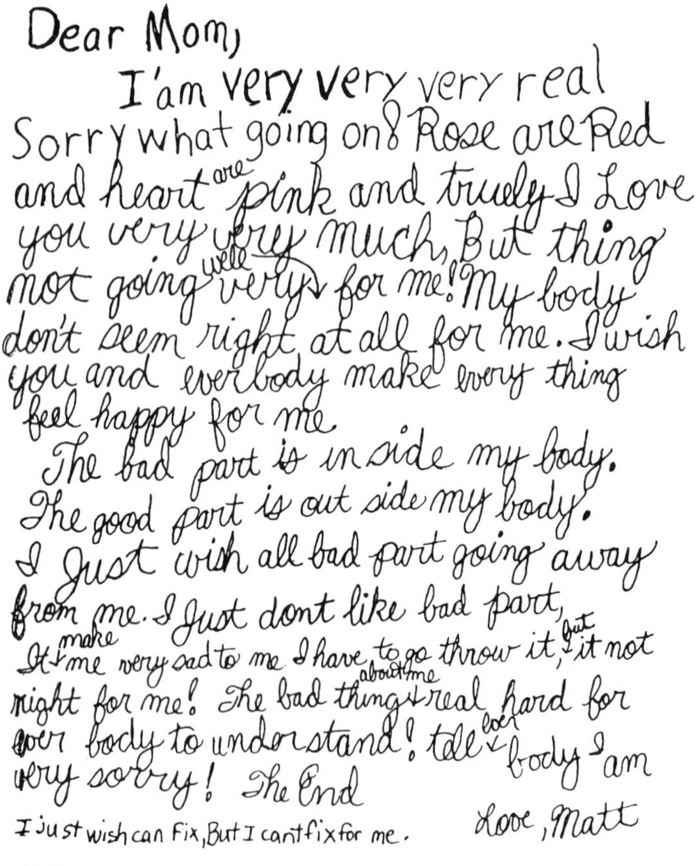

FIGURE 19.3.

Maybe we don't want to hear "beyond the tantrum" for fear of the pain we might see. In a recent crying spell, the lowest rating on the tantrum scale, we worked very hard to hear what Matt had to say. Matt tends to fixate on an issue for a while, then changes topics, but mostly his thoughts deal with the unfairness of having PWS. Once, after finding an article on PWS, he said that when he sees something written about PWS, it reminds him that he has "it," and said.

it goes over and over in my brain. I can't help read about it because I curious. It [the written information] say I always be short and I never [have sex . . . it say I never be normal. It hurt in my heart and in my head . . . It say about what between my legs [small penis and undescended testicles]. I never have a girlfriend. I be embarrassed she see me. It say I die before I get old . . . I think about food all the time. [When] I see food I can't have, I feel anxious. I want it real bad and it make me mad. . . . You don't know what it's like. You don't know what I feel!

We often wonder how much of Matt's rage is due to a chemical/ neurological dysfunction and how much is justified anger at the world. Being aware of his tortured mind is sometimes more than we (or he) can bear. You're right Matt, we don't know what it's like. If we let ourselves feel what you feel, we wouldn't be strong enough to lift you up when it was over, give you a hug, and say, "Let's go on from here."

The Teen Years

How do you keep a teenager from walking to a McDonald's that is just five blocks from home? Keeping Matt from finding extra food became even a greater challenge and, typical of teenagers with PWS, behavior problems certainly seemed to accelerate. But the struggles go far beyond dealing with food issues and temper tantrums.

There was the Matt who wanted desperately to learn to drive. He faithfully studied the "rules of the road," book then had to come to grips with the fact that his younger sister got her license and he could not. There was the Matt that wanted to be independent, take care of himself, and make money, who had to deal with rejection after rejection, after spending hours circling job wanted ads and making calls. There was the Matt who thought Richard was his "best friend in the whole world" and then sadly discovered that Richard, who did get his license and a job, said he was embarrassed by Matt and wanted nothing to do with him anymore. There was the Matt who wanted a girlfriend, but unfortunately longed for a "normal" one and just ended up looking at the girls longingly. He tried to be cool, flirted a bit, and dreamed.

There was the Matt, who as a teenager, wanted very much to be "cool," but didn't quite know how. He would ask his sister, Sarah, her advice about clothes, then not follow it. He would buy popular tapes yet never play them. He tried hard to walk, talk, and joke like a teen, but could never quite pull it off. There was the Matt who registered to vote so he could assume some political respnsibility. He studied the issues seriously and came to his own conclusions on how to save the world from crime and corruption. Some of his thoughts were rather profound and others were "out in left field." For example, he thought we should ban people from wearing shoes, because he thought drug dealers hid drugs in shoes!

There was the Matt who searched for a relationship with God and tried hard to figure out how to deal with good and evil. In some of the notes he gave us, he wrote,

I have a lot of questions to ask Jesus. . . . Did God make desserts?. . . . Did God make growth hormones?. . . . Is it a sin to pick?. . . . I want to wear clothes in heaven. [he worries about being seen naked]. . . . Tad [Matt's older step-brother] is always right about God and Jesus. I should listen to him. I always mess up. Maybe Tad should be God. . . . I want to be happy. . . . I don't want to do wrong things. . . . I'm thinking if I don't have a girlfriend or not get married, I pray I have one in heaven.

We think there are two very different parts to Matt and that if it is difficult for parents and caregivers to accept, how much more of a challenge it must be for an outsider to understand. The same Matt who cut up all his new clothes, also graciously thanked us for buying him a shirt. The Matt that can spew verbal abuse for hours during a tantrum will also tell us how much he loves us and hugs us goodnight. The Matt who can embarrass us to tears by creating a scene at one time may surprise us by being exceptionally charming and polite at the next event.

Which is the real Matt? We think it's the loving, gentle side that struggles in an unfair world of things beyond his reach. His teen years accentuated his dilemma. Matt hates the other side as much as we do. As he once wrote, "I just wish can fix, but can't fix for me." Someday we hope "it" can be fixed for Matt and all people with PWS.

The images of chained refrigerators and destructive temper tantrums tend to overshadow the gentler, sensitive side of our children. But the warmth that we know is there reminds us of how much we love them—and sometimes breaks our hearts. We watched out teenage son trying his very best to be a good person and find his place in the world while struggling against incredible odds. Unfortunately, because the kindness and love these young people often display are not actions that grab media attention or help get residential programs approved, we parents have to focus on the traumas arising from the more bizarre characteristics of PWS in order to get the services so desperately needed.

The Adult Years

Janalee and Al

When Matt no longer fit into the school system and our other children were not around to help keep an eye on him, how to care for Matt became a major issue. We began a two year battle to get a supportive living program opened. In the interim, we converted our home to meet his needs.

Our split-level home has sliding glass doors both on the top deck and on the bottom level that lead to the backyard and pool. Inside, we enclosed the stairway and made the lower level a separate (and temporary) apartment for Matt where he had his own access to the outdoors. He had his own bedroom, living room, bathroom, and phone line (with no long distance access) so could call us upstairs. Flip locks were installed on the inside door to prevent him from coming upstairs but allowed us to open it up at times. He had a small refrigerator for diet soda and could all us to check on meal times, which he did often. One weekend when all of us except Matt were gone, a friend stayed at the house. Because we forgot to forewarn her, she was awakened every hour starting at 4:00 AM by Matt asking, "Is it breakfast time yet?" We forgot to tell her that Matt must be told that "tomorrow is Saturday and we are sleeping in, so don't you *dare* call before 9:00"!

The "voice from below" became a source of irritation or humor—depending on what mood Matt or we were in. Our "tenant" would call and say, "I smell popcorn"? or "I hear Dad say, 'canned food'?" There were embarrassing moments too. Sarah brought a new boyfriend home to meet us and suddenly a voice from below said, "Can I come up?" When we went and flipped the lock, Matt came bouncing upstairs and hugged the young man with his elbows (he kept his hands in the air because he had been picking his fingernails and they were bleeding) and asked him, "Are you an Indian?" Sarah's boyfriends either came with a sense of humor—or left quickly!

Although Matt's life was "on hold" during this time, he was content. Matt would sleep all morning and then a respite provider would come at noon and take him out to lunch, after which they would go to the museum, zoo, show, or wherever Matt chose to go. We tried leaving his lunch in his refrigerator, but found that he would eat it five minutes after we left for work in the morning. The only productive activity he had was watering the plants in the back yard and cleaning his room under our supervision twice a week. Of course, he would stay up at night since he slept all morning, but usually after we went to bed he was content to watch TV, play Nintendo, or pick his nails and skin. Because of the complete lack of expectations from Matt, this was a quiet period and he seldom really "lost it." However, during one of those weeks when Matt was being lovable and profound, we got a call at 2:15 AM from a neighbor girl who said in a shaky voice, "Mrs. Heinemann? There is someone in your back yard hollering and talking to God." We looked at each other and our hearts sank. We threw on our robes and went outside where Matt was illuminated by the security light on the patio, waving his arms and hollering, "God! You need to help your son, Jesus. He's in trouble!" We convinced Matt that if he was worried about Jesus, he could pray quietly to God and God would hear him and that he was scaring the neighbors. We knew enough to not try to convince him Jesus was not in trouble. This was one of several brief episodes where Matt appeared delusional.

Moving Out

Janalee and Al

Matt had mixed feelings about moving out of our home. When he was younger, he knew we were involved in developing group homes for older persons, but he was bound and determined that he would never live in one. However, we were able to convince him that in a supported living program he could begin a new life where he could be more grown up and independent.

The agency that would be running the home included Matt in the planning stages and he wasn't about to let them pull anything over on him. He had 12 pages of questions for their first meeting. Typical of Matt, some of them were very perceptive, and some were very bizarre. The day the worker came to meet and interview Matt and us at our home happened to be one of his good days and some of his comments were,

I like to go to dance. . . . I stand by the food table—when a hot chick come along, I look at the food. . . . I look at the chick. . . . I look at the food again and I decide to go for the chick. . . . I believe God can make miracles and I can have a baby. . . . Life is complicated and confusing. . . . Two things you have to do in life—accept Jesus and accept yourself. . . . I think the world is funny and stupid and sad.

Unfortunately, the week that Matt and his two housemates, Timmy and Robert, were to move into the house, we got word that the neighbors were attempting to stop their move. This was particularly touching because Matt had just told us he would like to have a block party and invite all the neighbors to socialize and talk about keeping drugs out and protecting the neighborhood from crime. We explained the problem to him as best we could, but then the next night we overheard him saying in a phone conversation with his brother, "Hey, Tad, the neighbors scared of me that I'm moving in. I don't know why." Our hearts broke for the thousandth time.

Moving In

Janalee and Al

At the age of 19 years Matt moved into a beautiful red brick home in a suburb of St. Louis. He was a slim 135 pounds and stood 5'–10" tall thanks to growth hormones. The house was completely furnished with all new furniture and the necessary housekeeping items. His room was beautifully decorated with a display of his nice rock collection. We purchased him a new combination TV/VCR and set up his computer with Super Nintendo. All his clothes were placed neatly on the shelves, and several pictures were on his dresser. When we left, he was excited and hugged us good-bye several times.

Two days later the phone calls started. Matt was unhappy with the meals and the rules of the house. His behavior accelerated to the point where the police were called one night after he broke a window in his bedroom. At that time, the philosophy of the provider group managing the home was that Matt's things were his property and they would not stop him if he destroyed them. So, 2 weeks after we hugged him good-bye and breathed a sigh of relief, we walked back into a room that looked like it had been hit with a bomb. His new TV/VCR was destroyed, his computer broken, his furniture smashed, radio and tapes ruined, along with everything else except a silk plant on the top shelf. A relationship with a person with Prader–Willi syndrome is like being on a perpetual roller coaster, and we had just dropped to the bottom of the track at 100 miles per hour. As we cleaned up broken pieces of glass and pieces of wood that were once his drawers, all we could say over and over was, "How could you do this, Matt?" We were too stunned and devastated to even sound mad.

The next day a meeting was held with all the staff and Matt was included. We sat dumbfounded as all of the professionals from various disciplines carefully weighed each word they spoke for fear of setting Matt off. As the meeting progressed and Matt laid down all of his unrealistic demands, they appeared totally intimidated by him and he knew it. We didn't say much during the meeting but on the drive home we came to our senses, turned the car around, and went back. We took Matt into his room and chewed him out royally for destroying all of his things, then packed up the few usable things remaining and said we were taking them home until he could act like a decent human being. We also told him we would not take him anywhere until he could prove he could act appropriately at the house for at least 2 weeks. After we left we looked at each other and A1 said, "I still can't get over how satisfying that felt." We didn't agonize over hurting Matt's psyche either. We just took the reins of control again as parents and prayed the house staff would soon learn how to do that themselves—for all of our sakes.

And Life Goes On

Janalee and Al

Over the time that Matt has been living in this supportive living program, we have come to realize that the issues associated with PWS never are totally eliminated from our lives. Rather, for us, it merely means that the presence of the syndrome is no longer all consuming. Dealing with it intermittently gives us a new appreciation of just how frustrating and puzzling it can be at times.

Most of our visits with Matt have been positive and he is often sweet on the phone, but there are times he can still cause turmoil in our lives. For example, we took a trip one summer weekend to a family wedding. Our traveling companions were Matt and our two grandsons.

The first issue we had to deal with before we even left town had to do with Matt's attire. In his house Matt is given more freedom to decide what he wants to wear than what we allowed while he lived with us. Our point of view is that if he wants to be treated as normal, he must look normal. In anticipation of this trip, a special effort was made to tell staff that Matt would need appropriate clothes. We cringed when Matt walked out wearing white shorts, red and blue socks with Christmas trees on them, a wrinkled green tee-shirt, and carrying his winter jacket over his shoulder. He added an extra flair to his appearance by havng shaved the sides of his head with his electric shaver. Al leaned over and whispered, "Cool misses Matt by a mile." His suitcase and bag had what seemed like a year's worth of clothing stuffed into them. Our first challenge was to get him to change his outfit and leave three-fourths of what he had packed behind. Fortunately he was so eager to go that the necessary changes went better than expected.

The trip went smoothly until wedding reception time where, as expected, food was an issue. Problems developed because we tried to allow Matt some independence. We let him roam on his own at the reception hall after the food was cleared from the tables. What we didn't know was that food was still accessible and that Matt made many clandestine trips to the kitchen, then slipped out the back door. We were embarrassed because we had let down our guard and also disappointed that none of the relatives who saw Matt sneak the food bothered to alert us. Actually, we were oblivious to all his sneaking and had a wonderful evening dancing and visiting while Matt had a great evening stuffing himself.

The next morning an irritable Matt pushed for more food at breakfast. Due to Matt's testy mood, and the severe gas he had from eating all the food the night before at the wedding reception, the eight and a half hour drive home was a real "treat." We used an old ploy and had him sit in the back seat of the van where we could pretend not to hear him, but we couldn't avoid his odor. Matt continued to be pushy and argumentative about food all day but managed to keep his composure in front of his nephews. Interestingly, he seems to have the ability to control himself enough not to "loose it" in front of them. However, when we got close to home, Matt did get on the car phone and talked the staff into having a second supper ready for him when he returned. We called them back and explained that he had already eaten. Once Matt got into his house and his nephews were back in the van, he unleashed a verbal barrage toward the staff and us as we walked out the door. The difference now is that we could shut the door behind us on the torrent of abusive ranting and raving that was likely to last all evening. God bless the staff for being there in our place. We pray every day for their health, understanding, and fortitude.

Overall, we have found that if given too much latitude with his eating, Matt only presses for more. Once, at another party when Matt was very slim and doing exceptionally well on his diet, we decided this just this once we would give him free reign to eat with the only restriction being that he drink the diet soda we had brought (Matt had never been allowed regular soda pop). Unfortunately, having access to more food than ever before was not enough. He insisted that he was not going to drink the diet soda, got upset, hollered, and took off down the street. We left the party having learned the lesson that small, limited, prearranged diet exceptions work out as a special treat, but too much freedom seems to have a negative impact.

A Word about Siblings

Janalee and Al

Normal brothers and sisters of children with PWS are like siblings of children with other developmental disabilities and their actions and reactions are almost always age-related. These sibling issues are not discussed to attach more guilt to parents but to emphasize that, as with other disabilities, PWS does have an impact on other children in the family and that their lives will be both enriched and marred. They are entitled to their faults and feelings. They feel resentment, guilt, love, jealousy, anger, compassion, embarrassment, and loneliness. They fear isolation and worry that PWS may be catching or inherited. They wonder if their parents love their disabled sibling "more" and even feign illness to get attention. Our objective is to emphasize the importance of nurturing the positive effects and minimizing the negatives of the presence of PWS.

When Matt's sister Sarah was asked if any of her "feelings" had been overlooked, she said that sometimes she just felt downright miserable. But at the same time she became very protective. Among some old mementos we found a Christmas card that Sarah wrote when she was a third grader. Included in the card was a list of jobs she would perform as a gift to us. And, along with the usual "I will clean my room and I will take Lambi [our dog] for a daily walk," was "I will help when Matt has a tantrum." What seemed like a normal life to Sarah, at that time, was really far from that of the average 8 year old. By the time she was 12, she became even more aware of and sensitive to what her peers considered as OK or not OK. She really wanted to be just like all the other kids, but when the refrigerator and cupboards were locked and her brother would act "weird," she was embarrassed and uncomfortable. She once mentioned an incident where the Special Education Bus passed by and some boys began to mock and make fun of the special ed. children. Sarah said "I was mad at them and wanted to tell them, 'Stop! How would you feel if someone did that to you?' But, I didn't because I was afraid they would turn on me and make fun of me because of Matt."

As a lovely, young woman, Sarah now looks back on her life with Matt and exclaims, "What an experience! I often think of the times as a child when I ate cookies in my closet after Matt went to bed. How normal that seemed to me then. Now that I'm older, I realize what a strange life we led. Matt's syndrome engulfed much of my life." Sarah speaks of the need she felt to shelter Matt from the real world that was so cold to special people. She says, "We all tried to protect him from the harsh realities of his limitations, so Matt exists in an unrealistic world that we helped create. He desperately wants to be a normal person. What he doesn't realize is that normal people aren't as cool as he thinks they are and that many would be cruel and vicious to him. Yet he continues to live on the fringe of their world, longing to be part of it."

Does a Disabled Child Mean a Disabled Marriage?

Janalee and Al

"Don't let one tragedy multiply into others!" This remark was part of a speech given at a genetics conference. The point was that when other life stressors can be reduced and a good support system exists, coping with a child's disability will be less difficult. Unfortunately, a "domino effect" can begin when a child with a disability is born. Over time, the personal trauma to each parent, stress in the marital relationship, and an on-going state of anxiety and tension lead to shattered relationships and a dysfunctional family system. We have created our own techniques for survival as a couple.

We absolved ourselves of guilt. We recognize that we are not only parents but have a right to our own lives. We struggle with on-going stress and need to replenish our strengths. In other words, we "make time" not "find time." With other children, a large extended family, full time work, plus volunteering, we have had to be conscientious about prioritizing our time. The car may not get waxed, the oven is seldom cleaned, and we watch little TV. Occasionally the rest of the family is ignored so we can have our personal time together. If we don't nuture ourselves as individuals and as a couple, we cannot joyfully give to our children.

We work hard to avoid taking our relationship for granted, knowing that it takes time and effort to keep it good. It is too easy to get wrapped up in Matt and let everyone and everything take second place. Besides prioritizing our time, we have made a pact never to go to bed angry. This may mean long, late night discussions, but little hurts can build into major problems if avoided (the alternative is to be in bad marriage and a bad marriage can be the loneliest place in the world).

We keep an eye on our stress factors. It helps to be able to identify them rather than just have vague uneasy feelings. Periodically, we take a look at what is stressing us. One year when we had any number of unforeseen crises, we were able to stand back and say, "No wonder we're feeling stressed!" When life is going more smoothly, we look back and realize that we are often uptight about minor issues that are just not worth the bother. We also savor the good times. It is too easy to get into an "ain't life awful" frame of mind and miss the pleasant things. Today is to be appreciated. Will that cleaning project be left undone on a beautiful day in order to take a walk in the woods with all the children? Can a favorite TV program be skipped for an hour in the bedroom where you can talk over the day? Sometimes we have to remind each other what we are thankful for. Of course this is easier to do when we are out to dinner alone while the children, the house, and the bills are miles away.

We have also discovered that getting physically active helps. We work out and swim and feel better when we do it on a regular basis. Admittedly, this is hard to fit into our busy lives. Once I (Janalee) was away from the health club so long, I forgot my locker combination. For us, "getting physical" also means making time for personal closeness and intimacy.

When life seems overwhelming and you are hurting for your child *and* for yourself, it is OK to let go. Take time to cry a little, laugh a lot, and be a bit crazy. Even in the worst of situations, events can be funny. What is so funny about PWS? Come to parent's meeting and listen to the anecdotes. Humor is an important tactic for survival.

There are choices to be made . . . we can wallow in self pity or pick ourselves up and make the best of a given situation. We are not here to suffer with our child but to accept the challenge to reach beyond the suffering. Our personal strengths and relationship can grow out of difficult situations. Having a child with PWS does not have to mean that a relationship will automatically deteriorate. It does mean that only a conscious and daily effort will keep it alive and whole. Like a beautiful garden, it takes daily attention. We have a favorite quote from an unknown author that says it all.

The most important thing a father can do for his children is to love their mother.

Coming Out of the Closet

Janalee and Al

People often say to us, "How do you deal with locks on your kitchen?" We have lived with PWS so long that we have almost forgotten how bizarre the syndrome must seem to others and what a difference it has made in the way we live. We also realize, like other parents dealing with PWS, that we have hidden our problems behind a well-developed facade. The true tragedy of PWS is that the serious behavior issues are often kept secret. Why? Perhaps we are ashamed. Perhaps we are afraid the behaviors will reflect on our ability to parent appropriately. So . . . we have decided to come out of the closet! We *know* that Matt's behavior problems are not the result of our lack of parenting skills; we feel we have done the right things. But we also have come to accept the fact that we can't solve all of the riddles associated with PWS behaviors.

The pain is still there . . . we sense it in other parents at local support group meetings and on a larger scale at national conferences. Some problems came "out-of-the-closet" at a meeting with professional providers who were talking about normalizing the environment and providing a home-like setting for persons with PWS. One parent described how she had to lock her 20-year-old son in the basement in order to keep him from running away and stealing food. Another said her daughter had broken all the windows in their home and attempted to put her hand down the garbage disposal when she was upset. We described an episode where Matt had cut up all his clothes, something we never dreamed he would do. Because of his child's behavior, one parent' desperate cry came across loud and clear. When asked what he would do if a group home wasn't started, he said, "I guess I would buy two guns, hand one to my wife and hope we have the nerve to pull the triggers at the same time." We could tell that the professionals were uncomfortable, but at least as parents, we had the courage to provide honest facts that gave a whole new meaning to the term normal.

Our message is not one of resignation, or we would have bought guns too. But, unless we are honest and come out of the closet, no one can help us reduce our personal nightmares. We are not ashamed and we don't feel guilty. We still believe in fighting for every ounce of control over the syndrome and in helping Matt to fight for every bit of control he can achieve. Like the other families dealing with PWS, despite our struggles, we have love, happiness, and many strengths.

Our Francie: A Younger Parent's Point of View: Linda Thornton

Francie is now in her twelfth year. She has been with us for nearly half of our married life. To me, this seems incredible! Looking back, these early years have been good. We enjoyed Francie as a baby and as a young child growing up (Figure 19.4). It really doesn't seem as if 11 years have passed, probably because she doesn't act that old. Some days are not so bad but some days there is a heavy weight on my heart as I contemplate the years to come. And there are always so many questions!

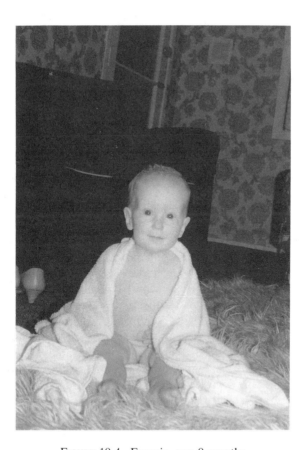

FIGURE 19.4. Francie, age 9-months.

What about Diagnosis?

Francie was not diagnosed until she was 3 years old, and only then because a friend gave me an Australian magazine article to read. It was all about a young teenager with something called "Prader–Willi syndrome." What struck me forcibly was the similarity in physical features between this person from another country and my own daughter. What terrified me was what these parents had been through. I survived the next 3 months by alternately not thinking about it and crying with rage and frustration. Everywhere I truned for help, there was none forthcoming. No one seemed to know about Prader–Willi syndrome. Our pediatrician did a blood test that came back normal. The advice that came with it was that I was an "overanxious mother" and to take things easy. This was not the sort of advice I needed—or perhaps it was. It made me determined to find out everything I could and to find a way to cope with what seemed at the time an insurmountable obstacle.

So, for a mother of a young child with what appeared to be an unknown illness that could possibly be something called Prader–Willi syndrome, what was I to do? First, it seemed, I should throw away any feeling of intimidation by medical professionals. Second, I should continue to ask, ask, ask. With a huge effort, I started. I asked my own general practitioner, I asked the speech therapist, the physiotherapist (all part of the Early Development Programme run here in New Zealand for preschool children with special or unidentified needs).

What about Support?

I asked anyone who would listen! Someone had seen an article and brought me the address of the PWS Association in the United States. I wrote and received the first understandable information I'd read. I decided for myself that Francie probably did have Prader–Willi syndrome and that I would follow up on four addresses in New Zealand that the American Association sent. How would I do this? I wrote to the IHC (New Zealand Society for the Intellectually Handicapped), wondering, since a low IQ was part of the syndrome, whether they could help. Daylight began to dawn for me and I was directed to the New Zealand Lottery Grants Board for financial help. I was able to visit the four families, all of whom had teenage boys. I saw firsthand the problems they were facing and I was devastated at the lack of information, support, and knowledge about this syndrome. Still reeling, I went back to the IHC and asked if I could set up a support group under their auspices. All this happened over 8 years ago and in 1989 the PWS Association (NZ) was formed. We started with five and now have 60 members.

What about Me? What about Our Family?

What about me, as a parent of a younger child with PWS? The first and most rapid thing that happened was that I developed a keen sense of trust in my own instincts. And, because I suddenly had to rely on myself, I had to become very strong. That strength has had to carry the rest of my family: a husband and two older daughters, and our wider family of grandparents, aunts and uncles, nieces and nephews. It has had to be maintained in order to carry over to the people Francie comes in contact with everyday, both friends and strangers. And it has taken a special strength to face all those professional people who obviously know more than I do about their own specialties but know nothing about Prader–Willi syndrome.

What a burden! And what a way to find out who your friends are! But we have come through and have completed this first decade. There have been times of pain and hurt, mostly felt by me, and also times of anger and frustration, mostly felt by the rest of family. Enormous sibling jealousy has emerged when acts of parenting are perceived as favoritism.

There was the time the lock went on the cupboard. I'd been thinking about this move for some time. In the end I went out and bought a lock and fixed it myself while the children were at school. Oldest daughter came home, shrieked with horror, and said she'd never invite anyone home any more. Middle daughter had exactly the same reaction, but it was accompanied by tears and rage. On the other hand, Francie, came home and said, "Oh! What a bright, shiny lock! Where did you get it? Did you put it on, Mum? Oh! You are clever!" Of course, she thinks the lock is there just as much for the benefit of her older sisters as for her. She even locks it and brings me the key. The whole scene completely took the wind from my sails.

What about School?

I remember the day I went to Francie's first school to interview the principal (Figure 19.5). I took with me someone from the Department of Special Education as support. I told the principal all I knew about Prader–Willi syndrome and the interview took an hour. As a new parent, I was determined the school should know everything. As it turned out, I needn't have worried. For a start, Francie simply didn't act the way the book said children with PWS would act because she was way too young. Her only "problem" was that she tended to fall asleep in the classroom. Her teachers loved her. She was monitored during lunch and play breaks and her first few years were quite innocuous. It did change, though. Slowly as

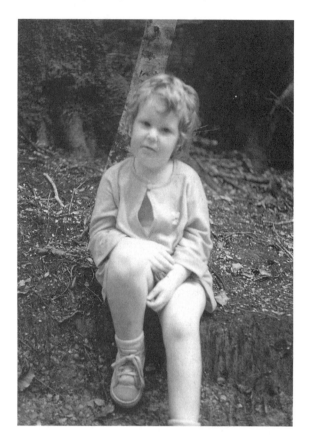

FIGURE 19.5. Francie, age 5 years.

she grew older and became more aware of things going on, she learned where the lunches were kept and just who was a "soft touch." To begin with, her classmates were told they had to keep their lunches "up high so the classroom was tidy." They didn't fall for that. And neither did Francie. She still took their lunches. Somehow this was inexcusable and instead of being seen as a child with a dysfunction, she was seen as a thief. So we decided to tell her class a little about PWS. This worked much better and now every new class gets some information about the syndrome—on a "need to know" basis. It takes time, effort, and diligence from her teachers, but it is working.

As for her school work, she is behind her peers. Probably on average she functions as a 7 year old. She initially had teacher-aide time and was helped on a one-to-one basis as needed. Her writing is very similar to others with PWS that I have seen. Her reading is at a good level and she enjoys the world of storytelling. Math is still very basic. She participates fairly well in the classroom with other activities and her classmates are very tolerant of her.

Socially, How Does It Work?

Francie doesn't have many friends. She still plays a lot with her dolls. They are very real to her and she will talk to them, answer for them, and play with them for hours. She still takes them to school, something I do try to dissuade. But she says she's lonely at school and needs something to talk to. Her friends are younger than she is; they seem to tolerate being told what to do! I like her to come to our annual PWS camps where she can meet her peers, and this generally works out very well. After all, these will probably be the people she ends up living with. Best of all, Francie likes to talk to adults. She perceives them as being able to communicate on her level; she likes to impress them with her good behavior and "intelligent" conversation. She likes to run a good conversation.

We try to keep life as "normal" as possible, but some things just aren't normal. It's not normal to lock cupboards. Francie's behavior is often not "normal" and in fact can be downright embarrassing. I guess it is the day-to-day handling that I find tough.

This last year Francie has put on weight that she shouldn't have. I really thought I was doing all I could, locking the pantry, checking her meals, etc. But what she was doing was stealing and sneaking. It has been an amazing transition from a child who was not a thief to one who brazenly goes through anyone's drawers for hidden goodies, who flatly lies, says that black is white, then rages and screams if I say I don't believe her.

I am missing my little girl and not enjoying this transition into "full-blown" PWS. She went out to play one day with a little girl who is her age but not particularly bright . . . they play well together. I thought I'd told the mother some time ago about PWS, so I didn't bother reminding her. I *knew* inside that I should have made the extra effort, had planned to phone around lunch time, but I was enjoying a Francie-free day and got lazy. I'd also primed Francie up to telling her playmate's mother what she normally had for lunch. I really thought she would do this! When she came home, the mother told me Francie had walked into the house and said, "Mum said I could eat anything I liked." She then ate four sandwiches ("Mum said I can have three pieces of luncheon per sandwich), four sausage rolls, a plate of rice bubbles, and four drinks. Well, I nearly dropped dead! As I said, I know I should have phoned and there was no one else to blane but myself! All the same, I had a go at Francie for lying, which to me is the worst thing, and sent her to bed with a plate of cucumber slices.

What about the Future?

Planning for the future is sometimes scary, but it has to be thought about. Schools have to be checked out. Will the schools be able to handle this unusual problem called PWS? Will we send Francie to a special residential secondary school, or will she go to a local secondary school that can cater to her special education needs?

What happens once school's out? Where will she go then? Will she be able to have a job? Where will she live? Will she be able to get a place in a residential home that will really know and understand the Francie we have raised? Are we doing the best we can for her?

There are many questions and sometimes not many answers. Most parents I know have the same questions for their "normal" children! As I

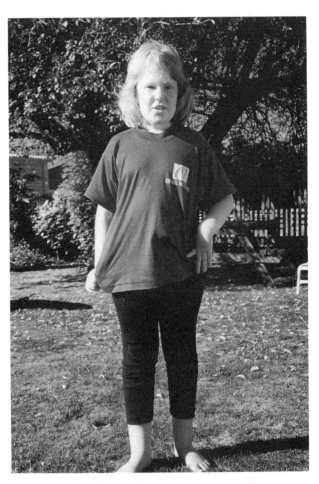

FIGURE 19.6. Francie age 11 years.

write this, I write both as a parent and also as the National Coordinator for the New Zealand PWS Association. I am aware of the special needs expressed by parents and am aware of the need for parent consolidation in order to get things moving: education, residential care, a wider knowledge of the syndrome, and so on. These days parents make a powerful group and the importance of working together to achieve goals cannot be stressed too greatly. As a single voice, I felt I was alone in the world. Working with a group, I know I have support, understanding, consolidation, and energy to overcome obstacles. The next years may hold different problems, but they may also hold new answers. The more we increase our knowledge and the more we share it, both nationally and internationally, the better we as parents will be able to cope with whatever the future holds.

There are days when I don't know how I'll survive the on-going battles—battles with bureaucracy, battles within the family, battles within myself. There are days when I feel quite lost, often because although I know the answers, I am at a loss when it comes to putting them into practice. Sometimes I feel I am failing everyone—all the parents who come to me for advice, my family who are really keen for things to be in harmony, myself when I lose my cool and know I shouldn't, and my daughter who relies on me more than she knows! Like the time she came to me, worried and concerned because she was starting to grow pubic hair at age nine. And all over again, those feelings of resentment, anger, and frustration with this wretchedly unfair syndrome that came rushing in on me. Why should this happen to my "little" daughter, Francie, who plays with dolls and talks to a fantasy friend called Janine. She is still intelligent (for her age), good company, and when she is with me by herself we have only minor alterations (Figure 19.6). Now she has to face something she knows nothing about. She will never be a mother and I will never get over being a mother, no matter how much knowledge I accumulate!

20
The Prader–Willi Syndrome Association (USA)

CURTIS J. SHACKLETT and STEWART MAURER

The Prader–Willi Syndrome Association (USA) is a viable source of information and support that has been built on an ongoing, collaborative relationship with its members. The vital importance of including parents of children with Prader–Willi syndrome (PWS) in all aspects of services for their offspring cannot be underestimated. Establishment of a viable relationship between knowledgeable professionals and parents who, early in the lives of their affected children feel bewildered and uninformed, is essential. Parents want to be provided with accurate information; they need to determine what can and should be done for their children immediately after diagnosis and what help is available on an as needed basis. They want to be linked to interdisciplinary resources that can serve their children and answer the questions that will arise only with time and experience. The Prader–Willi Syndrome Association (PWSA), known in the United States as PWSA (USA), provides a major link in the network of caring for persons with the syndrome and their families.

As with other, similar organizations, this association was established by highly motivated parents. In concert with its relationship with PWS associations throughout the world, PWSA (USA) exists solely to provide assistance to those affected by the syndrome. It encourages communication between parents and professionals, funds research, publishes educational literature for the purpose of promoting awareness of the syndrome, and is a resource for services that support the well-being of affected children and their families.

Historically, the PWSA (USA) was established by the singular efforts of Fausta and Gene Deterling, parents of a son with Prader–Willi syndrome. Following their son's diagnosis, the Deterlings were referred to the Child Development and Retardation Center in Seattle, Washington. There, together with other parents and professionals, along with the encouragement and support of Dr. Vanja Holm, they formed an organization called "Prader–Willi Syndrome Parents and Friends," which was soon renamed the Prader–Willi Syndrome Association. By late 1976, the membership numbered 140 and included representatives from England, Australia, Canada, Norway, and Germany. There are now over 1,500 members.

The association was incorporated as a nonprofit corporation in Minnesota the following year. As its first president, Gene Deterling did much to promote the association's initial growth and foster awareness of the syndrome among professionals and the general public.

Although founded primarily as a parents support organization, the association attracts medical and allied health care professionals, organizations, and other interested individuals to its membership. In keeping with its mission, PWSA (USA) provides parents and professionals with a national and international network of information, support services, and research endeavors. It also is committed to providing lifelong advocacy for affected individuals, maintaining crisis funds to temporarily assist PWS families in transition, and expanding its relationship with other national organizations that serve the developmentally disabled.

When the association first began, there was a dearth of accurate and relevant literature readily available about PWS that could help parents and providers. To overcome this lack of information a parent, Shirley Neason, established and initially edited the first newsletter, "*The Gathered View*," for the association's membership. It remains the official bimonthly publication of the Prader–Willi Syndrome Association. Content of this newsletter consists of contributions from both professional and lay authors that address current issues, offers a wealth of news from the membership, and frequently recounts personal experiences in a sensitive fashion.

In addition to the *Gathered View*, PWSA's initial publication, a booklet, *Prader-Willi Syndrome, A Handbook for Parents* (Neason, 1978), was made available. This booklet was a compilation of known facts and conclusions about PWS collected from parents and professionals at the original organizational meeting. PWSA (USA) now publishes and updates scores of booklets, articles, bibliographies, and medical and scientific papers, some of which have been translated into Spanish, French, and Dutch. A hardcover book *Prader-Willi Syndrome* (Holm, Sulzbacher, & Pipes, 1981) included information gathered at the first Parent Conference Workshop at the University of Washington in 1979, the first such meeting ever held in the United States. In 1988, PWSA partially funded the text *Management of Prader-Willi Syndrome* (Greenswag & Alexander, 1988). It was the first publication to provide a comprehensive source of knowledge about PWS and to offer commonsense guidelines for care.

In June 1979, a National conference supported by PWSA was held in Minneapolis, Minnesota, to disseminate information and provide support. Encouraged by parents and professionals, the Association began sponsoring annual national conferences with affiliated local organizations acting as hosts. Programming in the form of seminars, lectures, and discussion groups includes information on all aspects of PWS and available services. Professionals and parents participate in and collaborate on presentations and opportunities are provided for discussion of a variety of issues on a one-to-one basis. From an initial meeting of 25 families, attendance at the national conferences has increased to an average of 250 registrants each year. In addition, special youth programs provide all day activities for an average of 180 individuals with PWS of all ages who also attend. In recent years, due to increased incidence of early diagnosis, more young families are participating and every effort is made to meet their special needs when planning programs. PWSA also provided partial funding in support of The First International Conference on Prader–Willi Syndrome that was held in The Netherlands in 1991.

The day prior to the national conference is set aside for three symposiums. One, a Scientific Day meeting, provides scientists an occasion to report on current research. The second affords residential and other community providers the opportunity to exchange ideas and discuss issues associated with delivery of services. At the third gathering, chapter presidents meet with the national president and executive director to discuss program plans, chapter issues, and address Association concerns.

The association holds a general membership meeting at every annual conference where the board of directors are formally nominated and elected and reports of current projects and financial activities are presented. The 12 person volunteer Board, the corporate officers, and executive committee meet several times each year to ensure that the stated mission and the vision of PWSA (USA) are fulfilled. A Scientific Advisory Board reviews all requests for research grants and serves as a primary resource for funding scholarly investigations.

Shortly after the initial conference in Minnesota in 1979, the original founders determined that the organization required additional personnel to meet its growing needs. Marge Wett (the mother of a daughter with PWS) was appointed the associations' first executive director and through her tireless efforts, the National Office of PWSA was established in the Minneapolis/St. Paul area. Following her retirement in 1992, Theresa Schaffer assumed this position. Two years later, the national office moved to St. Louis, Missouri under the executive directorship of Russell Myler, MSW. Centrally located, this "Gateway City" is home to a significant number of parents and professional members and volunteers willing to assist office personnel.

Because primary services are often best provided at the local level, PWSA (USA) reaches out to its members through state chapters, the number of which continues to increase each year. Certainly, in terms of receiving services, the credibility of state groups is enhanced when they are formally linked to a credentialed, internationally recognized association (Wett, 1988). As the national organization continues to mature and reach out to affiliating groups, it increases its capacity to disseminate information and provide support. When families request assistance regarding educational, residential, and social services, state chapters are an excellent resource for information and individual support. For details regarding state organization call PWSA (USA) at 1-800-926-4797.

References

Greenswag, L.R., & Alexander, R.A. (Eds.). (1988). *Management of Prader-Willi syndrome*. New York: Springer-Velay.

Holm, V.A., Sulzbacher, S.J., & Pipes, P.L. (Eds.). (1981). *The Prader-Willi syndrome*. Baltimore: University Park Press.

Neason, S. (1978). *Prader-Willi syndrome—A handbook for parents*. Edina, MN: The Prader-Willi Syndrome Association.

Wett, M. (1988). A national parent network: The Prader-Willi Syndrome Association. In L.R. Greenswag & R.A. Alexander (Eds.), *Management of Prader-Willi syndrome* (p. 228). New York: Springer-Verlag.

Glossary

Adrenache: Pubic or axillary hair before 8 years of age.

Adrenal glands: They sit on top of the kidneys and regulate stress reactions and some minereal balance.

Adrenocorticotropic hormone (ACTH): A hormone secreted by the pituitary that acts upon the adrenal glands; part of the stress response system.

Amenorrhea: Lack of menstural flow.

Amniocentesis: A procedure in which a small amount of the amniotic fluid surrounding the fetus is drawn off and subjected to genetic and biochemical analysis.

Androgen: Any one of several male hormones.

Angelman syndrome: A syndrome with a similar chromosome deletion as PWS, but a different phenotype.

Chromosome: Carrier of hereditary material that appears in the nucleus of a cell. Each cell has a specific number of chromosomes; normal humans have 46.

Chromosome abnormality: Any variation from the normal chromosomal pattern. The common abnormalities found in Prader-Willi Syndrome are:

1. *Deletion*: a condition in which a piece of genetic material is lost or missing from a chromosome. Typically there is a small piece of the long arm of the 15th chromosome that is missing.
2. *Translocation*: a transfer of a fragment of one chromosome to another chromosome.

Cocontraction: The simultaneous contraction of all the muscles around a joint to stabilize it.

Cortisol: A hormone secreted by the adrenal glands in response to stress.

Cryptorchidism: Undescended testicles (testicles are not present in the scrotal sac).

de novo: New. Used in genetics to describe a structural alteration of the chromosomes that is present in a child but not in either parent.

Deletion: A missing piece of chromosomal material. In PWS, the deletion is in the proximal long arm of chromosome 15.

Down syndrome: A syndrome resulting from 3 (instead of the usual 2) copies of chromosome 21.

Dual-photon absorptiometry (DPA): A gamma radiation technique for measuring bone density.

FISH: Fluorescence *in situ* hybridization. A test using a fluorescence-tagged segment of DNA that combines with the DNA present in the normal PWS critical region and allows determination by its presence or absence as to whether a 15q deletion is present.

Gene: A unit of genetic information. Usually contains the genetic code for one protein.

Genetic imprinting: Differential modification of the expression of genes depending upon whether they are inherited from the mother or the father. This affects only certain segments of the human genetic complement, which require contributions from both mother and father for normal development, including PWS and Angelman syndrome on chromosome 15q.

Genetics counseling: Counseling that explains facts about genetics issues to parents/care providers. Emphasis is on clarification of information, possible recurrence risk, reproductive options, support to affected persons and their families, and follow-up services.

Glucocorticoid: Hormones secreted by the adrenal glands regulating sugar and energy availability.

Gonadotropin: A hormone acting upon the genital organs.

Growth hormone (GH):   A pituitary-secreted hormone that aids in growth.

Gynecomestia: Breast development—used in reference to male breast development.

Hyperphagia: Consumption of more than an optimal quantity of food.

Hypogenitalism: The genital organs are undersized or nonexistent.

Hypogonadism: A condition of abnormal decrease in the function of the ovaries and testes, causing retardation of growth and sexual development.

Hypogonadotropic hypogonadism: Hypogonadism resulting from a decrease in sex hormones released by the pituitary.

Hypopigmentation: Unusually fair hair, eyes, and skin for the family.

Hypothalamus: The part of the brain that controls appetite, body temperature, hormones, and other vital functions.

Hypotonia: Decreased muscle tone. The muscles are soft, weak, and flabby.

IGFBP-3:   A binding protein for IGF that carries it around the blood stream.

Insulin: A hormone secreted by the pancreas that regulates sugar in the body.

Insulin-like growth factor I and II (IGF-I, IGF-II):   Factors that act upon body tissues to stimulate growth.

Klinefelter's syndrome: XXY syndrome. Phenotypically a male.

Lability: Marked fluctuations in mood/disposition.

Learning disabled: A term applied to low-achieving children whose performance is inconsistent with overall intelligence. These children may be part of an identifiable group who are limited in their ability to process written or spoken language, which may result in limited capacity to master some basic academic tasks.

Luteinizing hormone (LH):   One of the pituitary-related hormones acting upon the genital organs.

Melatonin: A hormone secreted by the pineal gland in the brain.

Mental age: A measured level of cognitive function established by a test of intelligence.

Metabolism: Pertaining to the body's process of absorbing nourishment from food and turning it into energy or stored fat.

Motor planning: The ability of the brain to conceive of, organize, and carry out a sequence of unfamiliar activities. Also known as "praxis."

Narrow bifrontal diameter: A narrow forehead.

Normalization: The effort to make available activities and patterns of everyday life that are as close as possible to the habits of normal, mainstream individuals.

Obesity: A condition in which body weight is considerably (more than two standard deviations) above the range that is normal for body height.

Orchiopexy: Surgical lowering of the testicles into the scrotum.

Osteoporosis: Demineralization (thinning) of the bones.

Oxandrolone: An anabolic (mass-building) steroid.

Phenotype: The external appearance of an individual with a particular condition.

Pituitary: A gland at the base of the brain, stimulated by a portion of the brain called the hypothalamus, that secretes hormones that work elsewhere in the body (e.g., ACTH, FSH, LH, TSH, prolactin).

Polymorphism: Normal variation in genetic information. Used to describe minor variation in chromosome shape and normal or abnormal variation in molecular structure or content of genes.

Praxis: The capacity of the brain to integrate and carry out unfamiliar motor activities. Also known as motor planning.

Prolactin: A pituitary-secreted hormone acting upon the genital organs and breasts.

Proximal musculature: The muscles of the trunk, shoulder girdle, and hip girdle.

Rehabilitation: A dynamic process of continuing evaluation of disabled individuals in order to meet their needs and develop realistic methods of coping. This "process" acknowledges that one individual may have more than just one problem to confront and that the individual's ability to function cannot be separated from environmental concerns.

Sheltered workshop: A controlled work-oriented rehabilitation setting that utilizes work experiences and related services to assist handicapped individuals in making the maximum progress possible toward vocational productivity and normal living.

Strabismus: The condition of being "cross-eyed."

Syndrome: A term used to describe a symptom complex characterized by many medical signs. In many syndromes not all affected individuals will have every diagnostic sign.

System advocacy: Refers to actions taken by individuals or groups to influence policy making.

Tanner states: A five step staging of pubertal development: 1 = pre-puberty 5 = full adult breast (females), pubic hair, and genital development.

Thyroid-releasing hormone (TRH):   A hypothalamic hormone that stimulates the release of TSH from the pitutary.

Thyroid-stimulating hormone (TSH):   A pituitary hormone that stimulates the thyroid leading to increases in metabolism and heart rate.

Turner: A syndrome with only one sex chromosome (XO), but phenotypically appearance of a female.

Uniparental disomy: A situation in which both members of a chromosome pair are derived from a single parent. In some people with PWS, both chromosome 15s are maternal in origin, and no paternal chromosome 15 is present in the affected individual.

Suggested Readings

Alexander, R., Greenswag, L., & Nowak, A. (1987). Rumination and vomiting in Prader-Willi syndrome. *American Journal of Medical Genetics, 28,* 889–895.

Berg, J.M. et al. (1990). Specific mental retardation disorders and problem behaviors. *International Review of Psychiatry, 2,* 53–60.

Bottel, H. (1977, May). The eating disorder. *Good Housekeeping,* p. 176.

Bray, G.A., Dahms, W.T., Swerdloff, R.S., Fisher, R.H., Atkinson, R.L., & Carrel, R.E. (1983). The Prader-Willi syndrome: A study of 42 patients and review of the literature. *Medicine, 62,* 59–80.

Cassidy, S.B. (1984). Prader-Willi syndrome. *Current Problems in Pediatrics, 14,* 5–55.

Clarren, S.K., & Smith, D.W. (1977). Prader-Willi syndrome: Variable severity and recurrence risk. *American Journal of Diseases of Children, 131,* 798–800.

Curfs, L.M.G., Verhulst, F.C., & Fryns, J.P. (1992). Behavioral and emotional problems in youngsters with Prader-Willi syndrome. *Genetic Counseling, 2*(1), 33–41.

Donaldson, M., Chu, C., Cooke, A., Wilson, A., Greene, S., & Stephenson, J. (1994). The Prader-Willi syndrome. *Archives of Disease in Childhood, 70,* 58–63.

Dunn, H.G., Tze, W.J., Alisharan, R.M., & Schulzer, M. (1981). Clinical experience with 23 cases of Prader-Willi syndrome. In V.A. Holm, S.J. Sulzbacher, & P.L. Pipes (Eds.), *The Prader-Willi syndrome* (pp. 69–88). Baltimore: University Park Press.

Dykens, E.M., Hodapp, R.M., Walsh, K., & Nash, L.J. (1992). Adaptive and maladaptive behavior in Prader-Willi syndrome. *Journal of the American Academy of Child and Adolescent Psychiatry, 31*(6), 1131–1136.

Edmonston, N.K. (1983). Management of speech and language in a case of Prader-Willi syndrome. *Language, Speech and Hearing Services in Schools, 13,* 241–245.

Greenswag, L. (1984). *The adult with Prader-Willi syndrome: A descriptive investigation.* Unpublished doctoral thesis, University of Iowa. (DA 056952, University Microfilms International, Ann Arbor, MI.)

Greenswag, L. (1987). Adults with Prader-Willi syndrome: A survey of 232 cases. *Developmental Medicine and Child Neurology, 29,* 145–152.

Hall, B.D., & Smith, D.W. (1972). Prader-Willi syndrome. A resume of 32 cases including an instance of affected first cousins, one of whom is of normal stature and intelligence. *The Journal of Pediatrics, 81,* 286–293.

Hanson, J.W. (1981). A view of the etiology and pathogenesis of Prader-Willi syndrome. In V.A. Holm, S.J. Sulzbacher, & P.L. Pipes (Eds.), *The Prader-Willi syndrome* (pp. 45–53). Baltimore: University Park Press.

Herrman, J. (1981). Implications of Prader-Willi syndrome for the individual and the family. In V.A. Holm, S.J. Sulzbacher, & P.L. Pipes (Eds.), *The Prader-Willi syndrome* (pp. 229–238). Baltimore: University Park Press.

Holm, V.A., & Nugent, J.K. (1982). Growth in the Prader-Willi syndrome. *Birth Defects: Original Article Series, 18* (No. 3B), 93–100.

Holm, V.A., Sulzbacher, S.J., & Pipes, P.L. (Eds.). (1984). *The Prader-Willi syndrome*. Baltimore: University Park Press.

Holm, V.A., Cassidy, S.B., Butler, M.G., Hanchett, J.M., Greenswag, L.R., Whitman, B.Y., & Greenberg, F. (1993). Prader-Willi syndrome: Consensus diagnostic criteria. *Pediatrics*, 398–402.

Kousseff, B.G. (1982). The cytogenetic controversy in the Prader-Labhart-Willi syndrome. *American Journal of Medical Genetics, 13*, 431–439.

LeConte, J.M. (1981). Social work intervention strategies for families with children with Prader-Willi syndrome. In V.A. Holm, S.J. Sulzbacher, & P.L. Pipes (Eds.), *The Prader-Willi syndrome* (pp. 245–257). Baltimore: University Park Press.

Ledbetter, D.H., Riccardi, V.M., Airhart, S.D., Strobel, R.J., Keenan, B.S., & Crawford, J.D. (1981). Deletions of chromosome 15 as a cause of Prader-Willi syndrome. *New England Journal of Medicine, 304*, 325–329.

Levine, K., & Wharton, R.H. (1993). *Children with Prader-Willi Syndrome: Information for School Staff* (revised edition). New York: Visible Ink, Inc.

Marshall, B.D., Jr., Elder, J., O'Bosky, D., Wallace, C.J., & Liberman, R.P. (1979). Behavioral treatment of Prader-Willi syndrome. *The Behavior Therapist, 2*, 22–23.

Mitchell, L. (1981). *An overview of Prader-Willi syndrome*. Edina, MN: The Prader-Willi Syndrome Association.

Nardella, M.T., Sulzbacher, S.J., & Worthington-Roberts, B.S. (1981). Activity levels of persons with Prader-Willi syndrome. *American Journal of Mental Deficiency, 87*, 498–505.

Neason, S. (1978). *Prader-Willi syndrome: A handbook for parents*. Edina, MN: The Prader-Willi Syndrome Association.

Prader, A. (1981). The Prader-Willi syndrome: An overview. *Acta Paediatrica Japonica, 23*, 307–311.

Prader, A., Labhart, A., & Willi, H. (1956). Ein Sydrom von Adipositas, Klein-wuchs, Kryptorchismus, und Oligophrenie nach myatonieartigem Zustand im Neugeborenenalter. *Schweizerische Medizinische Wochenschrift, 86*, 1260–1261.

Stephenson, J.B.P. (1980). Prader-Willi syndrome: Neonatal presentation and later development. *Developmental Medicine and Child Neurology, 22*, 792–795.

Thompson, T., Kodluboy, S., & Heston, L. (1980). Behavioral treatment of obesity in Prader-Willi syndrome. *Behavior Therapy, 11*, 588–593.

Wett, R.J. (1983). Prader-Willi syndrome: The disabled child. *The Journal of the American Medical Association, 249*, 1836.

Whitman, B., & Accardo, P. (1987). Emotional symptoms in Prader-Willi syndrome adolescents. *American Journal of Medical Genetics, 28*, 897–905.

Whitman, B., & Greenswag, L. (1992). *A survey of mediation usage and effectiveness in persons with Prader-Willi syndrome*. Paper presented at the PWSA-USA National Conference, Scottsdale, Arizona. July.

Whitman, B., & Greenswag, L. (1992). The use of psychotropic medications in persons with Prader-Willi syndrome. In S. Cassidy (Ed.), *Prader-Willi syndrome and other chromosome 15q deletion disorders* (pp. 223–231). Springer Verlag: New York.

Zellweger, H., & Schneider, H.J. (1968). Syndrome of hypotonia, hypomentia, hypogonadism, obesity (HHHO) or Prader-Willi syndrome. *American Journal of Diseases of Children, 115*, 588–598.

Appendices

Appendix A
Sleep Disorders in Prader–Willi Syndrome: Management Considerations

GILA HERTZ and MARY CATALETTO

Sleep difficulties and excessive daytime sleepiness (EDS) have been reported in over 90% of patients with PWS (Greenswag, 1987; Clarke, Waters, & Corbett, 1989; Cassidy, McKillop, & Morgan, 1990; Holm, Cassidy, Butler, et al., 1993). Caretakers describe long sleep periods exceeding 10 hrs, restless sleep and frequent napping during the day. Because of their obesity and daytime sleepiness, these patients have been considered at risk for sleep-disordered breathing, particularly sleep apnea, but until recently no sleep data from objective polysomnographic studies have been available to confirm these reports. Over the last few years, advanced technology and a growing number of sleep facilities available for sleep research have allowed scientists to use polysomnographic (sleep) studies to look into the unique physiological aspects of sleep in PWS and to gain more understanding of the spectrum of symptoms presented by these patients.

Sleep Evaluation: Polysomnography

Polysomnographic studies are continuous all night simultaneous recordings of multiple physiologic parameters that are essential in the assessment of sleep architecture and in the formulation of sleep disorders diagnoses. Most polysomnographic studies include the recording of electroencephalography (EEG), eye movements (EOG), and muscle activity (EMG) to determine sleep staging and evaluate sleep architecture. In addition, the concurrent measurement of respiratory airflow, respiratory muscle efforts, and pulse oximetry to determine the presence of sleep-disordered breathing is also included. The overnight recorded data are typically analyzed by inspecting every 30-sec epoch of recorded information to determine the presence of movements and/or breathing abnormalities and to score sleep stages. In many laboratories computerized systems aid in the preliminary overview of the sleep record. The results are summarized to give an overall impression of sleep architecture (hypnogram) and to determine a diagnosis.

When patients present with excessive daytime sleepiness, an additional daytime test, the Multiple Sleep Latency Test (MSLT), is indicated. This test is generally performed on the day following the nocturnal polysomnographic recording. It consists of four to five 20-min. scheduled naps, at 2-hr intervals, typically beginning at 2 hr after the end of the nocturnal recording. The time from lights out to the first epoch of sleep (sleep latency) as well as the occurrence of rapid eye movement (REM) sleep is determined for each nap. A report of MSLT scores usually includes the mean daily MSLT score and the presence of REM periods. A daily mean MSLT less than 5 min. indicates a pathological level of daytime sleepiness. The presence of sleep onset REM period (SOREMP) in two or more naps has been consistently shown in MSLT of patients with narcolepsy.

Polysomnographic Findings in PWS

Sleep Architecture

Disturbances in sleep architecture have been recently reported in both children and adults with PWS. These include delayed sleep onset, frequent arousals in sleep, and an increase in total waking after sleep onset (WASO). Specific REM sleep abnormalities in PWS have also been reported by several authors and can be summarized as follows: REM latency (time from sleep onset to first REM period) is often markedly shortened, total number of REM periods is higher and mean REM period duration is significantly shorter when compared to normal controls. REM sleep fragmentation is common. (Vela-Bueno, Kales, & Soldatos, 1984; Harris & Allen, 1985; Hertz & Cataletto, 1992). Sleep-disordered breathing and occasional drops in oxygen saturation, typically accompanied by arousals, may account for some sleep disturbances. However, sleep fragmentation and abnormal REM sleep have been observed in individuals with PWS who did not have disordered breathing. Thus, the observed sleep abnormalities seem independent of disordered breathing and might indicate deficits in the brain mechanisms involved in sleep/wake regulation.

Daytime Sleepiness

The results of MSLT testing (reported to date for adults with PWS only) confirm the presence of abnormal daytime sleepiness. In our group of patients, mean MSLT score was 6.3 min. (normal MSLT scores >

10 min.). A number of nocturnal sleep parameters were significantly correlated with MSLT scores: total waketime after sleep onset (WASO), AHI, and measures of nocturnal oxygen saturation.

In addition to the abnormal MSLT scores, some individuals in our group demonstrated REM sleep during naps, a finding typically associated with narcolepsy. However, most of our patients did not exhibit the other signs of narcolepsy e.g., cataplexy, hypnagogic hallucinations and sleep paralysis. Also, the presence of HLA DR2 antigen, found in virtually all patients with narcolepsy, has not been found in PWS (Helbing-Zwanenburg, Mourtazaer, d'Amoro, et al., 1993; Hertz, Cataletto, Feinsilver, 1994b). The evaluation of daytime sleepiness in children with PWS may be more difficult since children are often unable to cooperate with the test instruction. Alternative measures of alertness, which provide a continuous monitoring over longer periods of time, are currently evaluated in our laboratory.

Sleep Disordered Breathing

Despite the presence of obesity, hypotonia, and daytime hypersomnolence, sleep studies have shown that patients with PWS have relatively mild obstructive sleep apnea (OSA), mostly in the form of snoring and hypopneas (Vela-Bueno, Kales, & Soldatos, 1984; Kaplan, Fredrickson, & Richardson, 1991; Brooks & Owen, 1992; Hertz, Cataletto, Feinsilver, et al., 1993). The effects of age on the severity of OSA have been studied in PWS patients ranging in age from 2 to 25 years old. An analysis of the apnea/hypopnea index (AHI) revealed no age effect, although there was a trend for increased sleep apnea in the preadolescent group. These studies also found no significant difference in AHI between males and females across all age groups. (Hertz et al., 1993; Hertz, Cataletto, Feinsilver, et al., 1994a). This is in contrast to the general population, where sleep apnea is by far more prevalent in men as compared to women.

In contrast to lack of significant OSA, the presence of nocturnal oxygen desaturation during sleep is a consistent finding in PWS. The severity of oxygen desaturation is significantly correlated with increased body weight and is worse during REM sleep when muscle hypotonia is maximal. Cardiopulmonary complications, particularly pulmonary hypertension, resulting from nocturnal hypoxemia have been implicated in the morbidity and mortality of patients with PWS.

Management Considerations

Because of the potential cardiopulmonary complications of sleep-disordered breathing, attention should be directed first to findings of abnormal breathing patterns during sleep. Based on the results of the sleep study an individual treatment plan is formulated. Clinically, an AHI < 10 is considered mildly abnormal for adults but may be more significant in children. In the case of mild sleep apnea, management is generally targeted at preventing worsening of the symptoms. Weight control becomes even more important in the presence of OSA. Attention should also be given to contributory factors such as nasal allergies and upper airways infections. In more severe cases of OSA the administration of nasal continuous positive airways pressure (CPAP) may be considered (Sforza, Krieger, Geisert, et al., 1991). This portable and well-tolerated system consists of a generator that delivers air under pressure through a nasal mask. Benefits from nasal CPAP can be seen as soon as the morning after the CPAP trial, with patients reporting a general sense of well being and having slept well. Some minor side effects related to delivery of continuous air pressure or ill fitted masks have been reported, including air leaks, nasal and oral dryness, skin rashes, and patient anxiety. Most masks and their accessories can be customized to fit different facial sizes and configurations to maximize patient comfort and compliance. Recent improvements in design of nasal masks have made them softer, more contoured, and better tolerated. The development in the last few years of a bilevel positive pressure device (BiPAP) has made breathing patterns more physiologic and has reduced difficulties falling asleep because of excess pressure. In our experience, BiPAP has been found to be better tolerated and compliance improved (Cataletto & Hertz, 1992).

OSA was found more frequently in children with PWS when compared with adult patients. When accompanied by tonsilloadenoidal hypertrophy, tonsillectomy and/or adenoidectomy should be considered. Although the incidence of T&As has declined over recent years, OSA as an indication for this type of surgery has increased. Because of the higher incidence of nocturnal oxygen desaturation in PWS patients, close intra- and postoperative monitoring of oxygen saturation is recommended. Clinical improvement is almost always noted following T&A, although this has not yet been confirmed by objective studies.

The most frequently identified sleep abnormality in patients with PWS is sleep-related oxygen desaturation, particularly during REM sleep, when muscle tone is at its lowest levels. obesity has been found to be the most obvious correlate to the severity of oxygen desaturation and in morbidly obese patients oxygen levels may not return to normal levels even during NREM sleep. In such patients, weight control is a crucial factor in management. Indications for treatment with low flow supplemental oxygen during sleep is based on three criteria: the severity and duration of oxygen desaturation, the presence of apneas and the baseline respiratory status. In adult patients, when in addition to oxygen desaturation, frequent episodes of obstructive apneas are present, a combination of nasal

CPAP with supplemental low flow oxygen should be considered. Significant improvements have been noted on polysomnographic studies following combined treatment with oxygen and CPAP (Cataletto & Hertz, 1992). Surprisingly, however, in spite of the improvement noted in sleep disordered breathing, daytime sleepiness often remains a problem.

An alternative potential approach to the management of daytime sleepiness in patients with REM related nocturnal desaturation may be the use of non sedating tricyclic antidepressants drugs (TCA). Studies using TCA in obese non PWS patients with sleep apnea showed promising results with improvement of REM related breathing abnormalities as well in daytime functioning. The results may have been related to the suppressive effects of TCA drugs on REM sleep in addition to its daytime stimulating effects. To date, there is only one reported case of a patient with PWS treated with Protriptyline (Cataletto & Hertz, 1992). In this 19 year old patient, treatment with Protriptyline alone resulted in improved daytime functioning, but only minor changes were noted in sleep disordered breathing and oxygen desaturation. Nasal BiPAP therapy was then added to improve nocturnal breathing. The combination of these two treatments resulted in significant improvement in both nocturnal and daytime symptoms, allowing him to return to a work program.

The treatment of EDS in PWS has received very little attention in spite of its high prevalence. After the exclusion of sleep-disordered breathing, management in our patients is currently focused on improving sleep hygiene, monitoring worst sleepiness time during the day, and scheduling resting or napping periods accordingly. In the general population, children who are sleepy, often show lapses in concentration, easy distractibility, frustration and aggressive behavior (Sheldon, 1992). Anecdotal parental reports point to a positive correlation between daytime sleepiness and the frequency of temper tantrums in children with PWS, but no studies are available to confirm such data. It may be further hypothesized that sleep disturbances may actually be involved in promoting dysfunctional eating patterns and obesity in PWS. Thus, sleep abnormalities which result in daytime sleepiness may cause decreased daytime activity which in turn results in increased eating and weight gain. Increased weight further degrades ventilation during sleep causing more sleep fragmentation, which in turn makes daytime sleepiness worse.

Further investigation is warranted in the neuroregulatory and behavioral factors involved in PWS sleep as sleep qualities have an impact on learning, daytime functioning and cardiopulmonary well being. At this stage in our knowledge focus needs to be placed on early identification of patients with sleep disordered breathing, relief of hypoxemia and upper airways obstruction when present, and weight control. The role of pharmacologic therapy in PWS sleep is still in its early phases and treatment needs to be individually tailored.

References

Brooks, L., & Owens, R. (1992). Sleep and breathing patterns in patients with Prader Willi syndrome. *Sleep Research, 21,* 285.

Cassidy, S.B., McKillop, J.A., & Morgan, W.J. (1990). Sleep disorders in Prader Willi syndrome. *Dysmorphology and Clinical Genetics, 4*(1), 13–17.

Cataletto, M., & Hertz, G. (1992). Therapeutic modalities in the treatment of sleep-related breathing abnormalities in patients with Prader Willi syndrome. *Sleep Research, 21,* 287.

Clarke, D.J., Waters, J., & Corbett, J.A. (1989). Adults with Prader Willi syndrome: abnormalities of sleep and behavior. *Journal of the Royal Society of Medicine, 82,* 21–24.

Greenswag, L.R. (1987). Adults with Prader Willi syndrome: A survey of 232 cases. *Developmental Medicine and Child Neurology, 29,* 145–152.

Harris, J.C., & Allen, R.P. (1985). Sleep disordered breathing and circadian disturbances of REM sleep in Prader Willi syndrome. *Sleep Research, 14,* 235.

Helbing-Zwanenburg, B., Mourtazaer, M.S., d'Amaro, J., Dahlitz, M., Vaughan, R., Page, G., Cliff, S., Parks, J.D., & Kamphuisen, H.A.C. (1993). HLA types in the Prader Willi syndrome. *Journal of Sleep Research, 2*(2), 115.

Hertz, G., & Cataletto, M. (1992). REM sleep abnormalities in patients with Prader Willi syndrome. *Sleep Research, 21,* 295.

Hertz, G., Cataletto, M., Feinsilver, S.H., & Angulo, M. (1993). Sleep and breathing patterns in patients with Prader Willi syndrome (PWS): effects of age and gender. *Sleep, 16*(4), 366–371.

Hertz, G., Cataletto, M., Feinsilver, S.H., & Angulo, M. (1994a). Developmental trends in sleep related breathing disorders in patients with Prader Willi syndrome. *American Journal of Medical Genetics,* (in press).

Hertz, G., Cataletto, M., Feinsilver, S.H., & Angulo, M. (1994b). HLA typing in Prader Willi syndrome: lack of evidence for narcolepsy (letter). *Journal of Sleep Research, 3*(2), 127.

Holm, V.A., Cassidy, S.B., Butler, M.G., Hanchett, J.M., Greenswag, L.R., Whitman, B.Y., & Greenberg, F. (1993). Prader Willi syndrome: consensus diagnostic criteria. *Pediatrics, 91*(2), 398–402.

Kaplan, J., Fredrickson, P.A., & Richardson, J.W. (1991). Sleep and breathing in patients with Prader Willi syndrome. *Mayo Clinic Proceedings, 61,* 1124–1126.

Sforza, E., Krieger, J., Geisert, J., & Kurtz, D. (1991). Sleep and breathing abnormalities in a case of Prader Willi syndrome. The effects of acute continuous positive airways pressure treatment. *Acta Paediatric Scand, 80,* 80–85.

Sheldon, S. (1992). Disorders of excessive somnolence. In S. Sheldon, J.P. Spire, & H.B. Levy (Eds.), *Pediatric Sleep Medicine* (pp. 91–105). Philadelphia: W.B. Saunders.

Vela-Bueno, A., Kales, A., & Soldatos, C.R. (1984). Sleep in the Prader Willi syndrome: clinical and polygraphic findings. *Archives of Neurology, 41,* 294–296.

Appendix B
Growth Charts for Prader–Willi Syndrome

Vanja A. Holm

Short stature, considering genetic background, is one of the diagnostic hallmarks in the Prader-Willi syndrome (PWS) (Holm, Cassidy, Butler, et al., 1993). In a previous publication, the expected linear growth in this condition has been described (Holm & Nugent, 1982). In that study we plotted growth on standard U.S. growth charts (Hamill, Drizd, Johnson, et al., 1977) from a mixture of cross-sectional and longitudinal data from 92 subjects, 56 males and 36 females (Figures B.1 and B.2).

From the height data obtained from age 3 years to early adulthood, growth curves were fitted for males and females that encompassed most of the data points. From these data, growth charts specific for PWS, age 3 to early adulthood, have been developed. Growth during the first 36 months of life is too unpredictable in this condition—it is characterized by a fall-off in growth—to lend itself to the development of a special growth chart for that age. The growth curves from the childhood, adolescence, and early adulthood years have been made into graphs for easy charting (Figures B.3 and B.4).

These PWS-specific growth charts can be used to clinically follow the growth of individuals with this condition. The growth of adolescents with PWS is often worrisome because their adolescent growth spurt is considerably less than expected (Holm & Nugent, 1982). Plotting the growth on these charts might be reassuring for the physician, the parents, and the adolescent. On the other hand, if a child with PWS shows a fall-off in growth during childhood, which is not typical, the physician using these syndrome-specific growth charts will easily spot this child, who needs further endocrinological workups.

Research exploring growth-promoting regimens can also benefit from these specific growth charts. They have been used in a study of the effects of oxandrolone therapy in males with this syndrome (Holm, Nugent, Ruvalcaba, et al., 1989). Synthetic growth, hormone is now becoming widely available, and growth hormone therapy is used where growth

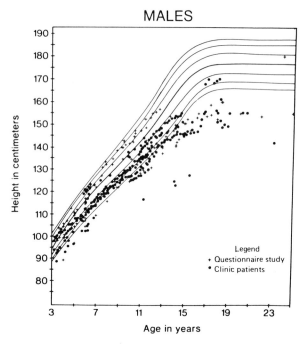

FIGURE B.1. Growth data from 56 male subjects with PWS, plotted on standard U.S. growth charts.

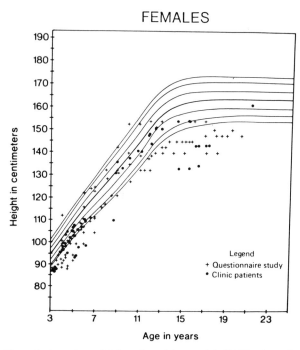

FIGURE B.2. Growth data from 36 female subjects with PWS, plotted on standard U.S. growth charts.

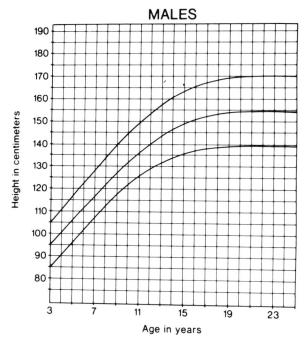

FIGURE B.3. Blank chart with growth curves for PWS males from age 3 to early adulthood.

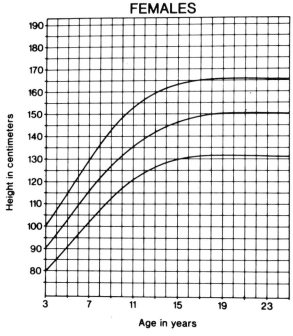

FIGURE B.4. Blank chart with growth curves for PWS females from age 3 to early adulthood.

hormone deficiency has been demonstrated. These syndrome-specific growth charts are useful in evaluating the effects of such treatment.

References

Hamill, P.V., Drizd, T.A., Johnson, C.L., Reed, R., & Roche, A.F. (1977). NCHS growth curves for children birth-18 years, United States. *Vital and Health Statistics Series 11*, Number 165. U.S. Department of Health, Education, and Welfare, Pub. No (PHS) 78-1650. Washington, D.C.: U.S. Government Printing Office.

Holm, V.A., Cassidy, S.B., Butler, M.G., Hanchett, J.M., Greenswag, L.R., Whitman, B.Y., & Greenberg, F. (1993). Prader-Willi syndrome: Consensus Diaguastic Giteria. *Pediatrics, 91*, 398–402.

Holm, V.A., & Nugent, J.K. (1982). Growth in the Prader-Willi syndrome. *Birth Defects: Original Article Series, 18*, 93–100.

Holm, V.A., Nugent, J.K., Ruvalcaba, R.H.A., & Costeff, H. (1989). Oxandrolone therapy in six males with the Prader-Willi syndrome. *Journal of Pediatrics, 114*, 325–327.

Appendix C
Food Exchange Guidelines

TABLE C.1. Sample Menu.[a]

	Monday	Tuesday	Wednesday	Thursday	Friday	Saturday	Sunday
BREAKFAST	Milk, skim Pancake Diet syrup Bacon slice Peaches, sliced Orange juice Coffee Diet sweetener	Milk, skim Omelet Dry cereal Banana Tomato juice Toast Margarine Coffee Diet sweetener	Milk, skim Cottage cheese Dark toast Margarine Diet jelly Grapefruit juice Prunes Coffee Diet sweetener	Milk, skim Scrambled egg Malt-O-Meal Toast Margarine Orange juice Pears Coffee Diet sweetener	Milk, skim Cinnamon toast Dry cereal Apple juice Orange Coffee Diet sweetener	Milk, skim Boiled egg English muffin (½) Diet jelly Margarine Grapefruit juice Applesauce Coffee Diet sweeteneer	Milk, skim Scrambled egg Raisin toast Pineapple juice Grapefruit (½) Coffee Diet sweetener
LUNCH	Milk, skim Peanut butter Whole wheat bread Diet jelly Celery sticks Orange Graham cracker	Milk, skim Turkey slices Whole wheat bread Carrot coins Red apple Vanilla wafers Mayonnaise	Milk, skim Tuna salad Rye bread Radishes Seasonal fruit Crackers	Milk, skim Turkey ham Pumpernickel Cauliflower Raisins Mayonnaise Vanilla wafers	Milk, skim Sliced cheese Whole wheat bread Sliced tomato w/lettuce Mayonnaise Red apple Graham cracker	Milk, skim Cottage cheese salad Curried slaw Blueberry muffin Seasonal fruit Ice milk	Milk, skim French bread pizza Dzerta Tossed salad Seasonal fruit

Ice water ——→

	Monday	Tuesday	Wednesday	Thursday	Friday	Saturday	Sunday
DINNER	Milk, skim BBQ chicken Rice Broccoli Peas Marsh mallow crispies Tea Diet sweetener	Milk, skim Cheeseburger Dinner roll String bean salad Sauerkraut Potato salad Seasonal fruit Tea Diet sweetener	Milk, skim Baked pork chop Pasta/vegetable salad Beets/orange salad Dinner roll Margarine Seasonal fruit Tea Diet sweetener	Milk, skim Chicken Waldorf salad Dilled carrots Bread sticks Dzerta Seasonal fruit Chocolate pudding Tea Diet sweetener	Milk, skim Broiled fish w/lemon Oriental mixed vegetables Orange wheat salad Whole kernel corn Tossed salad Juice sicle Tea Diet sweetener	Milk, skim Roast beef Baked potato Mixed vegetables Spinach salad lemon dressing Margarine Bread Peach yogurt freezee Tea Diet sweetener	Milk, skim Ham slices Sweet potatoes/ apples Seasoned rice Steamed broccoli Fruit ice Margarine Relish sticks Tea Diet sweetener

Ice water ——→

	Monday	Tuesday	Wednesday	Thursday	Friday	Saturday	Sunday
PM SNACK	Popcorn (5 c) Lemonade	Cookies (2) Apple/tea cooler	Angel food cake Frozen strawberries	Vanilla wafers (5) Applesauce	Popcorn (5 c)	Cookies (2) Grape sparkle	Graham crackers Seasonal fruit

[a] Adapted from nutritional program at Oakwood Residence, Minnetonka, MN, 1986.

TABLE C.2. Example of diet based on food exchange system.[a]

Monday—Week 1								
	Portion/		Energy content of diet					
Meal	amount	Exchange	900	1,000	1,200	1,500	1,800	2,000
Breakfast								
Milk, skim	1 c	1 milk	x	x	x	x	x	x
Pancake	1	1 bread/1 fat	x	x	x	2x	2x	2x
Diet syrup	—	Free	x	x	x	x	x	x
Bacon	1 slice	1 fat	x	x	x	x	x	x
Peaches, sliced	½ c	1 fruit	0	0	0	x	x	x
Orange juice	½ c	1 fruit	x	x	x	x	x	x
Coffee	—	Free	x	x	x	x	x	x
Diet sweetener	—	Free	x	x	x	x	x	x
Lunch								
Milk, skim	1 c	1 milk	x	x	x	x	x	x
Peanut butter	2 tbsp	1 meat/1 fat	x	x	x	x	x	x
Whole wheat bread	1 slice	1 bread	x	x	x	2x	2x	2x
Diet jelly	—	Free	x	x	x	x	x	x
Celery sticks	8 sticks	1 vegetable	x	x	x	x	x	x
Orange	1	1 fruit	x	x	x	x	x	2x
Graham cracker	2 squares	1 bread	0	0	0	0	0	x
Dinner								
Milk, skim	1 c	1 milk	½x	x	x	x	x	x
BBQ chicken	1 oz	1 meat	2 oz	2 oz	3 oz	3 oz	3 oz	5 oz
Rice	½ c	1 staroh	x	x	x	x	x	x
Broccoli	½ c	1 veg	x	x	x	2x	2x	2x
Peas	½ c	1 starch	0	0	0	0	x	x
Marsh mallow crispies	1 square	1 fruit	x	x	x	x	x	x
Margarine	1 tsp	1 fat	0	0	x	2x	2x	2x
Tea	Free	Free	x	x	x	x	x	x
Diet sweetener	—	Free	x	x	x	x	x	x

[a] Adapted from nutritional program at Oakwood Residence, Minnetonka, MN, 1986. X, Inclusion in diet; 2x, inclusion of twice the portion size in the daily intake; 0, do not include in diet.

TABLE C.2. *Continued*

Meal	Portion/ amount	Exchange	Energy content of diet					
			900	1,000	1,200	1,500	1,800	2,000
Breakfast								
Milk, skim	1 c	1 milk	x	x	x	x	x	x
Omelet	1 egg	1 meat	x	x	x	x	x	x
Dry cereal	¾ c	1 bread	x	x	x	x	x	x
Banana	½	1 fruit	0	0	0	x	x	x
Tomato juice	6 oz	1 fruit	x	x	x	x	x	x
Toast	1 slice	1 bread	0	0	0	0	x	x
Margarine	1 tsp	1 fat	0	0	0	0	x	x
Coffee	—	Free	x	x	x	x	x	x
Diet sweetener	—	Free	x	x	x	x	x	x
Lunch								
Milk, skim	1 c	1 milk	x	x	x	x	x	x
Turkey slices	1 oz	1 meat	2x	2x	2x	3x	3x	3x
Whole wheat bread	1 slice	1 bread	x	x	x	2x	2x	2x
Carrot coins	½ c	1 veg	x	x	x	x	x	x
Red apple	1 small	1 fruit	x	x	x	x	x	2x
Vanilla wafers	5	1 bread	0	0	0	0	0	x
Mayonnaise	1 tsp	1 fat	—	x	x	x	x	2x
Dinner								
Milk, skim	1 c	1 milk	½x	x	x	x	x	x
Cheeseburger	1	3 oz (3 meat)	x	x	x	x	x	½x
Dinner roll	1	1 starch	0	0	0	0	x	x
String bean salad	½ c	1 veg	x	x	x	2x	2x	2x
Sauerkraut	¼ c	Free	x	x	x	x	x	x
Potato salad	½ c	1 starch	x	x	x	x	x	x
Seasonal fruit	1 or ½ c	1 fruit	x	x	x	x	x	x
Tea	Free	Free	x	x	x	x	x	x
Diet sweetener	Free	Free	x	x	x	x	x	x

Tuesday—Week 1

TABLE C.2. *Continued*

			Wednesday—Week 1					
	Portion/		Energy content of diet					
Meal	amount	Exchange	900	1,000	1,200	1,500	1,800	2,000
Breakfast								
Milk, skim	1 c	1 milk	x	x	x	x	x	x
Cottage cheese	¼ c	1 oz meat	x	x	x	x	x	x
Dark toast	1 slice	1 bread	x	x	x	x	2x	2x
Margarine	1 tsp	1 fat	x	x	x	x	x	x
Diet jelly	—	Free	x	x	x	x	x	x
Grapefruit juice	½ c	1 fruit	x	x	x	x	x	x
Prunes	2 medium	1 fruit	0	0	0	x	x	x
Coffee	—	Free	x	x	x	x	x	x
Diet sweetener	—	Free	x	x	x	x	x	x
Lunch								
Milk, skim	1 c	1 milk	x	x	x	x	x	x
Tuna salad	¼ c	1 meat/1 fat	x	x	x	2x	2x	2x
Rye bread	1 slice	1 bread	x	x	x	2x	2x	2x
Radishes	6 pieces	1 veg	x	x	x	x	x	2x
Seasonal fruit	1	1 fruit	x	x	x	x	x	x
Crackers	6	1 bread	0	0	0	0	0	x
Dinner								
Milk, skim	1 c	1 milk	½x	x	x	x	x	x
Baked pork chop	1 chop	3 oz	x	x	x	x	x	½x
Pasta/vegetable salad	½ c	1 starch	x	x	x	x	x	x
Beets/orange salad	½ c	1 veg	x	x	x	2x	2x	2x
Dinner roll	1	1 starch	0	0	0	0	x	x
Margarine	1 tsp	1 fat	0	0	x	x	x	x
Seasonal fruit	1 or ½ c	1 fruit	—	—	x	x	—	—
Tea	Free	Free	x	x	x	x	x	x
Diet sweetener	Free	Free	x	x	x	x	x	x

TABLE C.2. *Continued*

			Thursday—Week 1					
	Portion/		Energy content of diet					
Meal	amount	Exchange	900	1,000	1,200	1,500	1,800	2,000
Breakfast								
Milk, skim	1 c	1 milk	x	x	x	x	x	x
Scrambled egg	1	1 meat	x	x	x	x	x	x
Malt-O-Meal	½ c	1 bread	x	x	x	x	x	x
Toast	1 slice	1 bread	0	0	0	0	x	x
Margarine	1 tsp	1 fat	0	0	0	0	x	x
Orange juice	½ c	1 fruit	x	x	x	x	x	x
Pears	2 halves	1 fruit	0	0	0	x	x	x
Coffee	—	Free	x	x	x	x	x	x
Diet sweetener	—	Free	x	x	x	x	x	x
Lunch								
Milk, skim	1 c	1 milk	x	x	x	x	x	x
Turkey ham	1 oz	1 meat	x	x	2x	2x	2x	3x
Pumpernickel	1 slice	1 bread	x	x	x	2x	2x	2x
Cauliflower	½ c	1 veg	x	x	x	x	x	x
Raisins	¼ c	1 fruit	x	x	x	x	x	x
Mayonnaise	1 tsp	1 fat	0	0	x	x	2x	2x
Vanilla wafers	5	1 bread	0	0	0	0	0	x
Dinner								
Milk, skim								
Chicken Waldorf salad	¾ c	3 meat/1 fat	½ c	½ c	½ c	x	x	1 c
Dilled carrots	½ oz	1 veg	—	—	x	2x	2x	2x
Bread sticks	2	1 starch	x	x	x	x	3 sticks	3 sticks
Dzerta	Free	Free	x	x	x	x	x	x
Seasonal fruit	1 or ½ c	1 fruit	x	x	x	x	x	x
Chocolate pudding	½ c	1 milk	x	x	x	x	x	x
Tea	Free	Free	x	x	x	x	x	x
Diet sweetener	Free	Free	x	x	x	x	x	x

TABLE C.2. *Continued*

Friday—Week 1								
Meal	Portion/ amount	Exchange	Energy content of diet					
			900	1,000	1,200	1,500	1,800	2,000
Breakfast								
Milk, skim	1 c	1 milk	x	x	x	x	x	x
Cinnamon toast	1 slice	1 bread/1 fat	x	x	x	x	x	x
Dry cereal	¾ c	1 bread	x	x	x	x	x	x
Apple juice	½ c	1 fruit	x	x	0	x	x	x
Orange	1	1 fruit	0	0	x	x	x	x
Coffee	x	Free	x	x	x	x	x	x
Diet sweetener	x	Free	x	x	x	x	x	x
Lunch								
Milk, skim	1 c	1 milk	x	x	x	x	x	x
Sliced cheese	1 slice	1 meat	2x	2x	2x	2x	2x	3x
Whole wheat bread	1 slice	1 bread	x	x	x	2x	2x	2x
Sliced tomato w/ lettuce	1 slice	1 veg	x	x	x	x	x	x
Mayonnaise	1 tsp	1 fat	0	x	x	x	2x	2x
Red apple	1 small	1 fruit	x	x	x	x	x	x
Graham cracker	2 squares	1 bread	0	0	0	0	0	x
Dinner								
Milk, skim	1 c	1 milk	½x	x	x	x	x	x
Broiled fish w/lemon	3 oz	3 meat	x	x	x	x	x	5 oz
Oriental mixed vegetables	½ c	1 veg	x	x	x	2x	2x	2x
Orange wheat salad	½ c	1 starch	x	x	x	x	x	x
Whole kernel corn	½ c	1 starch	0	0	0	0	x	x
Tossed salad	Free	Free	x	x	x	x	x	x
Juice sicle	1	1 fruit	x	x	x	x	x	x
Tea	Free	Free	x	x	x	x	x	x
Diet sweetener	Free	Free	x	x	x	x	x	x

TABLE C.2. *Continued*

			Saturday—Week 1					
	Portion/		Energy content of diet					
Meal	amount	Exchange	900	1,000	1,200	1,500	1,800	2,000
Breakfast								
Milk, skim	1 c	1 milk	x	x	x	x	x	x
Boiled egg	1 egg	1 meat	x	x	x	x	x	x
English muffin	½ muffin	1 bread	x	x	x	x	2x	2x
Diet jelly	—	Free	x	x	x	x	x	x
Margarine	1 tsp	1 fat	x	x	x	x	x	2x
Grapefruit juice	½ c	1 fruit	x	x	x	x	x	x
Applesauce	½ c	1 fruit	0	0	0	x	x	x
Coffee	—	Free	x	x	x	x	x	x
Diet sweetener	—	Free	x	x	x	x	x	x
Lunch								
Milk, skim	1 c	1 milk	x	x	x	x	x	x
Cottage cheese salad	½ c	2 meat	x	x	x	x	x	¾ c
Curried slaw	½ c	1 veg	x	x	x	x	x	x
Buleberry muffin	1	1 starch, 1 fat	x	x	x	x	x	x
Seasonal fruit	1 or ½ c	1 fruit	x	x	x	x	x	x
Ice milk	½ c	1 starch, 1 fat	x	x	x	x	x	x
Dinner								
Milk, skim	1 c	1 milk	½x	x	x	x	x	x
Roast beef	2 oz	2 meat	x	x	x	x	3 oz	4 oz
Baked potato	1 small	1 starch	x	x	x	x	x	x
Mixed vegetables	½ c	1 veg	x	x	x	2x	2x	2x
Spinach salad, lemon dressing	Free	Free	x	x	x	x	x	x
Margarine	1 tsp	1 fat	x	x	x	2x	2x	2x
Bread	1 slice	1 starch	0	0	0	x	x	x
Peach yogurt freeze	1 c	1 fruit	x	x	x	x	x	x
Tea	Free	Free	x	x	x	x	x	x
Diet sweetener	Free	Free	x	x	x	x	x	x

TABLE C.2. *Continued*

			Sunday—Week 1					
	Portion/		Energy content of diet					
Meal	amount	Exchange	900	1,000	1,200	1,500	1,800	2,000
Breakfast								
Milk, skim	1 c	1 milk	x	x	x	x	x	x
Scrambled egg	—	1 meat	x	x	x	x	x	x
Raisin toast	1 slice	1 bread	x	x	x	x	2x	2x
Margarine	1 tsp	1 fat	x	x	x	x	x	2x
Pineapple juice	½ c	1 fruit	x	x	0	x	x	x
Grapefruit	½ c	1 fruit	0	0	x	x	x	x
Coffee	—	Free	x	x	x	x	x	x
Diet sweetener	—	Free	x	x	x	x	x	x
Lunch								
Milk, skim	1 c	1 milk	x	x	x	x	x	x
French bread pizza	6 inch	2 meat, 2 bread	x	x	x	x	x	x
Dzerta	Free	1 veg, 1 fat	x	x	x	x	x	x
Tossed salad	Free	Free	x	x	x	x	x	x
Seasonal fruit	1 or ½ c	Free 1 fruit	x	x	x	x	x	x
Dinner								
Milk, skim	1 c	1 milk	½x	x	x	x	x	x
Ham slices	2 oz	2 meat	x	x	x	x	3 oz	4 oz
Sweet potatoes/apples	⅓ c	1 starch	x	x	x	x	x	x
Seasoned rice	½ c	1 starch	0	0	0	x	x	x
Steamed broccoli	½ c	1 veg	x	x	x	2x	2x	2x
Fruit ice	½ c	1 fruit	x	x	x	x	x	x
Margarine	1 tsp	1 fat	0	0	x	x	x	x
Relish sticks	Free	Free	x	x	x	x	x	x
Tea	Free	Free	x	x	x	x	x	x
Diet sweetener	Free	Free	x	x	x	x	x	x

[a] Adapted from nutritional program at Oakwood Residence, Minnetonka, MN, 1986. X, Inclusion in diet; 2x, inclusion of twice the portion size in the daily intake; 0, do not include in diet.

Appendix D
Activity Therapy Guidelines

Section 1: Annotated Bibliography of Evaluation Tools for Occupational Therapists

Evaluation

1. *Human Figure Drawing* (Florence L. Goodenough, Ph.D.). Assesses body scheme awareness in children ages 3–13.

2. *Developmental Test of Visual-Motor Integration (VMI)* (Keith E. Beery). A sequence of 24 geometric forms to be copied with pencil on paper and designed for use with students ages 3–15.

3. *The University of Kansas Fine Motor Evaluation.* An adapted instrument comprised of items selected from four standardized references, including manipulation skills in developmental sequence as well as many visual motor items and items that look at motor planning and bilateral integration. This test yields two scores, an age-equivalent score, and a score of functional level of accomplishment. Covers ages 0–72 months.

4. *Erhardt Developmental Prehension Assessment* (Rhoda Priest Erhardt). Measures prehension from the fetal and neonatal period to 15 months (which is considered the maturity level of prehension). Also measures pencil grasp and drawings for ages 1–6 years.

5. *Bruininks–Oseretsky Test of Motor Proficiency.* Fine motor component. Assesses these areas of fine motor function: (1) speed of response to a moving visual stimulus (untimed); (2) visual motor control (untimed); and (3) upper limb speed and dexterity (timed). Covers ages 4 years 11 months to 15 years 11 months. Cannot be used with children below the mild range of mental retardation.

6. *Motor Free Visual Perception Test (MVPT).* A test of visual perception that avoids motor involvement. The five categories of visual perception assessed are visual discrimination, figure/ground, visual closure, visual memory, and spatial relationships. Covers ages 4 years to 8 years 11 months.

7. *Jebsen Test of Hand Function.* Consists of 7 subtests designed to be representative of various hand activities and standardized for individuals ages 6–19 years.

8. *Clinical Observations* (A. Jean Ayres). A systematic nonstandardized assessment that looks at various components of sensorimotor development: muscle tone, kinesthesia, eye movements, balance and equilibrium, reflexes, motor planning, cocontractions (ability of the body to stabilize itself), and tremors.

Resources

1. *Sensorimotor Integration for Developmentally Disabled Children: A Handbook*, Patricia Montgomery, M.A., R.P.T., and Eileen Richter, O.T.R. Western Psychological Services, 12031 Wilshire Boulevard, Los Angeles, California 90025.

Section 2: Sample Low-Impact Aerobic Activity Protocols for Individuals with Prader–Willi Syndrome[1]

Name: _____   Date: _____   Therapist: _____

Routine low-impact aerobic exercise may contribute to weight loss in Prader–Willi syndrome (PWS) while improving general cardiovascular fitness. General fitness, including flexibility and strength, may also improve when low-impact aerobic conditioning program is performed regularly.

Aerobic conditioning is achieved by increasing the heart rate (HR) to an appropriate level for individuals with PWS 20 min every other day. The HR increases in response to exercise. The appropriate level of HR is called the *target heart rate*. The target heart rate is 85% of the maximum HR. The maximum HR is determined by subtracting the individual's age from 220.

Maximum HR is 200 − _____ = _____
10-sec target HR is _____ = _____
Target HR is 85% of _____ = _____

Any aerobic conditioning program has three parts:

A. *Warm Up*: The warm up lasts 5 min. It should include two types of exercises:

1. Stretching activities appropriate to the aerobic exercise chosen to apperform.
2. Exercise to gradually increase HR. This is usually the aerobic exercise performed at a slower rate.

B. *Aerobic Conditioning Exercise*: The aerobic exercise should last 20 min. Examples of exercises that will increase the HR to the target HR are fast working, stationary cycling, tricycle riding, swimming, and rowing with low resistance.

C. *Cool Down*: The cool down should last 5 min. This can be done using the same aerobic conditioning exercise, but at a lower intensity. Once the aerobic conditioning exercise is complete, keep moving and active, at the lower level, to allow the HR to recover and keep the blood from pooling in the arms and legs.

---

[1] Duesterhaus-Minor, M. (1984). University of Iowa Hospital School, Iowa City.

General Rules

1. Exercise before meals, not immediately after eating.
2. The HR should be taken immediately after the aerobic exercise phase and again 5 min after stopping. The HR should decline rapidly.
3. Occasionally take pulse first thing in the morning before getting out of bed. This is called a resting heart rate. Over time, if aerobic fitness is improving, the resting heart rate will become lower.
4. The stretching exercises should help prevent injuries.
5. In the beginning it may not be possible to exercise at the target HR for 20 min. Gradually increase the amount of time every few days. However, keep exercising for the full 20 min, even if some of that is at less than target HR.
6. If there has been no exercise for a few days, reduce the level of intensity of exercise to below the level of last exercise day.
7. Do not exercise if a serious cold, flu, fever, or other illness is occurring. Wait until symptoms are gone before resuming activity.
8. Stop exercising for the day if nausea or faintness is noted. The next time, exercise at a slightly lower intensity.
9. In extreme temperatures (hot or cold) reduce the intensity of exercise.

Exercise Prescription

A. Type of aerobic exercise
   _____ walking
   _____ swimming
   _____ stationary bike riding
   _____ riding a tricycle
   _____ rowing
   _____ other:
B. Time
   _____ as soon as home from school/work
   _____ just before supper
   _____ 1–2 hours after supper
C. Type of stretching
   _____ hamstring   _____ rectus femoris
   _____ gastrocnemius   _____ trunk extensors
   _____ trunk rotators   _____ shoulder

Section 3: A Sensorimotor Program for Individuals with Prader–Willi Syndrome[2]

Section 3

Purpose	Activity
Enhance tactile discrimination	*Carpet sample erase*—draw picture letter or numbers on carpet sample (or play tic-tac-toe) and have student erase with hands, feet, forearms.
Enhance tactile discrimination (good group game)	*Dried parts*—using towel or yarn ball, have child dry and name body parts.
Enhance tactile discrimination	*Inch Worm*—lying on side, have student move himself *slowly* forward and back from one spot to another, like an inch-worm. Demonstration may be necessary.
Enhance tactile discrimination (good group game; may be adapted by having a student match the object to a picture)	*Feely-Meely*—the Feely-Meely box has a hole in the side large enough to put a hand in and remove objects. The objects are everyday items. Student reaches in, feels, names object, then brings it out. If wrong guess, object goes back in box.
Gross motor planning Bilateral motor integration	*Many Balls*—may be done in group or one-to-one. Seated on floor, child is given a utility ball that is held with both hands. Roll utility ball toward student, and student will return the ball by hitting it with the ball he or she is holding.
Reflex inhibition Bilateral motor integration Kinesthetic awareness	*Blast Off*—lying stomach down on scooter board, student places feet on wall and pushes off into a glide. He or she may need assistance with placing feet and bending knees (try it yourself to "get the idea") prior to pushing. A nice adaptation is to place a target to elicit stronger push and longer glide. It is also fun to suspend a beach or Nerf ball so the student can tag it as he or she glides past. Tag with one hand, both hands, or head.
Reflex inhibition Bilateral motor integration	*Surfing*—seated, kneeling or on stomach, lying on scooter board, student propels himself or herself simultaneously.
Reflex inhibition Motor planning Kinesthetic awareness	*Wheelbarrow*—using a utility ball, have student kneel over ball (4-point kneel) then "walk out" using hands (legs stay together). Ball will roll back as student moves forward. Try to get ball to ankles. Next step is to reverse the process ending in kneeling position.

(Continued)

---

[2] Adapted from Fink, B. (1977). *Sensory-motor integration—an activities curricula* (3rd ed.). Lowell, MI, published by the author.

Section 3 *Continued*

Purpose	Activity
Motor planning	*Obstacle Course*—stomach lying or kneeling on scooter board, student propels himself or herself through obstacle course.
Bilateral motor integration Postural adjustments Motor planning	*Body Ball*—seated on the floor, roll ball back and forth using both feet. Ask for other ideas of what body parts to use. If done in group, encourage naming the person to whom the ball is to be rolled.
Reflex inhibition	*Statue*—with student on all fours, place a beanbag or stuffed toy between right shoulder and chin. Student places right hand on hip. Student should "freeze" and hold object without dropping it while you attempt to gently push or pull student out of position. Do the same with left hand on hip. After strength is gained, downgrade items to be held (i.e., a potholder to sheet of paper).
Develop righting and equilibrium responses	*Rolling*—always roll both directions; roll with arms stretched over head (may need to hold scarf or length of rope). Encourage tucking chin down and flexing hips to initiate roll.
Encourage balance and motor planning Kinesthetic awareness	*Bean Bag Walk*—student knee-walks while balancing bean bag on head. It helps to give student a target to look at while walking (colored circle of tape on wall at eye level).
Motor planning Postural adjustments	*Stoop Tag*—tape "X"s on floor. One person is "it." He or she chases others, who must stop on X before being tagged. If tagged before stopping, that person becomes "it."
Motor planning Postural adjustments	*Kick Ball*—with a 12″ utility ball, student uses forward, backward, then sideways (to both sides) kick. Ask student to name the place or person he or she is going to kick to.
Bilateral coordination Motor planning	*Catch It*—make a catcher by cutting the bottom end out of a plastic Clorox bottle or milk carton and attach a ball on a string to it (the shorter the easier). The object is to catch the ball in the catcher with a catcher in each hand.

Section 4: Short Motor Program for Individuals with Prader–Willi Syndrome[3]

Equipment Needed: Gymnastics ball (or cage ball), scooter board, rope, two Indian clubs.

General Directions: Start with scooter board activities, then follow with ball activities. Instructor needs to try each activity before working with student.

Scooter Board Activities

1. Lie in prone position. Move to wall and push off with feet. Fly like a plane (arms outstretched).
2. Lie in prone position. Scooter stays in one spot on the floor. Student uses arms to rotate self in circle (helicopter). (Arms should cross midline and legs go out straight for good form.)
3. Sit on scooter. Teacher holds rope and student pulls hands to chest (avoid hand-over-hand patterns) moving in direction of teacher. (Teacher positions self in direct line and on either side of the student.)
4. Lie in prone position. Tie long rope to doorknob and have teacher hold free end. Have student pull self toward door, using rope and hand-over-hand pattern.
5. Lie in prone position. Move to wall and push off wall with feet (airplane). Have all on floor several feet from wall and direct student to try to push ball with hand after "blast off."
6. Lie in prone position. Move to wall and push off with both feet. Student holds an Indian club in both hands and tries to hit ball thrown by teacher during "blast off."

Gymnastic Ball Activities

1. Lie in prone position with stomach on top of ball. Student places hands on ground and walks out using arms so knees move to top of ball and stomach is suspended in the air. Student continues walking to ankles so that knees and stomach are both suspended. Reverse procedure, so that student ends up back in prone position with stomach on top of ball.
2. Lie in prone position with stomach on top of ball. Student places hands on ground and uses legs to pull ball, so knees are positioned on top. Student then moves to balance on knees with arms out to sides like an airplane.
3. Sit on ball. Student extends legs to teacher (legs stiff). Teacher gets between student's calves and moves student to the right and left, while student shifts body weight to maintain balance.

---

[3] Carr, T. (1981). University of Iowa Hospital School, Iowa City.

4. Sit on ball. Place hands on floor. Keep hands stationary and rotate trunk around ball. Go from sitting position to stomach and back to sitting.

Small Ball Activities

1. Student on hands and knees. Teacher tosses ball and student attempts to use forehead to direct ball back to teacher.
2. Student on back with knees bent and legs in the air. Teacher tosses ball toward student and student extends legs and attempts to direct ball back to teacher.

Section 5: Sample Postural Control Exercises

These exercises have been adapted and sequenced for therapeutic purposes. It is recommended that they be demonstrated and monitored by a qualified occupational or physical therapist. Adults who carry out this program should be familiar with correct body alignment in order to avoid use of compensated postures and movement.

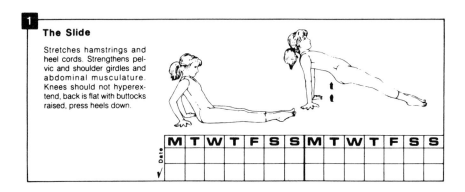

1

The Slide

Stretches hamstrings and heel cords. Strengthens pelvic and shoulder girdles and abdominal musculature. Knees should not hyperextend, back is flat with buttocks raised, press heels down.

Date	M	T	W	T	F	S	S	M	T	W	T	F	S	S
✓														

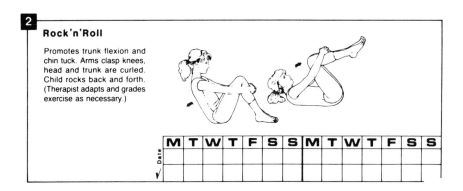

2

Rock'n'Roll

Promotes trunk flexion and chin tuck. Arms clasp knees, head and trunk are curled. Child rocks back and forth. (Therapist adapts and grades exercise as necessary.)

Date	M	T	W	T	F	S	S	M	T	W	T	F	S	S
✓														

3

Side-Lying Leg Lift

Strengthens pelvic girdle musculature. Promotes co-contractions of trunk. Body is in side-lying position, legs are stacked vertically. Arm on bottom cushions head, arm on top is used for support. Leg lift is done in neutral (without hip flexion or extension.)

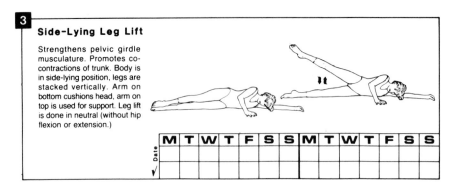

Date ✓	M	T	W	T	F	S	S	M	T	W	T	F	S	S

4

Swallow

Stretches back and hip extensors.

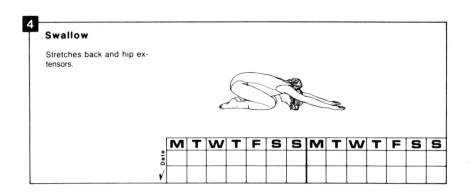

Date ✓	M	T	W	T	F	S	S	M	T	W	T	F	S	S

5

Cat Stretch

Stretches back extensors. Strengthens abdominal muscles, promotes co-contractions of trunk, pelvic and shoulder girdle musculature. Precaution—do not permit back to sway, back is either curled into flexion or flat.

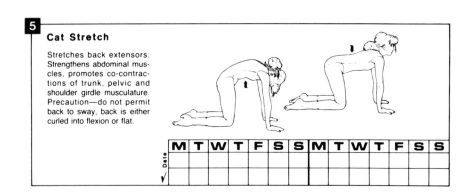

Date ✓	M	T	W	T	F	S	S	M	T	W	T	F	S	S

6

Kneeling Leg Stretch

Gives total body stretch. Promotes co-contraction. Exercise begins on all fours. Curl one knee toward chest then extend the leg back. Extended leg should be at hip height. Hips should be level. Alternate right and left.

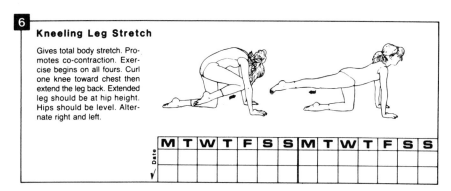

	M	T	W	T	F	S	S	M	T	W	T	F	S	S
Date														

7

Dog Stretch

Improves pelvic, trunk, and shoulder girdle stability. Chin is tucked, feet are flat on the floor, knees are straight, hands are in alignment with shoulders, elbows do not hyperextend.

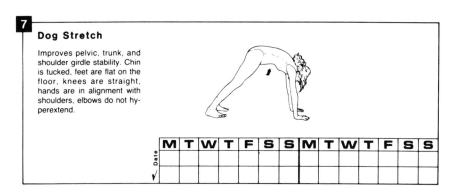

	M	T	W	T	F	S	S	M	T	W	T	F	S	S
Date														

Section 6: Sample Postural Tone Exercises[4]

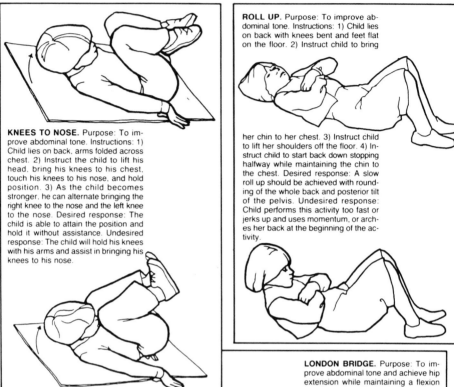

KNEES TO NOSE. Purpose: To improve abdominal tone. Instructions: 1) Child lies on back, arms folded across chest. 2) Instruct the child to lift his head, bring his knees to his chest, touch his knees to his nose, and hold position. 3) As the child becomes stronger, he can alternate bringing the right knee to the nose and the left knee to the nose. Desired response: The child is able to attain the position and hold it without assistance. Undesired response: The child will hold his knees with his arms and assist in bringing his knees to his nose.

ROLL UP. Purpose: To improve abdominal tone. Instructions: 1) Child lies on back with knees bent and feet flat on the floor. 2) Instruct child to bring her chin to her chest. 3) Instruct child to lift her shoulders off the floor. 4) Instruct child to start back down stopping halfway while maintaining the chin to the chest. Desired response: A slow roll up should be achieved with rounding of the whole back and posterior tilt of the pelvis. Undesired response: Child performs this activity too fast or jerks up and uses momentum, or arches her back at the beginning of the activity.

LONDON BRIDGE. Purpose: To improve abdominal tone and achieve hip extension while maintaining a flexion tone throughout the trunk. Instructions: 1) Child lies on back with knees bent and feet flat on the floor. 2) Instruct the child to raise his chin to his chest and then push with his legs in order to make a bridge. Desired response: Full hip extension while maintaining chin tuck and therefore good abdominal tone. Undesired response: The child may perform the hip extension with the head extended, which increases extension throughout the trunk, or the child may not be able to lift the pelvis off the supporting surface with the bottom while the head is flexed.

---

[4] Reprinted from Embrey, D., Endicott, J., Temple, G., & Jarger, D.L. (1983). Developing better postural tone in grade school children. *Clinical Management in Physical Therapy*, *3*, 6–10, by permission of the American Physical Therapy Association.

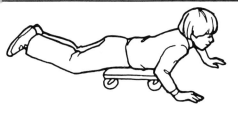

BACK-UP. Purpose: To improve shoulder stability. Instructions: 1) Child lies on stomach on a scooter board. 2) Instruct him to push with his hands on the floor to propel himself backwards while keeping his head up. Desired response: The child is able to keep the head and shoulders stable while pushing with the hands. Undesired response: The child is unable to keep the head up, or lacks the necessary shoulder stability or coordination to push backwards.

ROW YOUR BOAT. Purpose: To elongate the pectoral muscles. Instructions: 1) Two children sit erect in a ring-sitting position back to back. 2) Each pair holds a hula-hoop or dowel over their heads. 3) Instruct one child to move the hoop forward bringing the other child's arms into shoulder flexion while sitting erect. 4) Instruct the children to take turns moving the hoop. Desired response: The child whose arms are being pulled into flexion should keep the arms straight, and the pectoralis major and minor muscles should be elongated. Undesired response: The children may lean forward and backward rather than elongating the pectoral muscles.

HEEL WALKING. Purpose: To improve abdominal tone. Instructions: 1) Instruct the child to walk on his heels backwards. Desired response: Posterior pelvic tilt with contraction of abdominal muscles. Undesired response: The child maintains an anterior pelvic tilt.

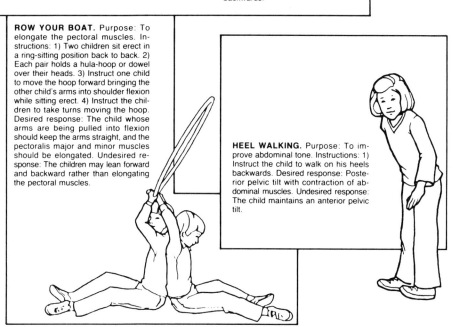

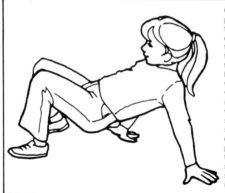

CRAB WALKING. Purpose: To improve shoulder stability and abdominal tone, and elongate the pectoral muscles. Instructions: 1) Child sits on the floor leaning back on her hands with feet flat on the floor. 2) Instruct the child to raise her bottom off the floor while her hands and feet maintain contact with the floor. 3) Instruct the child to walk backwards with the hands leading. 4) Instruct the child to walk forward with the feet leading. Desired response: The child is able to extend the shoulders sufficiently to get the pelvis off the floor and to walk in an all-fours position with only the hands and feet touching the support. Undesired response: The child drags her bottom or scoots on her bottom rather than walking with her hands and feet.

FEET OVER HEAD. Purpose: To improve abdominal tone. Instructions: 1) Child lies on back. 2) Instruct the child to bend his knees, lift his feet over his head, and touch his toes to the floor.

3) As the child returns to the starting position, instruct him to bend his knees as he slowly lowers his feet, keeping the lumbar spine flat on the floor. Desired response: The child should contract the abdominal muscles as the hips are lifted and as the feet are brought back down. Undesired response: The child may attempt to keep his knees straight and bring feet over his head without lifting the hips, or the child may arch the back as the legs are lowered.

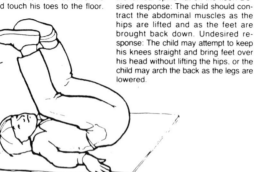

KING ON ONE KNEE. Purpose: To improve abdominal tone and balance reactions. Instructions: 1) Two children kneel facing each other, approximately two feet apart. 2) Instruct each child to raise the right knee so he is half-kneeling with the right foot forward. 3) Instruct the children to "shake hands" and try to pull each other off balance. 4) Change to the opposite foot and hand. Desired response: Children will stabilize the pelvis by bringing one leg up and maintaining a posterior pelvic tilt. This should improve balance reactions and abdominal tone. Undesired response: The children will arch the back rather than maintain a posterior pelvic tilt. Note: This activity should be done on a gymnastic mat.

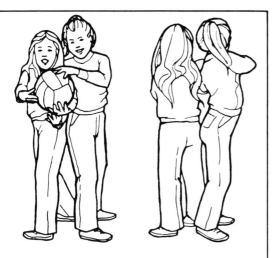

BACK-TO-BACK BALL PASS. Purpose: To improve tone of trunk musculature and range of trunk rotation. Instructions: 1) Two children stand back to back. 2) Give a ball to one child and instruct her to hand it to her partner who must then hand it back on the other side so the ball will go around in a circle. 3) Instruct the children to keep their feet stationary as they perform this activity. Desired response: The children should rotate the trunk Undesired response: Children move their feet in order to pass the ball. They lean backwards as they turn.

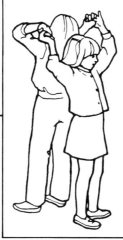

WASHING MACHINE. Purpose: To elongate the pectoral muscles. Instructions: 1) Two children face each other, holding both hands. 2) Instruct the children to turn their hands together so arms elevate as they turn. 3) Instruct the children to continue the movement until they are facing each other again. Desired response: Both children will elongate their pectoral muscles while holding hands. Undesired response: The children will not elevate their arms while they do this activity and thus will not elongate the pectoral muscles.

Section 7: Sample Occupational Therapy Evaluation and Recommendations

NAME:
B.D.:
DATE:
C.A.

Current Occupational Therapy Evaluation and Results

Feeding: Independent at age level
Undressing/Dressing: Cooperative at the 3-year level
Hand/Upper Extremity Function: Significantly delayed secondary to overall developmental delay
Adaptions/Equipment: Milwaukee brace—23 hours/day

_____ was accompanied by her parents and younger sister. Tests given today were the Kansas University Fine Motor Evaluation (KUFM), the Beery Developmental Test of Visual-Motor Integration, and the Draw-a-Person. The KUFM is an adapted instrument comprised of items selected from four standardized references and including manipulation skills in a developmental sequence, as well as many visual-motor items and some items that look at motor planning and bilateral integration. This test yields a functional level of accomplishment in fine motor development that covers ages 0–72 months. _____'s age equivalent score on the KUFM was 18¼ months with emerging skills at 20¼ months. The items with which she had best results were form boards and bilateral manipulation skills. She began to experience difficulty with items that required dynamic control of the shoulder and arm and good hand stability, as well as those that required depth perception, motor planning, and perceptual acuity. The Draw-a-Person is a normed assessment that looks at the individual's awareness of body scheme. _____'s age-equivalent score on this test was 2 years. The Developmental Test of Visual-Motor Integration is a sequence of geometric forms to be copied with pencil and paper and was designed for use with students from preschool through junior high. Her age-equivalent score was below 2 years, 11 months.

By observation, _____ displays low postural tone with deficits in cocontractions (ability of the body to stabilize itself) and with antigravity holding positions. A slight tremor was observed during testing, and overflow movement was present during mild resistive activities. Grasp and release patterns used in manipulation activities at the 1 to 1½ year level were good, with smooth release patterns and precise opposition being used functionally. Fingers are hypermobile, and _____ has a wavering approach to pick up or place an object that she is correcting with no difficulty or frustration at this point. Shoulder patterns are moderately immature, with excessive abduction being used to accomplish tasks. _____ has not established laterality at this point and does not have good bilateral assist when using either hand as the prime mover. For prewriting skills her pencil grasp is immature but appropriate for her developmental level (1–2 years), with the pencil being held primarily in the hand and occasionally shifting from a static tripod to a pronated grasp.

_____ is able to remove and put on socks and shoes and to assist with clothing for toileting as well as to remove most clothing. Behavior during resting was cooperative and pleasant. Although she demonstrates a short attention span, _____ has a good task persistence for activities in which she is interested. She enjoys movement-based activities and follows directions well.

Impressions

_____ has a number of subtle fine motor problems that are influencing hand/upper extremity function. In addition, she has significant perceptual deficits, including difficulties with depth perception and spatial relationships. With low postural tone and deficits in cocontractions, _____ lacks the trunk, shoulder, and head stability to form a solid physical base for moving into fine motor proficiency and dexterity. Optimal seating and appropriate level of work surface will be important in helping _____ compensate for low muscle tone and poor proximal stability.

Actions Taken

Evaluation results and recommendations were discussed with _____'s parent. They were given a copy of *Sensorimotor Inregration for Developmentally Disabled Children: A Handbook* by Patricia Montgomery, M.A., R.P.T., and Eileen Richter, O.T.R., to review for ideas for movement-based activities that they could incorporate into play-time at home.

Recommendations

1. A program of movement-based activities that includes rolling, crawling, and pushing objects with weight would be good for helping _____ to develop proximal stability. These activities would also work on the areas of bilateral integration and improved motor planning (ability to organize movement).

2. Resistive activities are appropriate for improving co-contractions and joint stability. Some examples are pushing a grocery cart or a doll

buggy with weight added, carrying a milk carton in from shopping, putting away canned goods, working with Play Dough.

3. Continue excellent programming at home with the "heavy work" activities that you have been providing, which include supervised climbing and swinging on playground equipment and a swim program.

4. Incorporate activities with a tactile base whenever possible to provide additional touch cues for position of hands and arms in space (examples are Play Dough, cornstarch play, fingerpaint, sand and water play).

5. Provide bilateral activities such as pushing a large ball from a seated or kneeling position, pushing a large ball with both feet from a seated position, stacking large cardboard boxes, pouring water or sand from one container to another, helping mix cookie dough.

6. Continue current excellent school program, with occupational therapist consulting to the classroom teacher regarding positioning and giving recommendations for activities that could be adapted to meet _____'s current developmental level.

_____   _____

Occupational Therapist/O.T.R./L   Date

Appendix E.1
Weight Loss Treatment in an Institutionalized Individual with Prader–Willi Syndrome: A Case Study

FRANZ KLUTSCHKOWSKI and IRA COLLERAIN

Weight reduction as a function of a behavior intervention program emphasizing self-reinforcement in conjunction with contingency management techniques were examined in an 32-year-old individual with Prader–Willi syndrome (PWS). Also examined were the collateral effects of a behavior intervention program on the rates of problem behaviors. No significant changes were noted in the rates of maladaptive behaviors. Behavioral techniques produced a substantial weight reduction relative to baseline levels over a 15-7 month time period.

Introduction

This study implies that there may be indicators for some PWS individuals who benefit from antidepressant psychotrophic medication. The Prader–Willi Syndrome Association (1991) has indicated that the use of fluoxetine has been helpful with some PWS individuals concerning behavioral improvement, although there has not been evidence of its efficacy relating to weight control. Along with the use of fluoxetine, an important component of this behavior intervention program is self-reinforcement. Self-reinforcement has long ago been shown to be a method of behavior change (Bandura, 1969, 1971; Kanfer, 1966, 1970, 1977; Rimm & Masters, 1979). Harchik, Sherman, & Sheldon (1992) reported a total of 59 studies using self-management procedures by individuals with developmental disabilities.

Behavior intervention programs are typically used with PWS individuals utilizing extrinsic and intrinsic reinforcement and contingencies for inappropriate behaviors (Sulzbacher, 1988). Environmental engineering is appropriate as well, although, in most living environments, this is difficult to accomplish (Martin, Harbeitner & DuPont, 1990). Treatment occurred within an institutional setting, specifically designed for individuals with PWS. (For a description of such a residential program, see Chapter 15.)

This report involves a 32-year-old, male diagnosed as having the Prader–Willi syndrome by a medical geneticist. He is mildly mentally retarded, severely obese, and resides at a state institution for the developmentally disabled (since 1971). He has a psychiatric diagnosis of organic personality disorder, with personality and mood aspects secondary to Prader–Willi syndrome, dysthymic disorder, early onset, primary, and secondary types to Prader–Willi syndrome, and major depression, recurrent (moderate but not psychotic). This study spans a 15-month time period, from 1992 through 1993, and involves the use of psychopharmacology, fluoxetine, environmental engineering (controlled access to his kitchen at his home), and a behavior intervention program that was developed with an interdisciplinary treatment team (physician, dietitian, psychologist, social worker, staff who work directly with the PWS individual, Qualified Mental Retardation Professional (QMRP), vocational staff, and his legal guardian).

Prior to the beginning of this study, this individual with PWS had been placed in the infirmary for several months during the previous 2 years. His infirmary placement was directly related to his obesity at one point up to 419 pounds. During his infirmary treatment, which consisted primarily of a strictly controlled diet and environment, he lost weight. However, after each infirmary treatment, he was returned to his apartment home at a state institution, and in a relatively short time he regained the lost weight.

T. was the first child of his 26-year-old mother. The pregnancy had some complications, which were not explained in the medical records, and he was a breech delivery and weighed 5 pounds and 11 ounces. His sucking reflex was reported as poor and other developmental milestones of childhood were reportedly delayed. Early descriptive characteristics described T. as a happy-go-lucky child until someone made him angry. He would then become explosive and prone to temper tantrums. At 9 years of age T. weighed 140 pounds, and his parents stated that he spent a lot of time devising methods of sneaking food from the refrigerator. He began school in a special education classroom of a major independent school district. He was later described as being lackadaisical and not enjoying most physical activities.

T.'s medication history includes the use of an antipsychotic agent, thioridazine, from 1985 through 1990. Molindone was introduced briefly in 1990. Later in 1991, molindone was discontinued and fluoxetine was started. From January until May 1992, T. was taking 20 mg/day of Prozac, and during this time his weight averaged at 397 pounds, which is considered to be the baseline weight for this study.

Method

A behavior intervention program was developed for T. that included the use of fluoxetine for depressive behaviors. Contingency management techniques and self-reinforcement were the primary methods for treating obesity. Weight loss was the dependent variable in this study. Self-reinforcement consisted of weighing himself twice a week in his apartment, and recording his weight on his own weight log book. If he forgot to weight himself, staff were instructed to remind him to weigh. Prior to the beginning of his behavior intervention program, T. was taken on a shopping trip where he purchased a weight log book of his choosing. Contingency management techniques consisted of the following: (1) Each weight loss resulted in verbal praise from staff. Verbal praise occurred immediately after weighing, later in the day from his psychologist, and also from staff at his workplace. (2) Each 5-pound weight loss resulted in receiving a diet caffeine-free drink, which was delivered during the same day of his weight loss. (3) Each 10-pound weight loss resulted in receiving a special shopping trip, whereby he would purchase nonfood items that he enjoyed (particularly art supplies). This reinforcement was delivered during the same week of this weight loss. (4) Each 15-pound weight loss resulted in receiving a salad lunch at a local restaurant of his choice. The use of food as a reinforcer for individuals with PWS has been used successfully by other researchers (Caldwell, Taylor, & Bloom, 1986). This reinforcer was also delivered the same week of losing the required weight. (5) Each 30-pound weight loss resulted in receiving a visit to a horse ranch along with his salad lunch. Response costs included very close supervision if he gained more than 5 pounds above his lowest baseline. Close supervision was for the purpose of preventing T. from obtaining unauthorized food. Environmental engineering consisted of T. living in an apartment with the kitchen locked. However, T. was able to freely move around the institution where there were numerous opportunities to obtain food elsewhere.

Results

Throughout the duration of this research study, the maladaptive behaviors related to his Axis I diagnoses (DSM III-R) generally remained stable at a low rate. However, a spike in depressive behaviors occurred in November 1992 and his fluoxetine was increased to 40 mg/day, which remains his current dosage. Because T. was taking fluoxetine for five months prior to the beginning of the behavioral interventions related to weight loss, this medication was not considered to be a factor relating to his obesity. However, fluoxetine was instrumental in controlling his

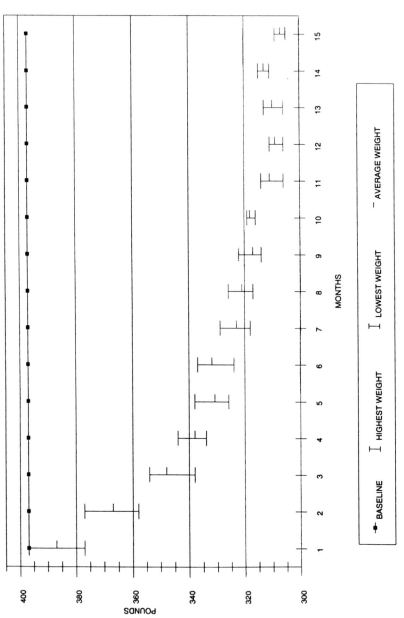

FIGURE E.1.1. Baseline and treatment weights.

depressive symptoms and was a likely intervening variable in facilitating T.'s cognitive functioning (Oliver, 1993).

The data presented in Figure E.1.1 indicate a clear downward trend. The baseline rate for his weight at the beginning of this intervention was 397 pounds. Baseline weight was calculated by taking the average weights from January through May 1992.

T.'s final weight at the conclusion of this study was 305 pounds as of August 1993. It should also be noted that the variability of his average weight for each month generally decreased during the 15 months.

Summary

An interdisciplinary treatment team was instrumental in the development of a behavior intervention program addressing the needs of an individual with Prader–Willi syndrome. Self-reinforcement and contingency management techniques were successfully utilized in the treatment of weight management. It appears that the use of fluoxetine was useful in controlling the symptoms of T.'s depression. However, the use of this antidepressant did not appear to be related to the identified weight loss. It should also be noted that substantial support and cooperation from his legal guardian were essential to the implementation of the behavioral interventions.

References

Bandura, A. (1969). *Principles of Behavior Modification*. New York: Holt, Rinehart & Winston.

Bandura, A. (1971). Self-Reinforcement Processes. In R. Glaser (Ed.), *The nature of reinforcement*. New York: Academic Press.

Caldwell, M.L., Taylor, R.L., & Bloom, S.R. (1986). An investigation of the use of high-and low-preference food as a reinforcer for increased activity of individuals with Prader-Willi syndrome. *Journal of Mental Deficiency Research*, *30*, 347–354.

Hanson, J.W. (1981). A view of etiology and pathogenesis of Prader-Willi syndrome. In V.A. Holm, S.J. Sulzbacher, & P. Pipes (Eds.), *Prader-Willi syndrome*. Baltimore: University Park Press.

Harchik, A.E., Sherman, J.A., & Sheldon, J.B. (1992). The use of self-management procedures by people with developmental disabilities: A brief review. *Research in Developmental Disabilities*, *13*, pp. 153–171.

Kanfer, F.H. (1966). Influence of age and incentive conditions on children's self-rewards. *Psychological Reports*, *19*, 263–274.

Kanfer, F.H. (1970). *Self-regulation: Research, issues and speculation in clinical psychology*. New York: Appleton-Century-Crofts.

Kanfer, F.H. (1977). Self-regulation and self-control. In H. Zeier (Ed.), *The psychology of the 20th century* (vol. 4). Zurich: Kindler Verlag.

Martin, S., Harbeitner, M.H., & DuPont, M. (1990). *Effect of self-reinforcement on weight loss and behavior change of a Prader-Willi client*. Paper presented at the Annual Convention of the TAMR, Beaumont, Texas.

Oliver, J.H. (1993). Personal communication.

Prader-Willi Syndrome Association. (1991). *The Gathered View*. Newsletter of the Prader-Willi Syndrome Association, *16*(2).

Rimm, D.C., & Masters, J.C. (1979). *Behavior therapy – Techniques and empirical Findings*. New York: Academic Press.

Appendix E.2
Sample of Token Economy/ House Guidelines Program Used with Individuals Who Have Prader–Willi Syndrome[1]

Jeanne Lehrer, Kathy Kobilis, and Scott Spreat

Individuals with Prader–Willi syndrome (PWS) generally achieve their greatest behavioral success when involved with a highly structured system. This prosthetic system must incorporate consistent consequences for behavior while teaching and reinforcing positive socialization skills. The token economy system, incorporated into an individualized behavioral program, is an effective tool to provide the consistent reinforcement necessary to meet the needs of individuals with PWS.

The general token economy system used with individuals who have PWS involves earning a "token" every 30 min for the absence of specific socially unacceptable behaviors. Individual needs are assessed in terms of which maladaptive behaviors should be prioritized as target behaviors, the function or reinforcement contingencies that maintain these behaviors, as well as the prosocial behavior that must be taught and/or reinforced to replace the maladaptive behaviors. Thus, in addition to earning tokens for the absence of specific socially unacceptable behaviors, individuals are reinforced for exhibiting specific prosocial behaviors. Individuals accumulate tokens throughout the day and into the early evening. Accumulated tokens are then used to "purchase" items at the token store. Individuals have the opportunity to trade in tokens on a daily basis or to save the tokens for future purchases of higher cost items. Items offered in the token store are selected with the input of individuals participating in the token economy.

In addition to individual programs, a general system of house guidelines was developed to provide structure and limits for those maladaptive

---

[1] Reprinted with permission of Woods Services, Langhorne, Pennsylvania 19047.

behaviors not addressed in individual programs. The guidelines were developed by the individuals who live in the house with the input of professional staff. They serve to provide clear expectations for appropriate social behavior in the residence and consistent consequences when this behavior does not occur. The guidelines are linked to the token economy system through the consequences for maladaptive behaviors. In general, if a specific guideline is broken, the consequence is an additional "cost" for items in the token store for that day. The amount of the increased "cost" depends on the seriousness of the maladaptive behavior. These guidelines are reviewed with the individuals who participate in the program every 6 months for the purpose of updating and revising them as necessary. Participation of the individuals for whom the program is applied is considered essential to the success of the program. These house guidelines are outlined below, along with examples of the consequences of specific behaviors.

In addition to the above procedures, there are several environmental considerations that contribute to the program success of individuals with PWS. Attempts are made to minimize the time that individuals spend in large groups. Several activities occur concurrently, which minimizes the number of persons participating in any one activity. Decreasing group size helps to decrease conflict and increase staff attention to individuals. In addition, a general increase in scheduled activities serves to reduce the opportunity for peer conflict, consequently contributing to the success of individual programs.

Token System

Tokens are awarded for each 30-min period that passes without occurrence of a maladaptive behavior. Tokens accumulate through the day and may be traded in for reinforcers at the token store after dinner. Typical objects in the token store include the following:

Decaffeinated coffee	20 tokens
Diet candy	5 tokens
1:1 trip	70 tokens
Stationery—2 sheets	5 tokens
Envelopes	10 tokens
Stamps	25 tokens
Pencil	5 tokens
Pen	10 tokens
Notebook	50 tokens
Batteries	50 tokens
Cassette tape	75 tokens
VCR tape	75 tokens
Movie rental	50 tokens

Puzzle book	40 tokens
Comic book	25 tokens
Magazine	40 tokens
Playing cards	30 tokens
Grab bag	50 tokens
Walkman	150 tokens

There are response costs for various forms of inappropriate social expression. These costs typically consist of an increase of the prices in the token store, however, for both aggression and food stealing, the individual loses the opportunity to purchase any items from the token store for one day. The individual can carry over one half of their tokens to the following day. Samples of response costs appear below:

Behavior	Costs increase by
Property destruction	25 tokens
Theft of property	20 tokens
Tantrums	10 tokens
Teasing others	5 tokens
Improper borrowing	5 tokens
Poor room maintenance	5 tokens
Not completing hygiene	2 tokens
Not doing own laundry	2 tokens
Not showering	2 tokens
Inappropriate noise levels	2 tokens
Interrupting/rude behavior	2 tokens

House Guidelines

1. Individuals will attempt to receive optimal benefit from programming:
   - Participate in individualized program
   - Attend scheduled day program
   - Maintain satisfactory personal hygiene
   - Get sufficient sleep
2. Individuals will show respect for each other and for property:
   - Maintain appearance of own room
   - Keep radios and TVs at reasonable level so as not to disturb others
   - Borrow items only with specific permission
   - Control behavior when upset and approach staff to discuss problems
   - Avoid teasing and speak respectfully to all
   - Enter the room of another only with permission
3. Individuals will exhibit appropriate table manners:
   - Comply with menu
   - Avoid taking the food of others
   - Discuss menu disputes calmly with staff

Appendix E.3
Sample Positive Reinforcements for Behavioral Management

Positive reinforcement (rewards) for individuals with Prader–Willi syndrome (PWS) is very effective where realistic expectations are clearly understood and consistency is maintained.

Positive reinforcement for persons with PWS should be appropriate to mental and emotional age. Rewards may need to be changed frequently and remain concrete.

Furthermore, unlike most other mentally retarded persons who tend to maintain a competency level once a task is learned, task performance of individuals with PWS tends to fluctuate broadly. They may demonstrate productivity and cooperation for a time, only to "lose it ." It is practical to set rather low expectations for behavior and allow for more successful experiences than to always strive for a higher plateau. Less complicated, less stressful activities make the relearning process easier. Where possible, input from the individual with PWS should be incorporated into the decision–making process.

Behavioral charting is best done on a daily as well as a weekly basis. In addition to praise, stickers, stars, or tokens work well as long as the amount earned for a reward is relatively small and the time element short. In other words, concrete evidence of success should be available more frequently than once a week. The token/reward system should be integrated into the entire day's activities, carrying over from school to home or vocational program to group residence. Families and other primary providers appreciate specific guidelines and when all are "playing with the same set of rules" it is easier to preserve the consistency of the behavioral guidelines. For example, following directions within a set time limit may earn a token regardless of the setting.

In general, individuals with PWS have very good fine motor skills and like sedentary activities. Because they need regular exercise, any reward system should be linked to participation in specific physical programming. Also, persons with PWS, regardless of their age, seem to prefer to relate on a one-to-one with older individuals (particularly teachers and staff). They also like playing with younger children because they get to be "in charge."

Samples:

1. Daily and weekly charts with age-appropriate stickers (such as stars) or tokens
2. Puzzles, books
3. Card games (this helps to develop interpersonal skills)
4. Workbooks: coloring (paint or crayon), "connect the numbers," or "paint by numbers"
5. Handcrafts: knitting, needlepoint (large canvas). cross-stitch, weaving, simple sewing (hand or machine), simple woodwork or leatherwork
6. Special rewards (PWS individuals are usually very well groomed):
   brush and comb
   perfume or men's cologne
   bubble bath, bath oil, bath powder
   jewelery (bracelets, earrings, neck chains)
   fancy soaps
   makeup
   special shampoo
   towels and washcloths
   manicure sets
   small radio
7. Food items: sugarless gum, diet soda, cut-up vegetables (good for field trips)
8. Group events:
   movies
   bowling
   swimming
   roller skating
   salad bar lunch as a group with staff
   holiday party celebrations and planned picnics or camp-outs
9. Special evens (PWS individuals like one-to-one interactions):
   shopping trip with a staff member
   manicure
   trip to beauty shop
   exclusive time with teacher/staff
   visit to home of staff
   extra visit with parents/family
   helping with pre-school, day care, or kindergarten activities

Appendix F.1
Communication Boards

Communication boards can be a helpful tool in aiding the PWS child/adult in achieving a more functional state of communication. Depending upon the level of the individual, communication boards should contain the vocabulary to do any or all of the following: ask questions, make requests, direct actions of others, direct the sequence of events, and/or make the choices within a specific situation. Boards can be elaborate or simple, large or small, using pictures or written words; however, all *must* be flexible, portable, and highly personalized.

Materials

Most communication boards can be made from inexpensive, readily available materials found at either a variety/discount store, i.e., Wal-Mart, K-Mart, Target, or a stationery store. The needed items are:

1. Photo album sheets that are laminated or clear vinyl contact paper.
2. Adhesive velcro dots or a glue stick (*not* liquid based glue, as that causes pictures to wrinkle).
3. Cardboard or oaktag file folders.
4. Pictures or photos of meaningful vocabulary.

Assembling the Board

1. Place the pictures, photos, or word cards onto your cardboard or oaktag file folder.
2. Use glue stick if items are to be permanent and cover with contact paper.
3. Use adhesive velcro dots if items are to be rearranged or changed and cover using the laminated photo sleeve.

When making "mini" communication boards, a small magnetic photo album holder or folded picture inserts from a wallet can be used. The contact paper and/or laminated photo sleeve help to protect items from moisture.

The communication board should be centered around themes, i.e., grooming, clothing, food items, leisure activities, job/school-related items, family members or events.

Remember, the key to making user-friendly communication boards is to keep them simple and *personalized* to meet the needs of each individual.

Appendix F.2
Product Information for Pragmatic Language Training

Companies dealing with special education materials for teachers, speech–language pathologists, and significant caretakers have tried to accommodate the demand to supply needed social skills training materials. The following list of suppliers and their relevant materials is not to be considered exhaustive or exclusive in selection. It is merely a point of reference for further exploration to aid in the critical decision-making process of purchasing specific materials for recognized needs in pragmatic language training.

Academic Communication Associates
Publications Division, Dept. 83-C
4149 Avenida de la Plata
PO Box 586249
Oceanside, CA 92058
  Knowing What to Say!
  Talking on Purpose!
  Conversation Express
  Situation Communication (SITCOM)
  Pragmatic Language Intervention Resource

Communication Skills Builders
3830 E Bellevue/PO Box 42050-E93
Tucson, AZ 85733
  Building Functional Social Skills, Group Activities for Adults
  INTERACT, A Social Skills Game
  A Sourcebook of Pragmatic Activities (Revised)
  A Sourcebook of Adolescent Pragmatic Activities
  Pragmatic Activities for Language Intervention
  Tackling Teen Topics
  Pragmatic-Language Trivia Junior

DLM
1 DLM Park
Allen, TX 75002
    CONVERSATIONS; Language Intervention for Adolescents
    Talk About It
    STARTLINE, Social Education/Communication

LinguiSystems
3100 4th Ave
PO Box 747
East Moline, IL 61244
    Life Skills Workshop
    On My Own with Language
    Communication Workshop
    RAPP (Resource of Activities for Peer Pragmatics)
    Room 14, A Social Language Program
    FriendZee, A Social Skills Game

PRO-ED
8700 Shoal Creek Blvd
Austin, TX 78758
    PALS: Pragmatic Activities in Language and Speech
    BEING ME A Social/Sexual Training Program
    Teaching the Moderately and Severely Handicapped, Vol II: Communication & Socialization (2nd Ed)
    The Walker Social Skills Curriculum
    The ACCEPTS Program: A Curriculum for Children's Effective Peer and Teacher Skills
    The ACCESS Program: Adolescent Curriculum for Communication and Effective Social Skills
    Peer Interaction Skills
    Talking, Listening, Communicating

The Psychological Corporation
555 Academic Ct
San Antonio, TX 78204
    Conversation Connections: A Whole Language Preschool Program
    Let's Talk: for Children (LTC)
    Let's Talk: for Intermediate Level
    Let's Talk: for Developing Prosocial Communication Skills

The Riverside Publishing Co
8420 Bryn Mawr Ave
Chicago, IL 60631
    SMALL TALK: Creating Conversation with Young Children

Thinking Publications
1713 Westgate Rd
PO Box 163
Eau Claire, WI 54702
  Scripting: Social Communication for Adolescents
  Skillstreaming the Adolescent
  Skillstreaming the Elementary School Child
  Skillstreaming in Early Childhood
  Daily Communication
  Communicate (game)
  Communicate Junior (game)
  Social Skill Strategies
  SOCIAL STAR, General Interaction Skills

Appendix G
Vocational Training Sample Task Performance Checklists[1]

These task performance checklists are examples of task breakdowns that a Prader–Willi syndrome individual would likely be able to manage. Further breakdown in components may be needed. In some cases, focusing on just one subtask may be required.

Gardening/Outdoor Maintenance Checklist

Fertilizes plants correctly and safely:

1. Identifies need for feeding/fertilizing
2. Demonstrates proper procedure for application of fertilizer using whirly-bird type applicator
3. Demonstrates proper procedure for application of fertilizer using hose sprayer
4. Demonstates proper procedure for application of fertilizer using spray tank
5. Follows safety precautions involved with agricultural chemicals

Plants/cultivates correctly:

1. Prepares soil properly prior to planting
2. Digs hole of proper depth
3. Places plant into hole
4. Packs dirt to proper consistency around plant
5. Uses hand shovel and cultivator properly around base of flowers, shrubs, trees, to afford better water intake

Prunes, shapes, weeds correctly:

1. Identifies need for pruning/shaping
2. Demonstrates proper technique for pruning/shaping common flowers, trees, shrubs (roses, fuchsias, junipers, etc.)

---

[1] From Copus, E. (1980). *The Melwood manual*. Menomonie, WI: The University of Wisconsin–Stout, Materials Development Center. Reprinted by permission.

3. Uses cutting tools safely
4. Identifies most common local weeds
5. Weeds area carefully
6. Discriminates between weeds which must be dug with tool (large root or stickers) or hand-pulled

Cleans up yard and gardening tools:

1. Determines need to sweep sidewalk, driveway, etc.
2. Selects proper broom for use
3. Sweeps sidewalk, walkway, driveway
4. Identifies properly swept sidewalk, walkway, etc.
5. Uses hose, if necessary, to wash away lawn clippings
6. Washes and wipes hand tools
7. Changes mower spark plugs monthly
8. Changes oil on mower monthly

Rakes lawn correctly:

1. Determines need to rake
2. Rakes lawn entirely free of debris
3. Removes and disposes of debris

Uses/maintains power mower correctly:

1. Determines need to mow lawn
2. Adjusts cutting height of mower properly
3. Checks gas in mower
4. Fills mower with gas
5. Checks oil in mower
6. Changes oil monthly
7. Transports mower to cutting area
8. Starts mower
9. Cuts lawn in straight line whenever possible, without missing spots
10. Recognizes completion of properly mown lawn
11. Shuts off mower
12. Follows safety procedures in use of lawn mower

Waters yard correctly:

1. Determines location to outside faucet
2. Attaches hose to outside faucet
3. Waters lawn correctly
4. Waters flowers correctly
5. Waters vegetables correctly
6. Waters trees/shrubs correctly
7. Identifies root feeder
8. Demonstrates proper use of root feeder
9. Demonstrates proper use of aerator

Identifies and demonstrates proper use/care of gardening tools:

1. Identifies and demonstrates proper use of rotary mower
2. Identifies and demonstrates proper use of gas can
3. Identifies and demonstrates proper use of spading fork
4. Identifies and demonstrates proper use of spade or shovel
5. Identifies and demonstrates proper use of hand shovel
6. Identifies and demonstrates proper use of Swedish tree saw
7. Identifies and demonstrates proper use of clippers
8. Identifies and demonstrates proper use of hoe
9. Identifies and demonstrates proper use of lawn edger
10. Identifies and demonstrates proper use of topping shears
11. Identifies and demonstrates proper use of pruning shears
12. Identifies and demonstrates proper use of broadcaster
13. Identifies and demonstrates proper use of hedge trimmer
14. Identifies and demonstrates proper use of spray atomizer
15. Identifies and demonstrates proper use of dustpan
16. Identifies and demonstrates proper use of cultivator
17. Identifies and demonstrates proper use of lawn rake
18. Identifies and demonstrates proper use of yard rake
19. Identifies and demonstrates proper use of pole pruner
20. Identifies and demonstrates proper use of mattock
21. Identifies and demonstrates proper use of wheelbarrow
22. Identifies and demonstrates proper use of soil test kit
23. Identifies and demonstrates proper use of folding tree saw
24. Identifies and demonstrates proper use of spray tank
25. Knows where tools are kept
26. Places tools in proper storage area
27. Discriminates between dull and sharp tools
28. Sharpens tools safely

Carpentry Procedures Checklist

Follows correct carpentry procedures:

1. Drives nail
2. Pulls nail
3. Identifies and demonstrates proper use of sandpaper
4. Sands with grain of wood
5. Uses correct grade of sandpaper for each job
6. Identifies need to replace sandpaper
7. Recognizes acceptably completed sanding procedure
8. Waxes wood following proper procedure
9. Stains items
10. Uses proper steps when gluing items
11. Returns items to proper storage place

Uses ladder correctly and safely:

1. Identifies and demonstrates proper use of ladder
2. Stores ladder correctly
3. Lifts ladder correctly

Identifies and demonstrates proper use of hand tools:

1. Identifies and demonstrates proper use of hammer
2. Returns hammer to proper storage place
3. Identifies and demonstrates proper use of saw
4. Returns saw to proper storage place
5. Identifies and demonstrates proper use of measure
6. Returns measure to proper storage place
7. Identifies and demonstrates proper use of screwdriver
8. Returns screwdriver to proper storage place
9. Identifies and demonstrates proper use of plane
10. Returns plane to proper storage place
11. Identifies and demonstrates proper use of pliers
12. Returns pliers to proper storage place
13. Identifies and demonstrates proper use of clamp
14. Returns clamp to proper storage place
15. Identifies and demonstrates proper use of vise
16. Returns vise to proper storage place
17. Identifies and demonstrates proper use of chisel
18. Returns chisel to proper storage place
19. Identifies and demonstrates proper use of file
20. Returns file to proper storage place

Uses power saw correctly and safely:

1. Verbalizes safety procedure for power saw
2. Identifies and demonstrates proper use of power saw under supervision
3. Feeds material to be sawed
4. Sets material to be sawed at desired point
5. Saws material accurately
6. Sets power saw to make special cut (i.e., halfway cut)
7. Identifies and demonstrates proper use of power saw independently
8. Disconnects plug when job is completed
9. Cleans area

Uses hand drill correctly and safely:

1. Identifies and demonstrates proper use of hand drill with supervision
2. Verbalizes safety procedure for using drill
3. Uses drill safely
4. Uses correct size drill bit for specific job
5. Changes drill bit

6. Recognizes dull drill bit
7. Drills to specific depth
8. Identifies and demonstrates proper use of hand drill independently
9. Stores drill properly

Uses drill press correctly and safely:

1. Follows safety measures for drill press
2. Loads material
3. Unloads material
4. Checks power switches and plugs in cord
5. Properly sets drill and table
6. Identifies and demonstrates proper use of jigs
7. Knows how to set a jig properly
8. Knows speed for separate drilling
9. Can adjust machine to separate speeds
10. Can identify drill bit
11. Uses correct size drill bit for specific job
12. Recognizes dull drill bit

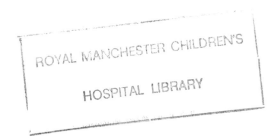

Index